Contemporary Nephrology and Kidney Transplantation

Contemporary Nephrology and Kidney Transplantation

Editor: Reagen Hu

FOSTER
ACADEMICS
www.fosteracademics.com

www.fosteracademics.com

FOSTER ACADEMICS

Cataloging-in-Publication Data

Contemporary nephrology and kidney transplantation / edited by Reagen Hu.
p. cm.
Includes bibliographical references and index.
ISBN 978-1-64646-609-2
1. Nephrology. 2. Kidneys--Transplantation. 3. Kidneys--Disease--Diagnosis.
4. Kidneys--Diseases--Treatment. I. Hu, Reagen.
RC902 .C66 2023
616.61--dc23

Foster Academics,
118-35 Queens Blvd., Suite 400,
Forest Hills, NY 11375, USA

ISBN 978-1-64646-609-2 (Hardback)

Contents

Preface

Over the recent decade, advancements and applications have progressed exponentially. This has led to the increased interest in this field and projects are being conducted to enhance knowledge. The main objective of this book is to present some of the critical challenges and provide insights into possible solutions. This book will answer the varied questions that arise in the field and also provide an increased scope for furthering studies.

Nephrology is the branch of science concerned with the diagnosis, prevention and treatment of kidney diseases. Renal replacement therapy, kidney transplantation and dialysis are a few common treatment methods to restore the normal functioning of kidneys. Kidney transplantation is a technique in which a healthy kidney of a donor is transplanted in place of a dysfunctional kidney. It can be classified into two types, namely, deceased donor kidney transplant and living donor kidney transplant. The process of surgically transplanting a deceased donor kidney into the body of a recipient whose original kidneys are unable to function normally is called deceased donor kidney transplant. A procedure in which a kidney is removed from a healthy donor and surgically placed in an individual with kidney failure is known as living donor kidney transplant. This book unravels the recent studies on nephrology and kidney transplantation. It strives to provide a fair idea about this discipline and to help develop a better understanding of the latest advances within this field. This book will serve as a valuable source of reference for graduate and postgraduate students.

I hope that this book, with its visionary approach, will be a valuable addition and will promote interest among readers. Each of the authors has provided their extraordinary competence in their specific fields by providing different perspectives as they come from diverse nations and regions. I thank them for their contributions.

Editor

1

Promises of Big Data and Artificial Intelligence in Nephrology and Transplantation

Charat Thongprayoon [1], Wisit Kaewput [2], Karthik Kovvuru [3], Panupong Hansrivijit [4], Swetha R. Kanduri [3], Tarun Bathini [5], Api Chewcharat [1], Napat Leeaphorn [6], Maria L. Gonzalez-Suarez [3] and Wisit Cheungpasitporn [3,*]

1 Division of Nephrology, Department of Medicine, Mayo Clinic, Rochester, MN 55905, USA; charat.thongprayoon@gmail.com (C.T.); api.che@hotmail.com (A.C.)
2 Department of Military and Community Medicine, Phramongkutklao College of Medicine, Bangkok 10400, Thailand; wisitnephro@gmail.com
3 Division of Nephrology, Department of Medicine, University of Mississippi Medical Center, Jackson, MS 39216, USA; kkovvuru@umc.edu (K.K.); skanduri@umc.edu (S.R.K.); mgonzalezsuarez@umc.edu (M.L.G.-S.)
4 Department of Internal Medicine, University of Pittsburgh Medical Center Pinnacle, Harrisburg, PA 17105, USA; hansrivijitp@upmc.edu
5 Department of Internal Medicine, University of Arizona, Tucson, AZ 85721, USA; tarunjacobb@gmail.com
6 Department of Nephrology, Department of Medicine, Saint Luke's Health System, Kansas City, MO 64111, USA; napat.leeaphorn@gmail.com
* Correspondence: wcheungpasitporn@gmail.com

Abstract: Kidney diseases form part of the major health burdens experienced all over the world. Kidney diseases are linked to high economic burden, deaths, and morbidity rates. The great importance of collecting a large quantity of health-related data among human cohorts, what scholars refer to as "big data", has increasingly been identified, with the establishment of a large group of cohorts and the usage of electronic health records (EHRs) in nephrology and transplantation. These data are valuable, and can potentially be utilized by researchers to advance knowledge in the field. Furthermore, progress in big data is stimulating the flourishing of artificial intelligence (AI), which is an excellent tool for handling, and subsequently processing, a great amount of data and may be applied to highlight more information on the effectiveness of medicine in kidney-related complications for the purpose of more precise phenotype and outcome prediction. In this article, we discuss the advances and challenges in big data, the use of EHRs and AI, with great emphasis on the usage of nephrology and transplantation.

Keywords: artificial intelligence; machine learning; big data; nephrology; transplantation; kidney transplantation; acute kidney injury; chronic kidney disease

---

1. Introduction

Kidney diseases, such as acute kidney injury (AKI) and chronic kidney disease (CKD) are major medical and public health issues worldwide, associated with high death and morbidity rates, together with great economic loss [1–6]. CKD is linked with a higher danger of argumentative outcomes, like cardiovascular complications, death, decreased quality of life, and substantial healthcare resource utilization [7–11], and it has been assessed that around 850 million individuals suffer different types of kidney diseases globally [12,13]. If left untreated, CKD may evolve into end-stage kidney disease (ESKD), which is associated with high mortality [14–16]. It is well-known that kidney diseases are very much multifactorial, with overlapping and complex clinical phenotypes, as well as morphologies [17].

The global distribution of nephrologists usually differs from one country to another, with bigger differences in its overall capacity [18]. Various nations across the world have established surveillance systems for kidney-related infections. Despite such attempts, the literature highlights that surveillance systems within third world countries are still not very strong [19]. In certain areas of some countries, basic records offices for transplantation and dialysis, as well as expert pathologists, are not even available [18,20]. Given how major gaps are always found in the main workforce in nephrology, the current eminence of kidney health management and research evidence in nephrology needs to be strengthened globally [21].

Traditionally, the randomized controlled trial (RCT) has always been used as the point of reference for offering evidence-based treatment. The numerical formulae applied in analyzing randomized control data have equally offered essential insights from numerous observational data. In the past few years, great emphasis has been placed on the pragmatic RCT, an essential component of real global research, which is applied when evaluating the great interventions within the actual clinical setting based on a great amount of samples so as to stimulate their individual practical value. A great amount of differences have been reported within nephrology, as well as some other relevant specialties. For instance, the literature indicates that nephrology trials were very limited in number and possessed minimally optimal features of high-quality designs [22]. Despite the fact that the already existing studies, as well as implemented works, have made major additions to a highly reliable prognostication, as well as an extensive understanding of the general histologic pathology, there is still a great amount of work which needs to be undertaken, as well as specific problems to be solved. The general capacity for undertaking cohort studies that involve a large sample size or Rapid Control trial is very much present across various parts of the globe, and has thereby resulted in the absence of research evidence within nephrology. In addition, limited activity in kidney research has impacted the evidence base for the treatment of kidney diseases, resulting in a lack of useful surrogate end-points for progression from the early stages of kidney disease-hindered trials [14,15]. On the same note, a great amount of cohort data could also be applied in generating relevant hypotheses and provide major insights into the etiology, pathogenesis, and prognosis of kidney diseases [23,24].

Those needs that are classified as unmet require provision of some ample spaces for the purpose of imagination in relation to leveraging the strength associated with big data, as well as relevant artificial intelligence (AI) to improve the overall status of patients with kidney diseases [25]. In this article, we discuss the big data concepts in nephrology, describe the potential use of AI in nephrology and transplantation, and also encourage researchers and clinicians to submit their invaluable research, including original clinical research studies [26–30], database studies from registries [31–33], meta-analyses [34–44], and artificial intelligence research [25,45–48] in nephrology and transplantation.

2. Big Data in Nephrology and Transplantation: Registries and Administrative Claims

Table 1 demonstrates known and commonly used databases that have provided big data in nephrology and transplantation [49–51]. For example, the United States Renal Data System (USRDS) is recognized as a state reconnaissance system that has the responsibility of collecting, analyzing, and subsequently distributing information regarding CKD and ESKD, all based on numerous big datasets. By delivering the yearly data report, the USRDS continuously tracks both the epidemiologic and economic burden linked to kidney diseases [52]. An important database in transplantation in the United States is the United Network for Organ Sharing (UNOS). The Organ Procurement and Transplantation Network (OPTN) data are linked by UNOS to the Social Security Death Master File for the purpose of augmenting ascertainment of different groups of candidates, as well as relevant deaths. The final data are attainable by different groups of researchers, and have always been applied in various studies regarding transplantation [50]. In addition to these databases in the United States, other countries worldwide also have big data within nephrology for researchers, such as the National Kidney Disease Surveillance Program in Ireland [53], the surveillance project on CKD management in

Canada [54], and the China Kidney Disease Network (CK-NET), a comprehensive CKD surveillance system for China [55].

Table 1. Nephrology and transplant databases and organizations.

Renal and Transplant Databases	Organizations
• United States Renal Data System (USRDS) (https://www.usrds.org) • Organ Procurement and Transplantation Network (OPTN) (https://optn.transplant.hrsa.gov) • United Network for Organ Sharing (UNOS) (https://unos.org) • Scientific Registry of Transplant Recipients (SRTR) (https://www.srtr.org) • National Health and Nutrition Examination Survey Database (NHANES) (https://www.cdc.gov/nchs/nhanes/index.htm) • Chronic kidney disease database (CKDd) (http://www.padb.org/ckddb/) • National Death Index (NDI) (https://www.cdc.gov/nchs/ndi/index.htm) • Nephrotic Syndrome Study Network (NEPTUNE) (https://nephcure.org/2015/12/nephrotic-syndrome-study-network-neptune/) • National Inpatient sample (NIS) (https://www.hcup-us.ahrq.gov/news/exhibit_booth/nis_brochure.jsp) • Polycystic Kidney Disease Consortium Data Base (PKD) (https://pkdcure.org/research-medical-professionals/pkdoc/) • Kidney Early Evaluation Program Data base (KEEP) (https://www.kidney.org/news/keep) • Diabetes mellitus Treatment for Renal Insufficiency Consortium Database (DIAMETRIC) (https://www.diametric.nl/diametric-database/) • Center for Medicare And Medicaid Services (CMS) (https://www.cms.gov) • Jackson Heart Study (JHS) (https://www.jacksonheartstudy.org) **Gene Based Databases:** • CKD- Gen Consortium Database (https://ckdgen.imbi.uni-freiburg.de) • Genome Wide Association Studies (GWAS) (https://dceg.cancer.gov/research/how-we-study/genomic-studies/gwas-overview) • Nephro Seq (https://www.nephroseq.org/resource/login.html) • Renal gene Expression Database (http://rged.wall-eva.net) • Humana Kidney and Urine Proteome Project (HKUPP) (http://www.hkupp.org) • Urine protein Biomarker Database (http://122.70.220.102/biomarker) • Urinary Peptidomics and Peak- maps (http://www.padb.org/updb/) • Kidney and Urinary Pathway Knowledge Database (KUPKB) (http://www.kupkb.org)	• ESRD Networks (https://esrdnetworks.org) • American Society of Nephrology (ASN) (https://www.asn-online.org) • National Kidney Foundation (NKF) (https://www.kidney.org) • International Society of Nephrology (ISN) (https://www.theisn.org) • American Transplant Congress (ATC) (https://atcmeeting.org) • Renal Physician Association (RPA) (https://www.renalmd.org) • International Society of Peritoneal Dialysis (ISPD) (https://ispd.org) • National Renal Administrators Association (NRAA) (https://www.nraa.org/home) • Kidney and Urology Foundation of America (http://www.kidneyurology.org) • American Kidney Fund (https://www.kidneyfund.org/about-us/) • American Society of Artificial Internal Organs (https://asaio.org/about/) • Organ Procurement Organization (OPO) (https://unos.org/transplant/opos-increasing-organ-donation) • Acute Dialysis Quality Initiative (ADQI) (http://www.adqi.net/) • National Institute of Health (NIH) (https://www.nih.gov) • National Institute of Diabetes and Digestive and Kidney Diseases (https://www.niddk.nih.gov) • National Center for Health Statistics (NCHS) (https://www.cdc.gov/nchs/about/index.htm)

Numerous networks of international collaboration, like the International Network of CKD cohorts [56], the Therapeutic Evaluation of Steroids in IgA Nephropathy Global study [57], and the Chronic Kidney Disease Prognosis Consortium [58] have grown immensely within the last few years. There are possible advantages of introducing a traditional data element that are linked to kidney infections, like escalating the overall power of the groups which are under-represented [59]. There is, however, great need to address numerous challenges, like standardization of data, identification of the patient, plus some other additional infrastructure-related challenges. Additionally, the cadre of genomics is developing at a very rapid rate towards realizing an analysis of single cells, and subsequent great advances within metabolomics and proteomics have been developed within the past few years.

A great amount of progress has equally been realized within technological developments within the areas of large-scale molecular data generation in various databases that are gene-based (Table 1). The most recent advancements in technology have made it possible for us to produce larger amounts of data, more specifically regarding the omics data. Further development of somehow less expensive genotype arrays and the subsequent presence of samples within biobanks made it possible to undertake genome-wide association studies among numerous groups of patients, offering highly essential insights into the great risk factors and the pathogenesis of multiple kidney diseases [60–63].

Within nephrology, numerous consortia-collecting biopsy biobanks of kidney tissue have been started to undertake such forms of collaborative study. Several initiatives that are aimed at extensive characterization of the relevant kidney biopsies for various groups of kidney diseases subtypes have subsequently been launched, comprising of the NEPTUNE (Nephrotic Syndrome STudy Network), ERCB (European Renal cDNA Bank), EURenOmics, C-PROBE (Clinical Phenotyping and Resource Biobank), PKU-IgAN, and more recently, TRIDENT (for diabetic nephropathy), CureGN (for glomerulopathies), and the NIDDK (National Institute of Diabetes and Digestive and Kidney Diseases) Kidney Precision Medicine Project (KPMP) [64].

Big data within the medicine field might offer the opportunity to envision patients suffering from kidney diseases in a more holistic manner, using numerous lenses, each of which adequately presents the great opportunity of studying various scientific queries. Such data within the big databases might subsequently comprise of the general administrative health-related data, biometric data, biomarker data, as well as imaging, and might subsequently come from various sources, comprising of electronic health records, biobanks, reports in the internet, and various clinical registries [65]. These data from the large databases are collected and updated overtime. These data are valuable and can be used by researchers to answer numerous research questions and advance knowledge in nephrology and transplantation [66–68].

3. Using Electronic Health Record Data in Nephrology

Two major events have been reported within the last 10 years that seem to have changed the whole situation. To begin with is making it possible to digitalize all relevant medical information—more specifically, the initiation of EHRs that have the medical histories of the patients—and facilitate the processing of medical information using computers. This helps to make information-processing become automated by the use of given specialized software. EHRs have been greatly utilized with major regularity, clinical informatics strategies have subsequently been refined, and subsequently, the EHR field enabled [69,70].

The wide application of EHRs, when put together with the relevant novel of big data, tends to create some forms of unique opportunities for the purpose of nephrology research, as well as improvement in care for individual patients who might be suffering from kidney complications and transplantation. The data which is there within the EHR is considered big insofar as its volume is concerned. Such interventions have resulted in a new era of big data which has subsequently fueled precision medicine. These types of approach have already indicated an improved level of diagnosis, risk assessment, as well as treatment and management of numerous health conditions. With medicine getting digitalized, a great amount of data has since been developed from all aspects of health care, comprising the laboratory tests, EHR, together with medical imaging.

For instance, in the instance of electronic AKI, the automated diagnostic strategy tends to create a great opportunity to initiate predictive strategies, optimize the relevant AKI alerts, and subsequently trace AKI events across various institutions, as well as administrative datasets. The growth in the adoption of EHR and subsequent maturation of the relevant clinical informatics techniques might provide some sort of unique opportunity to advance the general predictive capabilities. Immediately, AKI has been properly diagnosed within real time, and several EHR-enabled interventions have become so viable. One of such great prospects is actually the prediction of detecting events prior to their occurrence [71]. AKI events might temporarily get anchored within the EHR, which develops a pre-disease phase of care, having the information which had accumulated before the development of

AKI. With a greater amount of content, high-throughput strategies can be applied to such a group of data so as to help in identifying a form of pre-AKI signal, which can subsequently assist in discriminating between patients who are of high risk and low risk for the AKI. The capability to predict AKI risk in this manner might subsequently have some forms of dramatic impact, as presently there is no scientifically proven treatment for AKI once one develops such conditions [72]. As patients who are considered to be of high risk get identified, the extent of care can get modified, and further strategies for harm prevention implemented. In the long run, such groups of patients, institutions, and population-based techniques will result in better long- and short-term outcomes for the respective hospitals, patients, and the whole of the healthcare system. Despite the fact that potential barriers are always there, and several nuanced groups need to be taken into consideration, such approaches that are EHR-enabled have the ability to greatly improve AKI-associated knowledge and care.

Patients suffering from kidney complications are reported to have the highest level of heterogeneity in manifestation of the disease, treatment response, and overall progression. The growth in big data actually tends to stimulate the general boom of artificial intelligence that is a perfect tool that helps in handling, and also processing the big data. AI can assist in shedding light on the specific accuracy of medicines used to treat kidney diseases, for outcome prediction, and also to gain a more precise phenotype.

4. Artificial Intelligence in Nephrology and Transplantation

AI presently shows a very important function in nearly all areas of the day-to-day lives of human beings, as well as within different academic disciplines. Based on the fact that there has been growth in the power of computers, developments in techniques and methods, and the overall blast of the quantity of medicine, data has never been an exemption. Literature clarifies that artificial intelligence can be used in disease risk assessment. Actually, disease risk assessment has a very important influence on the general prognosis, as well as clinical intervention strategies. Accurate and rapid assessment can assist clinicians in determining the conditions of the patient, out of which optimal treatment strategies can be implemented. Links between prognosis and risk factors of the diseases are very complex. The same risk factors can be experienced within different groups of diseases, and a single disease can actually be composed of several risk factors. In such case, the links between the known risk factors and the disease has very strong correlativity, instead of simple causality. Artificial intelligence can hence be applied in doing disease risk assessment in order to understand the main factors linked to disease prognosis so as to offer effective treatment for tertiary prevention of the disease. One of the important sections of AI is machine learning, which is characterized as the study of algorithms and statistical models that computer systems utilize to learn from sample data and previous experience without being explicitly programmed to achieve particular assignments. With the ability to identify obscure patterns in the data, we can use machine learning to solve many problems, including assessing relationships of two variables, creating predictions based on baseline characteristics, identifying objects with comparable patterns, and incorporating subjects by specific criteria. Machine learning techniques have the capacities of managing complex datasets and tremendous numbers of variables that are exceeding the capability of classical statistical methods [17]—see Figure 1A. Machine learning algorithms are usually utilized without initiating as many presumptions of the underlying data. In addition, a machine-learning method can determine complex patterns of health trajectories of immense numbers of characteristics and patients, which has exhibited high predictive certainty, and been confirmed and replicated with various validation investigations [73]. Well-known machine-learning algorithms include the artificial neural network (ANN), random forest, gradient boosting trees, and support vector machine [17].

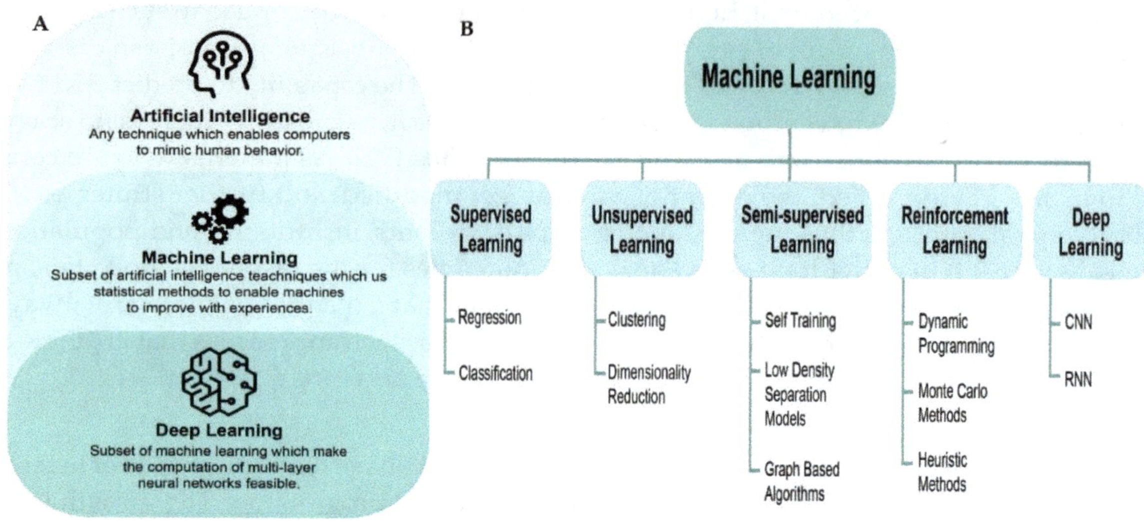

Figure 1. (**a**) Relationships between artificial intelligence, machine learning, and deep learning. (**b**) Types of machine learning. CNN, convolutional neural network; RNN, recurrent neural network.

Inspired by the idea of mimicking the biological structure of human brains, deep learning is a subfield of machine learning based on ANN [74]. Deep-learning models can learn many levels of data design with a multiple-processing-layers model structure, attaining more powerful model performance. This cutting-edge technology has significantly changed the paradigm of visual object recognition, speech recognition, and many other domains, such as genomics and drug discovery. Deep learning techniques are increasingly being applied to biomedical data, from image processing to genomic data analysis [75]. Such methods might outperform pathologists' fibrosis scores from histological renal biopsy images [76]. Well-known techniques include the convolutional neural network (CNN), fully connected neural network, generative adversarial network (GAN), deep reinforcement learning, and recurrent neural network (RNN) [17,77], shown in Figure 1B. AI-based clinical decision support systems (CDSS) can be implemented employing the expert system strategy, data-driven approach, or an ensemble approach by coupling both. An expert system consolidates a knowledge base containing a set of rules for specific clinical scenarios, and the initial rule set may be acquired from domain experts or learned from data through machine learning algorithms [72,78–80].

AI has recently been adopted for the prediction, diagnosis, and treatment of kidney diseases [76,81–85], as shown in Table 2. For example, a prediction model based on the combination of a machine learning algorithm and survival analysis has recently developed and can stratify risk for kidney disease progression among patients with IgA Nephropathy [86]. For AKI research, Tomasev et al. [83] recently used deep-learning methods to make a continuous prediction of AKI by developing a RNN model on the sequential health record data of >700,000 veterans, allowing physicians to practise with adequate data and sufficient time. In addition, regarding utilization of ANN and CNN methods, Kolachalama et al. [76] recently provided a perspicacity into the association of pathological fibrosis identified from histologic images with clinical phenotypes for patients with CKD, helping the diagnostics and prognostics of these phenotypes. Subsequently, there has been an increasing number of AI studies, with great emphasis on the usage of nephrology and transplantation [85,87–89].

Table 2. Selected articles reporting the utilization of artificial intelligence, machine learning, or deep learning in the field of nephrology and kidney transplantation.

Study	Country	Study Type	N	Subjects	Intervention
Zhou, 2020 [90]	China	R	212	Prediction of ARF and paraplegia after TAAAR	Machine learning classification models
Xu, 2020 [91]	USA	R	37,486	Identification the sub-phenotypes of AKI	Memory network-based deep learning approach
Song, 2020 [92]	USA	R	14,039	Longitudinal Risk Prediction of CKD in Diabetic Patients	Temporal-enhanced gradient boosting machine
Rashidi, 2020 [93]	USA	P, R	101	Early recognition of burn- and trauma-related AKI	Artificial intelligence /machine learning algorithms
Morid, 2020 [94]	USA	R	22,542	Prediction of adverse events in critical patients with AKI	Temporal pattern detection
Luo, 2020 [95]	China	R	519	Prediction of severe pneumonia during post-transplant hospitalization in recipients of a deceased-donor kidney transplant	Machine learning
Li, 2020 [96]	China	P	1952	Accuracy improvement of GFR estimation	Artificial neural network
Lei, 2020 [97]	China	R	1173	Prediction of AKI after liver cancer resection	Machine learning algorithms
Kate, 2020 [98]	USA	R	44,691	Prediction of AKI in hospitalized patients	Machine learning predictive models
Kang, 2020 [99]	South Korea	R	1571	Prediction of mortality in CRRT patients	Machine learning algorithms
Zimmerman, 2019 [100]	USA	R	23,950	Prediction of AKI following ICU admission	Machine learning models
Zhang, 2019 [101]	China	R	2456	Prediction of volume responsiveness in oliguric AKI	Machine learning models
Xu, 2019 [102]	USA	R	58,976	Prediction of mortality in patients with AKI in the ICU	Machine learning models
Xiao, 2019 [103]	China	R	551	Prediction of CKD progression	Machine learning tools
Mark, 2019 [104]	USA	R	100,000	Prediction of survival of kidney transplant recipients from UNOS	Machine learning models
Bae, 2019 [105]	USA	R	120,818	Prediction of survival after deceased donor kidney transplant from OPTN database	Machine learning methods

AKI, acute kidney injury; ARF, acute renal failure; AUC, area under curve; CKD, chronic kidney disease; CRRT, continuous renal replacement therapy; GFR, glomerular filtration rate; ICU, intensive care unit; OPTN, Organ Procurement and Transplantation Network; P, prospective; R, retrospective; TAAAR, thoracoabdominal aortic aneurysm repair; UNOS, United Network for Organ Sharing.

5. Potential Directions and Future Scope

In order to reinforce the usage and subsequent transformation of AI as well as data–based CDSSs in nephrology, AI, as well as big data, offers the chance to actually source knowledge from expert knowledge and big data and subsequently transform it into some form of intelligent system, which can be applied in risk classification, disease diagnosis, drug discovery, and prognostic evaluation, among some other things. AI might be useful in establishing the type of kidney disease and subsequently help in solving problems related to survival analysis of the patients who have gone through kidney transplants [106–114]. Renal biopsy images may be a good data base for application of machine learning algorithms.

Despite having numerous imperfections, big data, as well as artificial intelligence have been applied in the field of medication from numerous parts [115,116]. There are numerous possible guidelines of using big data and artificial intelligence in nephrology that requires greater attention, as well as further consideration [74,78,117–125].

6. Conclusions

In summary, the present status of kidney health care, and subsequently, research evidence in nephrology requires strengthening. Big data research that is problem-driven in nephrology is very much essential in promoting the interdisciplinary incorporation and subsequent improvements in kidney disease, and it may subsequently offer some greater insights to further studies in the future. Within the present era of using big data, it is strongly believed that big data and artificial intelligence will greatly reshape research done on kidney disease and consequently improve the general clinical practice of nephrology in the near future.

References

1. Sutherland, S.M.; Goldstein, S.L.; Bagshaw, S.M. Leveraging Big Data and Electronic Health Records to Enhance Novel Approaches to Acute Kidney Injury Research and Care. *Blood Purif.* **2017**, *44*, 68–76. [CrossRef] [PubMed]
2. Kashani, K.; Cheungpasitporn, W.; Ronco, C. Biomarkers of acute kidney injury: The pathway from discovery to clinical adoption. *Clin. Chem. Lab. Med.* **2017**, *55*, 1074–1089. [CrossRef] [PubMed]
3. Srivali, N.; Thongprayoon, C.; Cheungpasitporn, W.; Ungprasert, P.; Caples, S.M. Unusual cause of pleural effusion: Ovarian hyperstimulation syndrome. *QJM* **2016**, *109*, 197–198. [CrossRef] [PubMed]
4. Sanguankeo, A.; Upala, S.; Cheungpasitporn, W.; Ungprasert, P.; Knight, E.L. Effects of Statins on Renal Outcome in Chronic Kidney Disease Patients: A Systematic Review and Meta-Analysis. *PLoS ONE* **2015**, *10*, e0132970. [CrossRef] [PubMed]
5. Cheungpasitporn, W.; Thongprayoon, C.; Kittanamongkolchai, W.; Sakhuja, A.; Mao, M.A.; Erickson, S.B. Impact of admission serum potassium on mortality in patients with chronic kidney disease and cardiovascular disease. *QJM* **2017**, *110*, 713–739. [CrossRef]
6. Jadlowiec, C.; Smith, M.; Neville, M.; Mao, S.; Abdelwahab, D.; Reddy, K.; Moss, A.; Aqel, B.; Taner, T. Acute Kidney Injury Patterns Following Transplantation of Steatotic Liver Allografts. *J. Clin. Med.* **2020**, *9*, 954. [CrossRef]
7. Cheungpasitporn, W.; Thongprayoon, C.; O'Corragain, O.A.; Edmonds, P.J.; Kittanamongkolchai, W.; Erickson, S.B. Associations of sugar-sweetened and artificially sweetened soda with chronic kidney disease: A systematic review and meta-analysis. *Nephrology* **2014**, *19*, 791–797. [CrossRef]
8. Wijarnpreecha, K.; Thongprayoon, C.; Chesdachai, S.; Panjawatanana, P.; Ungprasert, P.; Cheungpasitporn, W. Associations of Proton-Pump Inhibitors and H2 Receptor Antagonists with Chronic Kidney Disease: A Meta-Analysis. *Dig. Dis. Sci.* **2017**, *62*, 2821–2827. [CrossRef]

9. Wijarnpreecha, K.; Thongprayoon, C.; Thamcharoen, N.; Panjawatanan, P.; Cheungpasitporn, W. Association of coffee consumption and chronic kidney disease: A meta-analysis. *Int. J. Clin. Pr.* **2017**, *71*. [CrossRef]
10. Wijarnpreecha, K.; Thongprayoon, C.; Nissaisorakarn, P.; Jaruvongvanich, V.; Nakkala, K.; Rajapakse, R.; Cheungpasitporn, W. Association of Helicobacter pylori with Chronic Kidney Diseases: A Meta-Analysis. *Dig. Dis. Sci.* **2017**, *62*, 2045–2052. [CrossRef]
11. Wijarnpreecha, K.; Thongprayoon, C.; Scribani, M.; Ungprasert, P.; Cheungpasitporn, W. Noninvasive fibrosis markers and chronic kidney disease among adults with nonalcoholic fatty liver in USA. *Eur. J. Gastroenterol Hepatol.* **2018**, *30*, 404–410. [CrossRef]
12. Glassock, R.J.; Warnock, D.G.; Delanaye, P. The global burden of chronic kidney disease: Estimates, variability and pitfalls. *Nat. Rev. Nephrol.* **2017**, *13*, 104–114. [CrossRef]
13. Jha, V.; Garcia-Garcia, G.; Iseki, K.; Li, Z.; Naicker, S.; Plattner, B.; Saran, R.; Wang, A.Y.; Yang, C.W. Chronic kidney disease: global dimension and perspectives. Chronic kidney disease: Global dimension and perspectives. *Lancet* **2013**, *382*, 260–272. [CrossRef]
14. Kaewput, W.; Thongprayoon, C.; Rangsin, R.; Ruangkanchanasetr, P.; Bathini, T.; Mao, M.A.; Cheungpasitporn, W. Association between serum uric acid and chronic kidney disease in patients with hypertension: A multicenter nationwide cross-sectional study. *J. Evid. Based Med.* **2019**, *12*, 235–242. [CrossRef]
15. Piccoli, G.B.; Breuer, C.; Cabiddu, G.; Testa, A.; Jadeau, C.; Brunori, G. Where Are You Going, Nephrology? Considerations on Models of Care in an Evolving Discipline. *J. Clin. Med.* **2018**, *7*, 199. [CrossRef] [PubMed]
16. Kaewput, W.; Thongprayoon, C.; Chewcharat, A.; Rangsin, R.; Satirapoj, B.; Kaewput, C.; Suwannahitatorn, P.; Bathini, T.; Mao, M.A.; Cato, L.D.; et al. Rate of kidney function decline and factors predicting progression of kidney disease in type 2 diabetes mellitus patients with reduced kidney function: A nationwide retrospective cohort study. *Ther. Apher. Dial.* **2020**. [CrossRef] [PubMed]
17. Xie, G.; Chen, T.; Li, Y.; Chen, T.; Li, X.; Liu, Z. Artificial Intelligence in Nephrology: How Can Artificial Intelligence Augment Nephrologists' Intelligence? *Kidney Dis.* **2020**, *6*, 1–6. [CrossRef] [PubMed]
18. Levin, A. Global challenges in kidney diseases. *Nephrol Dial. Transpl.* **2018**, *33*, 371–372. [CrossRef]
19. Yang, C.; Kong, G.; Wang, L.; Zhang, L.; Zhao, M.-H. Big data in nephrology: Are we ready for the change? *Nephrology* **2019**, *24*, 1097–1102. [CrossRef]
20. Kolachalama, V.B.; Singh, P.; Lin, C.Q.; Mun, D.; Belghasem, M.E.; Henderson, J.M.; Francis, J.M.; Salant, D.J.; Chitalia, V.C. Association of Pathological Fibrosis With Renal Survival Using Deep Neural Networks. *Kidney Int. Rep.* **2018**, *3*, 464–475. [CrossRef]
21. Bello, A.K.; Levin, A.; Tonelli, M.; Okpechi, I.G.; Feehally, J.; Harris, D.; Jindal, K.; Salako, B.L.; Rateb, A.; Osman, M.A.; et al. Assessment of Global Kidney Health Care Status. *JAMA* **2017**, *317*, 1864–1881. [CrossRef] [PubMed]
22. Inrig, J.K.; Califf, R.M.; Tasneem, A.; Vegunta, R.K.; Molina, C.; Stanifer, J.W.; Chiswell, K.; Patel, U.D. The landscape of clinical trials in nephrology: A systematic review of Clinicaltrials.gov. *Am. J. Kidney Dis.* **2014**, *63*, 771–780. [CrossRef] [PubMed]
23. Hulsen, T.; Jamuar, S.S.; Moody, A.R.; Karnes, J.H.; Varga, O.; Hedensted, S.; Spreafico, R.; Hafler, D.A.; McKinney, E.F. From Big Data to Precision Medicine. *Front. Med.* **2019**, *6*, 34. [CrossRef] [PubMed]
24. Shilo, S.; Rossman, H.; Segal, E. Axes of a revolution: Challenges and promises of big data in healthcare. *Nat. Med.* **2020**, *26*, 29–38. [CrossRef]
25. Gameiro, J.; Branco, T.; Lopes, J.A. Artificial Intelligence in Acute Kidney Injury Risk Prediction. *J. Clin. Med.* **2020**, *9*, 678.
26. Gore, E.J.; Gomes-Neto, A.W.; Wang, L.; Bakker, S.; Niesters, H.; de Joode, A.; Verschuuren, E.; Westra, J.; Leer-Buter, C.V. Torquetenovirus Serum Load and Long-Term Outcomes in Renal Transplant Recipients. *J. Clin. Med.* **2020**, *9*, 440. [CrossRef]
27. Swarte, J.C.; Douwes, R.M.; Hu, S.; Vich Vila, A.; Eisenga, M.F.; van Londen, M.; Gomes-Neto, A.W.; Weersma, R.K.; Harmsen, H.; Bakker, S. Characteristics and Dysbiosis of the Gut Microbiome in Renal Transplant Recipients. *J. Clin. Med.* **2020**, *9*, 386. [CrossRef]
28. Thölking, G.; Gillhaus, N.H.; Schütte-Nütgen, K.; Pavenstädt, H.; Koch, R.; Suwelack, B.; Reuter, S. Conversion to Everolimus was Beneficial and Safe for Fast and Slow Tacrolimus Metabolizers After Renal Transplantation. *J. Clin. Med.* **2020**, *9*, 328. [CrossRef]

29. Cheungpasitporn, W.; Kremers, W.K.; Lorenz, E.; Amer, H.; Cosio, F.G.; Stegall, M.D.; Gandhi, M.J.; Schinstock, C.A. De novo donor-specific antibody following BK nephropathy: The incidence and association with antibody-mediated rejection. *Clin. Transpl.* **2018**, *32*, e13194. [CrossRef]
30. Chewcharat, A.; Thongprayoon, C.; Cheungpasitporn, W.; Mao, M.A.; Thirunavukkarasu, S.; Kashani, K.B. Trajectories of Serum Sodium on In-Hospital and 1-Year Survival among Hospitalized Patients. *Clin. J. Am. Soc. Nephrol.* **2020**. [CrossRef]
31. Kaewput, W.; Thongprayoon, C.; Boonpheng, B.; Ungprasert, P.; Bathini, T.; Chewcharat, A.; Srivali, N.; Vallabhajosyula, S.; Cheungpasitporn, W. Inpatient Burden and Mortality of Goodpasture's Syndrome in the United States: Nationwide Inpatient Sample 2003–2014. *J. Clin. Med.* **2020**, *9*, 455. [CrossRef] [PubMed]
32. Cheungpasitporn, W.; Thongprayoon, C.; Ungprasert, P.; Wijarnpreecha, K.; Kaewput, W.; Leeaphorn, N.; Bathini, T.; Chebib, F.T.; Kröner, P.T. Subarachnoid Hemorrhage in Hospitalized Renal Transplant Recipients with Autosomal Dominant Polycystic Kidney Disease: A Nationwide Analysis. *J. Clin. Med.* **2019**, *8*, 524. [CrossRef] [PubMed]
33. Leeaphorn, N.; Thongprayoon, C.; Chon, W.J.; Cummings, L.S.; Mao, M.A.; Cheungpasitporn, W. Outcomes of kidney retransplantation after graft loss as a result of BK virus nephropathy in the era of newer immunosuppressant agents. *Am. J. Transpl.* **2019**. [CrossRef] [PubMed]
34. Lertjitbanjong, P.; Thongprayoon, C.; Cheungpasitporn, W.; O'Corragain, O.A.; Srivali, N.; Bathini, T.; Watthanasuntorn, K.; Aeddula, N.R.; Salim, S.A.; Ungprasert, P.; et al. Acute Kidney Injury after Lung Transplantation: A Systematic Review and Meta-Analysis. *J. Clin. Med.* **2019**, *8*, 1713. [CrossRef] [PubMed]
35. Thongprayoon, C.; Kaewput, W.; Thamcharoen, N.; Bathini, T.; Watthanasuntorn, K.; Lertjitbanjong, P.; Sharma, K.; Salim, S.A.; Ungprasert, P.; Wijarnpreecha, K.; et al. Incidence and Impact of Acute Kidney Injury after Liver Transplantation: A Meta-Analysis. *J. Clin. Med.* **2019**, *8*, 372. [CrossRef] [PubMed]
36. Wongboonsin, J.; Thongprayoon, C.; Bathini, T.; Ungprasert, P.; Aeddula, N.R.; Mao, M.A.; Cheungpasitporn, W. Acetazolamide Therapy in Patients with Heart Failure: A Meta-Analysis. *J. Clin. Med.* **2019**, *8*, 349. [CrossRef]
37. Gonzalez Suarez, M.L.; Thongprayoon, C.; Mao, M.A.; Leeaphorn, N.; Bathini, T.; Cheungpasitporn, W. Outcomes of Kidney Transplant Patients with Atypical Hemolytic Uremic Syndrome Treated with Eculizumab: A Systematic Review and Meta-Analysis. *J. Clin. Med.* **2019**, *8*, 919. [CrossRef]
38. Chewcharat, A.; Thongprayoon, C.; Bathini, T.; Aeddula, N.R.; Boonpheng, B.; Kaewput, W.; Watthanasuntorn, K.; Lertjitbanjong, P.; Sharma, K.; Torres-Ortiz, A.; et al. Incidence and Mortality of Renal Cell Carcinoma after Kidney Transplantation: A Meta-Analysis. *J. Clin. Med.* **2019**, *8*, 530. [CrossRef]
39. Cheungpasitporn, W.; Thongprayoon, C.; Craici, I.M.; Sharma, K.; Chesdachai, S.; Khoury, N.J.; Ettore, A.S. Reactivation of BK polyomavirus during pregnancy, vertical transmission, and clinical significance: A meta-analysis. *J. Clin. Virol.* **2018**, *102*, 56–62. [CrossRef]
40. Thongprayoon, C.; Cheungpasitporn, W.; Lertjitbanjong, P.; Aeddula, N.R.; Bathini, T.; Watthanasuntorn, K.; Srivali, N.; Mao, M.A.; Kashani, K. Incidence and Impact of Acute Kidney Injury in Patients Receiving Extracorporeal Membrane Oxygenation: A Meta-Analysis. *J. Clin. Med.* **2019**, *8*, 981. [CrossRef]
41. Thongprayoon, C.; Kaewput, W.; Thamcharoen, N.; Bathini, T.; Watthanasuntorn, K.; Salim, S.A.; Ungprasert, P.; Lertjitbanjong, P.; Aeddula, N.R.; Torres-Ortiz, A.; et al. Acute Kidney Injury in Patients Undergoing Total Hip Arthroplasty: A Systematic Review and Meta-Analysis. *J. Clin. Med.* **2019**, *8*, 66. [CrossRef]
42. Kanduri, S.R.; Cheungpasitporn, W.; Thongprayoon, C.; Bathini, T.; Kovvuru, K.; Garla, V.; Medaura, J.; Vaitla, P.; Kashani, K.B. Incidence and Mortality of Acute Kidney Injury in Patients Undergoing Hematopoietic Stem Cell Transplantation: A Systematic Review and Meta-analysis. *QJM* **2020**. [CrossRef] [PubMed]
43. Thongprayoon, C.; Cheungpasitporn, W.; Mao, M.A.; Sakhuja, A.; Erickson, S.B. Admission calcium levels and risk of acute kidney injury in hospitalised patients. *Int. J. Clin. Pr.* **2018**, *72*, e13057. [CrossRef] [PubMed]
44. Thongprayoon, C.; Khoury, N.J.; Bathini, T.; Aeddula, N.R.; Boonpheng, B.; Leeaphorn, N.; Ungprasert, P.; Bruminhent, J.; Lertjitbanjong, P.; Watthanasuntorn, K.; et al. BK polyomavirus genotypes in renal transplant recipients in the United States: A meta-analysis. *J. Evid. Based Med.* **2019**, *12*, 291–299. [CrossRef] [PubMed]
45. Lin, S.Y.; Hsieh, M.H.; Lin, C.L.; Hsieh, M.J.; Hsu, W.H.; Lin, C.C.; Hsu, C.Y.; Kao, C.H. Artificial Intelligence Prediction Model for the Cost and Mortality of Renal Replacement Therapy in Aged and Super-Aged Populations in Taiwan. *J. Clin. Med.* **2019**, *8*, 995. [CrossRef] [PubMed]

46. Díez-Sanmartín, C.; Sarasa Cabezuelo, A. Application of Artificial Intelligence Techniques to Predict Survival in Kidney Transplantation: A Review. *J. Clin. Med.* **2020**, *9*, 572. [CrossRef]
47. Azuaje, F.; Kim, S.Y.; Perez Hernandez, D.; Dittmar, G. Connecting Histopathology Imaging and Proteomics in Kidney Cancer through Machine Learning. *J. Clin. Med.* **2019**, *8*, 1535. [CrossRef]
48. Hsiao, C.C.; Tu, H.T.; Lin, C.H.; Chen, K.H.; Yeh, Y.H.; See, L.C. Temporal Trends of Severe Hypoglycemia and Subsequent Mortality in Patients with Advanced Diabetic Kidney Diseases Transitioning to Dialysis. *J. Clin. Med.* **2019**, *8*, 420. [CrossRef]
49. Gout, A.M.; Martin, N.C.; Brown, A.F.; Ravine, D. PKDB: Polycystic Kidney Disease Mutation Database—A gene variant database for autosomal dominant polycystic kidney disease. *Hum. Mutat.* **2007**, *28*, 654–659. [CrossRef]
50. Massie, A.B.; Kucirka, L.M.; Segev, D.L. Big data in organ transplantation: Registries and administrative claims. *Am. J. Transpl.* **2014**, *14*, 1723–1730. [CrossRef]
51. Papadopoulos, T.; Krochmal, M.; Cisek, K.; Fernandes, M.; Husi, H.; Stevens, R.; Bascands, J.L.; Schanstra, J.P.; Klein, J. Omics databases on kidney disease: Where they can be found and how to benefit from them. *Clin. Kidney J.* **2016**, *9*, 343–352. [CrossRef] [PubMed]
52. Port, F.K.; Held, P.J. The US Renal Data System at 30 Years: A Historical Perspective. *Am. J. Kidney Dis.* **2019**, *73*, 459–461. [CrossRef] [PubMed]
53. Stack, A.G.; Casserly, L.F.; Cronin, C.J.; Chernenko, T.; Cullen, W.; Hannigan, A.; Saran, R.; Johnson, H.; Browne, G.; Ferguson, J.P. Prevalence and variation of Chronic Kidney Disease in the Irish health system: Initial findings from the National Kidney Disease Surveillance Programme. *Bmc Nephrol.* **2014**, *15*, 185. [CrossRef] [PubMed]
54. Bello, A.K.; Ronksley, P.E.; Tangri, N.; Singer, A.; Grill, A.; Nitsch, D.; Queenan, J.A.; Lindeman, C.; Soos, B.; Freiheit, E.; et al. A national surveillance project on chronic kidney disease management in Canadian primary care: A study protocol. *BMJ Open* **2017**, *7*, e016267. [CrossRef] [PubMed]
55. Saran, R.; Steffick, D.; Bragg-Gresham, J. The China Kidney Disease Network (CK-NET): "Big Data-Big Dreams". *Am. J. Kidney Dis.* **2017**, *69*, 713–716. [CrossRef]
56. Dienemann, T.; Fujii, N.; Orlandi, P.; Nessel, L.; Furth, S.L.; Hoy, W.E.; Matsuo, S.; Mayer, G.; Methven, S.; Schaefer, F.; et al. International Network of Chronic Kidney Disease cohort studies (iNET-CKD): A global network of chronic kidney disease cohorts. *BMC Nephrol.* **2016**, *17*, 121. [CrossRef]
57. Lv, J.; Zhang, H.; Wong, M.G.; Jardine, M.J.; Hladunewich, M.; Jha, V.; Monaghan, H.; Zhao, M.; Barbour, S.; Reich, H.; et al. Effect of Oral Methylprednisolone on Clinical Outcomes in Patients With IgA Nephropathy: The TESTING Randomized Clinical Trial. *JAMA* **2017**, *318*, 432–442. [CrossRef]
58. Matsushita, K.; Ballew, S.H.; Astor, B.C.; Jong, P.E.d.; Gansevoort, R.T.; Hemmelgarn, B.R.; Levey, A.S.; Levin, A.; Wen, C.-P.; Woodward, M.; et al. Cohort profile: The chronic kidney disease prognosis consortium. *Int. J. Epidemiol.* **2013**, *42*, 1660–1668. [CrossRef]
59. Levin, A.; Tonelli, M.; Bonventre, J.; Coresh, J.; Donner, J.-A.; Fogo, A.B.; Fox, C.S.; Gansevoort, R.T.; Heerspink, H.J.L.; Jardine, M.; et al. Global kidney health 2017 and beyond: A roadmap for closing gaps in care, research, and policy. *Lancet* **2017**, *390*, 1888–1917. [CrossRef]
60. O'Seaghdha, C.M.; Fox, C.S. Genome-wide association studies of chronic kidney disease: What have we learned? *Nat. Rev. Nephrol.* **2011**, *8*, 89–99. [CrossRef]
61. Wuttke, M.; Köttgen, A. Insights into kidney diseases from genome-wide association studies. *Nat. Rev. Nephrol.* **2016**, *12*, 549–562. [CrossRef]
62. Ahlqvist, E.; van Zuydam, N.R.; Groop, L.C.; McCarthy, M.I. The genetics of diabetic complications. *Nat. Rev. Nephrol.* **2015**, *11*, 277–287. [CrossRef] [PubMed]
63. Mohan, C.; Putterman, C. Genetics and pathogenesis of systemic lupus erythematosus and lupus nephritis. *Nat. Rev. Nephrol.* **2015**, *11*, 329–341. [CrossRef] [PubMed]
64. Lindenmeyer, M.T.; Kretzler, M. Renal biopsy-driven molecular target identification in glomerular disease. *Pflug. Arch.* **2017**, *469*, 1021–1028. [CrossRef] [PubMed]
65. Rumsfeld, J.S.; Joynt, K.E.; Maddox, T.M. Big data analytics to improve cardiovascular care: Promise and challenges. *Nat. Rev. Cardiol.* **2016**, *13*, 350–359. [CrossRef]
66. Cheungpasitporn, W.; Thongprayoon, C.; Ungprasert, P.; Wijarnpreecha, K.; Raimondo, M.; Kroner, P.T. Acute pancreatitis in end-stage renal disease patients in the USA: A nationwide, propensity score-matched analysis. *Eur. J. Gastroenterol. Hepatol.* **2019**, *31*, 968–972. [CrossRef]

67. Thongprayoon, C.; Kaewput, W.; Boonpheng, B.; Ungprasert, P.; Bathini, T.; Srivali, N.; Vallabhajosyula, S.; Castaneda, J.L.; Monga, D.; Kanduri, S.R.; et al. Impact of ANCA-Associated Vasculitis on Outcomes of Hospitalizations for Goodpasture's Syndrome in the United States: Nationwide Inpatient Sample 2003-2014. *Medicina* **2020**, *56*, 103. [CrossRef]
68. Ungprasert, P.; Koster, M.J.; Cheungpasitporn, W.; Wijarnpreecha, K.; Thongprayoon, C.; Kroner, P.T. Inpatient epidemiology and economic burden of granulomatosis with polyangiitis: A 10-year study of the national inpatient sample. *Rheumatology* **2020**. [CrossRef]
69. Evans, R.S. Electronic Health Records: Then, Now, and in the Future. *Yearb. Med. Inform.* **2016**, *25* (Suppl. 1), S48–S61. [CrossRef]
70. Sutherland, S.M.; Goldstein, S.L.; Bagshaw, S.M. Acute Kidney Injury and Big Data. *Contrib. Nephrol.* **2018**, *193*, 55–67.
71. Sutherland, S.M. Electronic Health Record-Enabled Big-Data Approaches to Nephrotoxin-Associated Acute Kidney Injury Risk Prediction. *Pharmacotherapy* **2018**, *38*, 804–812. [CrossRef] [PubMed]
72. Sutherland, S.M. Big Data and Pediatric Acute Kidney Injury: The Promise of Electronic Health Record Systems. *Front. Pediatr.* **2019**, *7*, 536. [CrossRef] [PubMed]
73. Shipp, M.A.; Ross, K.N.; Tamayo, P.; Weng, A.P.; Kutok, J.L.; Aguiar, R.C.; Gaasenbeek, M.; Angelo, M.; Reich, M.; Pinkus, G.S.; et al. Diffuse large B-cell lymphoma outcome prediction by gene-expression profiling and supervised machine learning. *Nat. Med.* **2002**, *8*, 68–74. [CrossRef]
74. Saez-Rodriguez, J.; Rinschen, M.M.; Floege, J.; Kramann, R. Big science and big data in nephrology. *Kidney Int.* **2019**, *95*, 1326–1337. [CrossRef] [PubMed]
75. Angermueller, C.; Pärnamaa, T.; Parts, L.; Stegle, O. Deep learning for computational biology. *Mol. Syst Biol.* **2016**, *12*, 878. [CrossRef] [PubMed]
76. SGarcelon, N.; Burgun, A.; Salomon, R.; Neuraz, A. Electronic health records for the diagnosis of rare diseases. *Kidney Int.* **2020**, *97*, 676–686. [CrossRef]
77. Stead, W.W. Clinical Implications and Challenges of Artificial Intelligence and Deep Learning. *JAMA* **2018**, *320*, 1107–1108. [CrossRef]
78. Obermeyer, Z.; Emanuel, E.J. Predicting the Future—Big Data, Machine Learning, and Clinical Medicine. *N. Engl. J. Med.* **2016**, *375*, 1216–1219. [CrossRef]
79. Russakovsky, O.; Deng, J.; Su, H.; Krause, J.; Satheesh, S.; Ma, S.; Huang, Z.; Karpathy, A.; Khosla, A.; Bernstein, M. Imagenet large scale visual recognition challenge. *Int. J. Comput. Vis.* **2015**, *115*, 211–252. [CrossRef]
80. Pennington, J.; Socher, R.; Manning, C.D. (Eds.) Glove: Global vectors for word representation. In Proceedings of the 2014 Conference on Empirical Methods in Natural Language Processing (EMNLP), Doha, Qatar, 25–29 October 2014.
81. Hermsen, M.; de Bel, T.; den Boer, M.; Steenbergen, E.J.; Kers, J.; Florquin, S.; Roelofs, J.; Stegall, M.D.; Alexander, M.P.; Smith, B.H.; et al. Deep Learning-Based Histopathologic Assessment of Kidney Tissue. *J. Am. Soc. Nephrol.* **2019**, *30*, 1968–1979. [CrossRef]
82. Ginley, B.; Lutnick, B.; Jen, K.Y.; Fogo, A.B.; Jain, S.; Rosenberg, A.; Walavalkar, V.; Wilding, G.; Tomaszewski, J.E.; Yacoub, R.; et al. Computational Segmentation and Classification of Diabetic Glomerulosclerosis. *J. Am. Soc. Nephrol.* **2019**, *30*, 1953–1967. [CrossRef] [PubMed]
83. Tomašev, N.; Glorot, X.; Rae, J.W.; Zielinski, M.; Askham, H.; Saraiva, A.; et al. A clinically applicable approach to continuous prediction of future acute kidney injury. *Nature* **2019**, *572*, 116–119. [CrossRef] [PubMed]
84. Escandell-Montero, P.; Chermisi, M.; Martínez-Martínez, J.M.; Gómez-Sanchis, J.; Barbieri, C.; Soria-Olivas, E.; Mari, F.; Vila-Francés, J.; Stopper, A.; Gatti, E.; et al. Optimization of anemia treatment in hemodialysis patients via reinforcement learning. *Artif. Intell. Med.* **2014**, *62*, 47–60. [CrossRef] [PubMed]
85. Barbieri, C.; Molina, M.; Ponce, P.; Tothova, M.; Cattinelli, I.; Ion Titapiccolo, J.; Mari, F.; Amato, C.; Leipold, F.; Wehmeyer, W.; et al. An international observational study suggests that artificial intelligence for clinical decision support optimizes anemia management in hemodialysis patients. *Kidney Int.* **2016**, *90*, 422–429. [CrossRef] [PubMed]
86. Chen, T.; Li, X.; Li, Y.; Xia, E.; Qin, Y.; Liang, S.; Xu, F.; Liang, D.; Zeng, C.; Liu, Z. Prediction and Risk Stratification of Kidney Outcomes in IgA Nephropathy. *Am. J. Kidney Dis.* **2019**, *74*, 300–309. [CrossRef]

87. Samal, L.; D'Amore, J.D.; Bates, D.W.; Wright, A. Implementation of a scalable, web-based, automated clinical decision support risk-prediction tool for chronic kidney disease using C-CDA and application programming interfaces. *J. Am. Med. Inf. Assoc.* **2017**, *24*, 1111–1115. [CrossRef]
88. Tangri, N.; Stevens, L.A.; Griffith, J.; Tighiouart, H.; Djurdjev, O.; Naimark, D.; Levin, A.; Levey, A.S. A predictive model for progression of chronic kidney disease to kidney failure. *JAMA* **2011**, *305*, 1553–1559. [CrossRef]
89. Ravizza, S.; Huschto, T.; Adamov, A.; Böhm, L.; Büsser, A.; Flöther, F.F.; Hinzmann, R.; König, H.; McAhren, S.M.; Robertson, D.H.; et al. Predicting the early risk of chronic kidney disease in patients with diabetes using real-world data. *Nat. Med.* **2019**, *25*, 57–59. [CrossRef]
90. Zhou, C.; Wang, R.; Jiang, W.; Zhu, J.; Liu, Y.; Zheng, J.; et al. Machine learning for the prediction of acute kidney injury and paraplegia after thoracoabdominal aortic aneurysm repair. *J. Card. Surg.* **2020**, *35*, 89–99. [CrossRef]
91. Xu, Z.; Chou, J.; Zhang, X.S.; Luo, Y.; Isakova, T.; Adekkanattu, P.; Ancker, J.S.; Jiang, G.; Kiefer, R.C.; Pacheco, J.A.; et al. Identifying sub-phenotypes of acute kidney injury using structured and unstructured electronic health record data with memory networks. *J. Biomed. Inform.* **2020**, *102*, 103361. [CrossRef]
92. Song, X.; Waitman, L.R.; Yu, A.S.; Robbins, D.C.; Hu, Y.; Liu, M. Longitudinal Risk Prediction of Chronic Kidney Disease in Diabetic Patients Using a Temporal-Enhanced Gradient Boosting Machine: Retrospective Cohort Study. *JMIR Med. Inform.* **2020**, *8*, e15510. [CrossRef] [PubMed]
93. Rashidi, H.H.; Sen, S.; Palmieri, T.L.; Blackmon, T.; Wajda, J.; Tran, N.K. Early Recognition of Burn- and Trauma-Related Acute Kidney Injury: A Pilot Comparison of Machine Learning Techniques. *Sci. Rep.* **2020**, *10*, 205. [CrossRef] [PubMed]
94. Morid, M.A.; Sheng, O.R.L.; Del Fiol, G.; Facelli, J.C.; Bray, B.E.; Abdelrahman, S. Temporal Pattern Detection to Predict Adverse Events in Critical Care: Case Study With Acute Kidney Injury. *JMIR Med. Inform.* **2020**, *8*, e14272. [CrossRef] [PubMed]
95. Luo, Y.; Tang, Z.; Hu, X.; Lu, S.; Miao, B.; Hong, S.; Bai, H.; Sun, C.; Qiu, J.; Liang, H.; et al. Machine learning for the prediction of severe pneumonia during posttransplant hospitalization in recipients of a deceased-donor kidney transplant. *Ann. Transl. Med.* **2020**, *8*, 82. [CrossRef]
96. Li, N.; Huang, H.; Qian, H.-Z.; Liu, P.; Lu, H.; Liu, X. Improving accuracy of estimating glomerular filtration rate using artificial neural network: Model development and validation. *J. Transl. Med.* **2020**, *18*, 120. [CrossRef]
97. Lei, L.; Wang, Y.; Xue, Q.; Tong, J.; Zhou, C.-M.; Yang, J.-J. A comparative study of machine learning algorithms for predicting acute kidney injury after liver cancer resection. *PeerJ* **2020**, *8*, e8583. [CrossRef]
98. Kate, R.J.; Pearce, N.; Mazumdar, D.; Nilakantan, V. A continual prediction model for inpatient acute kidney injury. *Comput. Biol. Med.* **2020**, *116*, 103580. [CrossRef]
99. Kang, M.W.; Kim, J.; Kim, D.K.; Oh, K.-H.; Joo, K.W.; Kim, Y.S.; Han, S.S. Machine learning algorithm to predict mortality in patients undergoing continuous renal replacement therapy. *Crit. Care* **2020**, *24*, 42. [CrossRef]
100. Zimmerman, L.P.; Reyfman, P.A.; Smith, A.D.R.; Zeng, Z.; Kho, A.; Sanchez-Pinto, L.N.; Luo, Y. Early prediction of acute kidney injury following ICU admission using a multivariate panel of physiological measurements. *Bmc Med. Inform. Decis. Mak.* **2019**, *19* (Suppl. 1), 16. [CrossRef]
101. Zhang, Z.; Ho, K.M.; Hong, Y. Machine learning for the prediction of volume responsiveness in patients with oliguric acute kidney injury in critical care. *Crit. Care* **2019**, *23*, 112. [CrossRef]
102. Xu, Z.; Luo, Y.; Adekkanattu, P.; Ancker, J.S.; Jiang, G.; Kiefer, R.C.; Pacheco, J.A.; Rasmussen, L.V.; Pathak, J.; Wang, F. Stratified Mortality Prediction of Patients with Acute Kidney Injury in Critical Care. *Stud. Health Technol. Inform.* **2019**, *264*, 462–466. [PubMed]
103. Xiao, J.; Ding, R.; Xu, X.; Guan, H.; Feng, X.; Sun, T.; Zhu, S.; Ye, Z. Comparison and development of machine learning tools in the prediction of chronic kidney disease progression. *J. Transl. Med.* **2019**, *17*, 119. [CrossRef]
104. Mark, E.; Goldsman, D.; Gurbaxani, B.; Keskinocak, P.; Sokol, J. Using machine learning and an ensemble of methods to predict kidney transplant survival. *PLoS ONE* **2019**, *14*, e0209068. [CrossRef] [PubMed]
105. Bae, S.; Massie, A.B.; Thomas, A.G.; Bahn, G.; Luo, X.; Jackson, K.R.; Ottmann, S.E.; Brennan, D.C.; Desai, N.M.; Coresh, J.; et al. Who can tolerate a marginal kidney? Predicting survival after deceased donor kidney transplant by donor-recipient combination. *Am. J. Transpl.* **2019**, *19*, 425–433. [CrossRef] [PubMed]

106. Yoo, K.D.; Noh, J.; Lee, H.; Kim, D.K.; Lim, C.S.; Kim, Y.H.; Lee, J.P.; Kim, G.; Kim, Y.S. A Machine Learning Approach Using Survival Statistics to Predict Graft Survival in Kidney Transplant Recipients: A Multicenter Cohort Study. *Sci. Rep.* **2017**, *7*, 8904. [CrossRef] [PubMed]
107. Niel, O.; Bastard, P. Artificial Intelligence in Nephrology: Core Concepts, Clinical Applications, and Perspectives. *Am. J. Kidney Dis.* **2019**, *74*, 803–810. [CrossRef] [PubMed]
108. Improta, G.; Mazzella, V.; Vecchione, D.; Santini, S.; Triassi, M. Fuzzy logic-based clinical decision support system for the evaluation of renal function in post-Transplant Patients [published online ahead of print, 2019 Nov 12]. *J. Eval. Clin. Pract.* **2019**. [CrossRef]
109. Atallah, D.M.; Badawy, M.; El-Sayed, A.; Ghoneim, M.A. Predicting kidney transplantation outcome based on hybrid feature selection and KNN classifier. *Multimed. Tools Appl.* **2019**, *78*, 20383–20407. [CrossRef]
110. Nematollahi, M.; Akbari, R.; Nikeghbalian, S.; Salehnasab, C. Classification Models to Predict Survival of Kidney Transplant Recipients Using Two Intelligent Techniques of Data Mining and Logistic Regression. *Int. J. Organ. Transpl. Med.* **2017**, *8*, 119–122.
111. Tapak, L.; Hamidi, O.; Amini, P.; Poorolajal, J. Prediction of Kidney Graft Rejection Using Artificial Neural Network. *Healthc Inf. Res.* **2017**, *23*, 277–284. [CrossRef]
112. Shahmoradi, L.; Langarizadeh, M.; Pourmand, G.; Fard, Z.A.; Borhani, A. Comparing Three Data Mining Methods to Predict Kidney Transplant Survival. *Acta Inf. Med.* **2016**, *24*, 322–327. [CrossRef] [PubMed]
113. Luck, M.; Sylvain, T.; Cardinal, H.; Lodi, A.; Bengio, Y. Deep learning for patient-specific kidney graft survival analysis. *arXiv* **2017**, arXiv:170510245.
114. Topuz, K.; Zengul, F.D.; Dag, A.; Almehmi, A.; Yildirim, M.B. Predicting graft survival among kidney transplant recipients: A Bayesian decision support model. *Decis. Support. Syst.* **2018**, *106*, 97–109. [CrossRef]
115. Lyell, D.; Coiera, E. Automation bias and verification complexity: A systematic review. *J. Am. Med. Inf. Assoc.* **2017**, *24*, 423–431. [CrossRef] [PubMed]
116. Agarwal, R.; Sinha, A.D. Big data in nephrology-a time to rethink. *Nephrol. Dial. Transpl.* **2018**, *33*, 1–3. [CrossRef]
117. Lee, C.H.; Yoon, H.-J. Medical big data: Promise and challenges. *Kidney Res. Clin. Pr.* **2017**, *36*, 3–11. [CrossRef]
118. Calvert, J.; Saber, N.; Hoffman, J.; Das, R. Machine-Learning-Based Laboratory Developed Test for the Diagnosis of Sepsis in High-Risk Patients. *Diagnostics* **2019**, *9*, 20. [CrossRef]
119. Lim, E.-C.; Park, J.H.; Jeon, H.J.; Kim, H.-J.; Lee, H.-J.; Song, C.-G.; Hong, S.K. Developing a Diagnostic Decision Support System for Benign Paroxysmal Positional Vertigo Using a Deep-Learning Model. *J. Clin. Med.* **2019**, *8*, 633. [CrossRef]
120. Heo, S.-J.; Kim, Y.; Yun, S.; Lim, S.-S.; Kim, J.; Nam, C.-M.; Park, E.-C.; Jung, I.; Yoon, J.-H. Deep Learning Algorithms with Demographic Information Help to Detect Tuberculosis in Chest Radiographs in Annual Workers' Health Examination Data. *Int. J. Env. Res. Public Health* **2019**, *16*, 250. [CrossRef]
121. Kooman, J.P.; Wieringa, F.P.; Han, M.; Chaudhuri, S.; van der Sande, F.M.; Usvyat, L.A.; Kotanko, P. Wearable health devices and personal area networks: can they improve outcomes in haemodialysis patients? *Nephrol. Dial. Transplant.* **2020**, *35* (Suppl. 2), ii43–ii50. [CrossRef]
122. Shortliffe, E.H.; Sepúlveda, M.J. Clinical Decision Support in the Era of Artificial Intelligence. *JAMA* **2018**, *320*, 2199–2200. [CrossRef] [PubMed]
123. Santo, B.A.; Rosenberg, A.Z.; Sarder, P. Artificial intelligence driven next-generation renal histomorphometry. *Curr. Opin. Nephrol. Hypertens.* **2020**, *29*, 265–272. [CrossRef] [PubMed]
124. Na, L.; Yang, C.; Lo, C.C.; Zhao, F.; Fukuoka, Y.; Aswani, A. Feasibility of Reidentifying Individuals in Large National Physical Activity Data Sets From Which Protected Health Information Has Been Removed With Use of Machine Learning. *JAMA Netw. Open* **2018**, *1*, e186040. [CrossRef] [PubMed]
125. Obermeyer, Z.; Lee, T.H. Lost in Thought—The Limits of the Human Mind and the Future of Medicine. *N. Engl. J. Med.* **2017**, *377*, 1209–1211. [CrossRef]

2

TRPC Channels in Proteinuric Kidney Diseases

Gentzon Hall, Liming Wang and Robert F. Spurney *

Division of Nephrology, Department of Medicine, Duke University; Durham, NC 27710, USA; gentzon.hall@duke.edu (G.H.); liming.wang@duke.edu (L.W.)
* Correspondence: robert.spurney@duke.edu

Abstract: Over a decade ago, mutations in the gene encoding *TRPC6* (transient receptor potential cation channel, subfamily C, member 6) were linked to development of familial forms of nephrosis. Since this discovery, TRPC6 has been implicated in the pathophysiology of non-genetic forms of kidney disease including focal segmental glomerulosclerosis (FSGS), diabetic nephropathy, immune-mediated kidney diseases, and renal fibrosis. On the basis of these findings, TRPC6 has become an important target for the development of therapeutic agents to treat diverse kidney diseases. Although TRPC6 has been a major focus for drug discovery, more recent studies suggest that other TRPC family members play a role in the pathogenesis of glomerular disease processes and chronic kidney disease (CKD). This review highlights the data implicating TRPC6 and other TRPC family members in both genetic and non-genetic forms of kidney disease, focusing on TRPC3, TRPC5, and TRPC6 in a cell type (glomerular podocytes) that plays a key role in proteinuric kidney diseases.

Keywords: transient receptor potential cation channel; transient receptor potential canonical channel; TRPC channel; focal segmental glomerulosclerosis; diabetic kidney disease; diabetic nephropathy; chronic kidney disease; TRPC6; TRPC5; TRPC3

---

1. The Burden of Chronic Kidney Disease (CKD)

CKD is a public health problem that affects more than 20 million Americans in the United States [1]. The disease is caused by a diverse group of primary, secondary, and genetic disorders that impair the ability of the kidney to remove waste, regulate intravascular volume, reclaim essential nutrients, and stimulate erythropoiesis [2]. As the disease progresses, these essential functions become increasingly impaired, eventually leading to end-stage kidney disease (ESKD). Of the ≈20 million Americans with CKD, almost 600,000 have irreversible kidney failure and require either renal transplantation or dialysis to sustain life [3]. The expense of providing ESKD care to this patient population costs ≈50 billion dollars per year in the United States [3]. Moreover, morbidity and mortality are markedly increased in CKD patients with lesser degrees of renal impairment, which is largely caused by an increased risk of cardiovascular events as renal function declines [1,4]. Although current treatments for CKD may slow disease progression, many patients progress to more advanced stages of CKD, and ESKD, despite available therapies [2]. As a result, there is a significant interest in developing new treatment approaches.

2. The Glomerular Podocyte Plays a Key Role in Proteinuric Kidney Diseases

Podocytes are highly differentiated, postmitotic cells that play a critical role in maintaining the integrity of the glomerular filtration barrier [5]. As shown in Figure 1A,B, their interdigitating foot processes (FPs) cover the exterior surface of the glomerular basement membrane (GBM), and form a specialized intercellular junction between adjacent FPs known as the slit diaphragm (SD) [6]. The SD is a sieve-like, size-selective filtration barrier, which prevents loss of cells and macromolecules into the glomerular ultrafiltrate [7,8]. It is composed of proteins commonly found in tight and adherens junctions such as P-cadherin, zonula occludens-1 (ZO-1), and catenin family members, as well as proteins predominantly expressed in podocytes including nephrin, neph1, and podocin [7,8]. Both nephrin and neph1 are members of the immunoglobulin (Ig) superfamily [7]. Their extracellular domains contain multiple IgG-like motifs, which can aggregate and form zipper-like structures that surround the glomerular capillaries, creating a sieve-like filtration barrier. Both nephrin and neph1 also have a single transmembrane domain and a short intracellular carboxy-terminus, which serves as a scaffold for assembling signaling complexes with other podocyte proteins such as CD2AP (CD2-associated protein) and podocin [8,9]. The carboxy-terminus of nephrin has conserved tyrosine residues that can be phosphorylated by Src family kinases [7,10–13]. Phosphorylated nephrin recruits additional signaling molecules to the scaffolding complex that, in turn, influence multiple downstream signaling pathways and modulate cytoskeletal reorganization, cellular survival, membrane trafficking, cellular adhesion, and mechano-signaling [7,10,14,15].

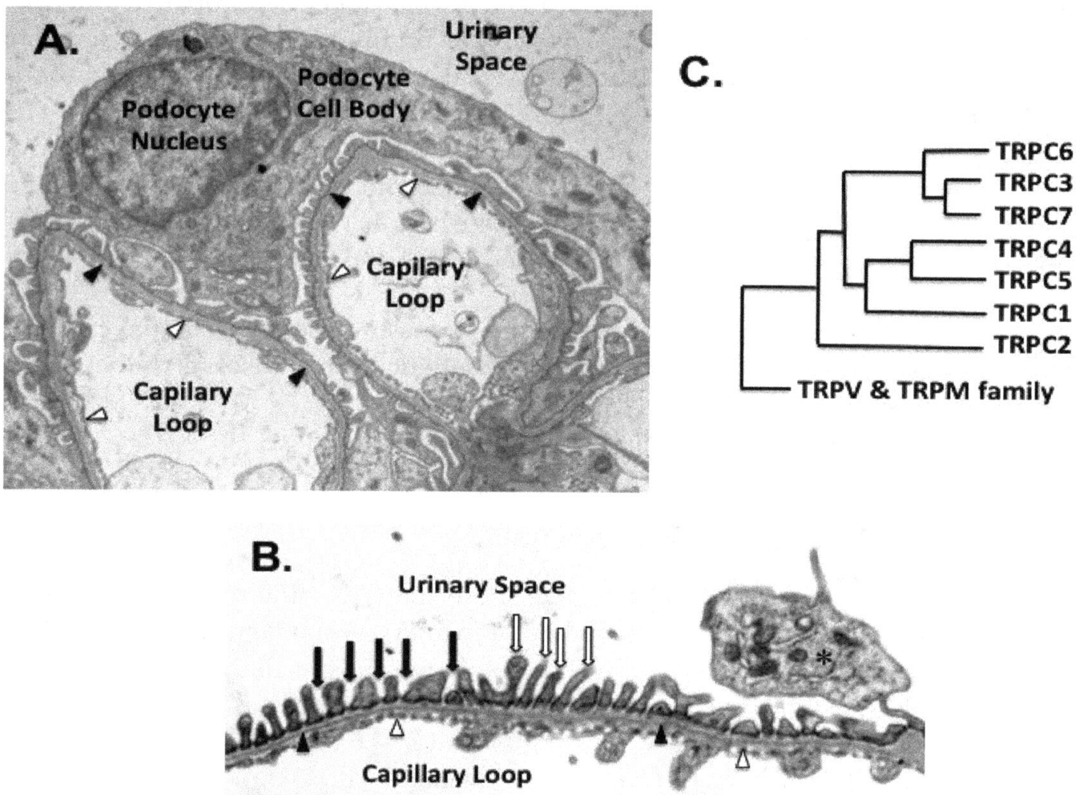

Figure 1. Glomerular ultrastructure and TRPC family members. (**A**) An electron micrograph of glomerular ultrastructure is presented. The podocyte cell body is located in the urinary space on the outer surface of the glomerular basement membrane (GBM). Primary processes extend from the cell body and branch into interdigitating foot processes (FPs) that cover the external surface to the GBM (black arrow heads) to form filtration slits and the specialized intercellular junction termed the slit diaphragm (SD). The glomerular filter is composed of the podocyte FPs with the intervening SDs, the GBM (black arrow heads), and a fenestrated endothelium (white arrowheads) that lines the capillary loops. (**B**) This high power view shows the three layers of the glomerular filter including the fenestrated endothelium (white arrowheads), GBM (black arrowheads), and the FPs (white arrows) with the interposed filtration slits (black arrows). An asterisk indicates a primary process (also termed a major process). (**C**) The phylogenetic tree of TRP family members is shown in panel C. The vertebrate TRPC family has seven members, which are divided into four subgroups: TRPC1, TRPC2, TRPC4/5, and TRPC3/6/7. The figure shows the relationship between TRPC family members and other members of the TRP family. In humans, TRPC2 is a pseudogene (see text).

In addition to their role in forming a size selective filtration barrier, podocytes stabilize the glomerular architecture by counteracting the elastic forces distending the GBM [6]. Indeed, the hydraulic pressure within glomerular capillaries is unusually high compared to other capillary beds [16]. It is estimated that podocytes are responsible for approximately 40% of the hydraulic resistance of the filtration barrier [6]. Moreover, accumulating evidence suggests that dynamic signaling between the SD and focal adhesions may promote both podocyte adherence to the GBM and maintenance of glomerular filtration barrier function [7,17,18]. In support of this hypothesis, lamellipodia formation at focal adhesions are necessary for cell migration and are induced downstream of nephrin phosphorylation in cultured podocytes [19,20]; conversely, β1 integrin activation induces tyrosine phosphorylation of nephrin [21]. This crosstalk between the SD and focal adhesions may help podocytes adapt to changes in the microenvironment including alterations in glomerular filtration rate or glomerular pressure. In addition, disruption of these signaling pathways in glomerular diseases may contribute to the loss of glomerular filtration barrier function, causing proteinuria. As the disease progresses, podocytes detach from the GBM due either to reduced cellular adhesion or cell death. Because podocytes are terminally differentiated, postmitotic cells, podocytes that are lost, cannot be effectively replaced [22,23]. As a result, a decrease in podocyte number of greater than ≈20–40% [24,25] leads to the collapse of the glomerular tuft, glomerulosclerosis, and disease progression [22,23]. On the basis of these observations, the current review focuses on the role of podocyte TRPC channels in proteinuric kidney diseases, but we acknowledge that expression of TRPC channels in other kidney cell types are likely to play a role in these disease processes.

3. TRPC Family Members

TRPC channels are part of a larger TRP family, which was first discovered in *Drosophila melanogaster* [26,27]. As shown in Figure 1C, the vertebrate TRPC family has seven members, which can be divided into four subgroups: TRPC1, TRPC2, TRPC4/5, and TRPC3/6/7 (G) [26,27]. In humans, TRPC2 is a pseudogene, although the channel plays a role in pheromone signaling in rodents [26]. All TRPC ion channels are calcium permeable, but the channels are poorly selective, with permeability ratios (PCa/PNa) that vary significantly between family members [26]. The calcium influx is stimulated following receptor-induced phospholipase C (PLC) activation in response to both tyrosine kinase receptors (TKRs) and G protein coupled receptors (GPCRs) [27]. PLC catalyzes hydrolysis of phosphatidylinositol 4,5-bisphosphate (PIP2) and generates the second messengers diacylglycerol (DAG) and inositol 1,4,5 trisphosphate (IP3) [28] that differentially affect TRPC activation, as reviewed elsewhere [27].

Several members of the TRPC family may be activated by additional mechanisms that are distinct from receptor operated channel (ROC) activation. For example, mechanical stretch was reported to activate TRPC1 in 2005 [29]. More recent studies suggest that other TRPC family members may also be responsive to mechanical stress, including TRPC3, TRPC5, and TRPC6 [30–35]. For example, TRPC6 was found to induce cationic currents in podocytes following mechanical stimulation, which persisted in the presence of either PLC inhibitors or blockade of G-protein activation, but was inhibited by TRPC6 knockdown as well as by pharmacologic blockade of TRPC6 [36]. Moreover, a point mutation in TRPC6 eliminates mechanical activation of cationic currents in podocytes without affecting activation by GPCRs or cell-permeable DAG analogs [34]. Although the role of mechanical stretch in activation of TRPC family members has recently been questioned [37], these data are consistent with the notion that stretch-induced TRPC6 activation in podocytes is mediated by both receptor-dependent and receptor-independent mechanisms.

A third mechanism of TRPC activation is oxidative stress, which is reported to activate TRPC5 and TRPC6 [38–40]. In podocytes, TRPC6 activation by angiotensin II and cell permeable DAG analogs is inhibited by both scavengers of reactive oxygen species (ROS) and by pharmacologic inhibition of NADPH oxidase 2 (NOX2) [41,42]. Similarly, ROS quenchers inhibit TRPC6 activation by ATP [43]. In addition, TRPC6 coimmunoprecipitates with the catalytic subunit of NOX2, and the

TRPC6–NOX2 interaction appears to require podocin because knockdown of the scaffolding protein podocin eliminates the TRPC6–NOX2 protein–protein interaction [42]. Taken together, these data suggest that localized production of ROS plays a key role in GPCR-induced TRPC6 activation.

4. TRPC6 in Familial Forms of Nephrosis

In 2005, Winn et al. identified a point mutation in *TRPC6*, which segregated with disease in a large family with autosomal dominant focal segmental glomerulosclerosis (FSGS) [44]. In heterologous expression systems, the mutant channel exhibited a gain-of-function in response to angiotensin II and to cell permeable DAG analogs [35,44]. Shortly after this initial report, Pollak and coworkers described five additional families with autosomal dominant FSGS caused by mutations in the *TRPC6* gene [45]. In this study, immuno-electron microscopy localized podocyte TRPC6 to the cell body, major processes, and foot processes adjacent to the slit diaphragm [45]. This group further demonstrated that TRPC6 co-immunoprecipitated with nephrin and podocin [45,46], raising the possibility that TRPC6, nephrin, and podocin physically interact and might form a signaling complex with TRPC6 at the SD [14,35,46]. In support of this view, the interaction between the cytosolic domains of TRPC6 and podocin regulate TRPC6 activity [35,36,45,46]. Moreover, podocyte FPs contain a contractile apparatus [45,47,48] that may be regulated by changes in calcium levels within the microenvironment [45,48]. These observations fit nicely with a role for TRPC6 as a mechanosensor that directly interacts with, and perhaps influences, the activity of the nephrin/podocin/CD2AP signaling complex at the SD.

Since the initial reports, multiple mutations in the *TRPC6* gene have been linked to familial forms of FSGS [49–57]. Examining the clinical characteristics of patients with these mutations has provided insights into the role of TRPC6 in glomerular diseases. For example, the majority of TRPC6 mutations causing FSGS promote a gain of channel function [49–57]. These data suggest that excessive intracellular calcium levels contribute to the pathophysiology of the disease in this patient population. Consistent with this hypothesis, a subset of these activating mutations causes large increases in channel currents, which leads to a more aggressive phenotype, with patients presenting in early childhood [54]. The majority of FSGS patients, however, with TRPC6 mutations present as young adults [49], although there is a wide age range between family members that carry the same causative mutation [49]. For example, in the large pedigree reported by Winn et al. [58], family members carrying the TRPC6 mutation presented at a mean age of 33, with an age range at presentation from 16 to 61 years of age. In a more recent study by Zhu et al. [55], the proband presented at age 35, and his sister was diagnosed with FSGS at age 41, but their father with the same activating mutation had normal renal function at age 75. Although the magnitude of the gain of function may lead to a more aggressive phenotype [54], it has been suggested that, in addition to the presence of the causative TRPC6 mutation, the development of disease may be precipitated by a "second hit" [59,60]. In support of this hypothesis, we developed a transgenic (TG) mouse model that promoted continuous activation of endogenous TRPC6, specifically in podocytes [61]. Surprisingly, this model did not exhibit a kidney phenotype at baseline. However, treatment with the podocyte toxin puromycin aminonucleoside (PAN) induced heavy proteinuria and glomerulosclerosis in TG mice, whereas PAN induced only mild disease in wild type mice [61]. Thus, a "second hit" with the podocyte toxin PAN induced a severe phenotype in the presence of persistent TRPC6 activation in the TG animals.

Although the majority of TRPC6 mutations that cause FSGS are activating, ≈25% of the reported mutations cause a loss of function [49], including a novel TRPC6 mutation (G757D) that acts as a dominant negative [49]. In contrast to patients with activating mutations (see above), the age at presentation for inactivating mutations tends to be in early childhood [49–53]. For example, the two patients with the dominant negative mutation (G757D) presented in early infancy [49]. In addition, most of these mutations are heterozygous missense mutations, which have been described in children with non-familial forms of steroid-resistant nephrotic syndrome [49–53]. These data suggest that some basal level of TRPC6 activity may be required to maintain normal glomerular function, which may be particularly important in early childhood.

5. TRPC Family Members in Glomerular Diseases: Mechanisms of Renal Injury

Familial forms of kidney disease account for only a small percentage of patients with CKD. The vast majority of kidney disease is caused by systemic disease processes, including diabetes mellitus; hypertension; autoimmune diseases such as lupus erythematosus; and, to a lesser extent, primary glomerular diseases including non-familial forms of FSGS, membranous glomerulonephritis (MGN), and minimal change disease (MCD). A role for TRPC6 in primary glomerular disease processes was first suggested by Reiser and colleagues [62], who demonstrated that TRPC6 was upregulated in microdissected glomeruli in human kidney biopsy specimens from patients with MGN and MCD, with a similar trend in patients with FSGS. Upregulation of TRPC6 in glomerular diseases likely plays a role in disease pathogenesis because overexpression of TRPC6 in heterologous expression systems causes enhanced intracellular calcium levels following TRPC6 activation compared to cells expressing their endogenous complement of TRPC6 channels [53,54]. These data suggest that enhanced expression of wild type TRPC6 channels in acquired proteinuric kidney diseases promote a similar pathology (enhanced intracellular calcium levels) as TRPC6 gain-of-function mutations in familial forms of FSGS. In support of this possibility, podocyte-specific overexpression of TRPC6 in vivo promotes proteinuria and modest glomerulosclerosis [63]. Since these initial observations, enhanced expression of TRPC6 has been demonstrated in other kidney diseases including rodent models of diabetic nephropathy [61,64–69], nephrotoxic serum nephritis [70,71], rodent models of FSGS [61,64,72–74], and ureteral obstruction [75,76]. Thus, increased expression of TRPC6 may be a common finding in a broad range of pathologic conditions affecting the kidney.

The molecular mechanisms regulating TRPC6 expression have been investigated in both renal and extrarenal disease processes [61,64,72,74,77,78]. An important observation was that activation of TRPC6 stimulated a positive feedback loop that promoted further expression of TRPC6 in the heart [77–79]. As shown in Figure 2, PLC-coupled receptors, such as GPCRs for angiotensin II or endothelin 1, activate TRPC6, which promotes calcium entry into the cell and stimulates the calcium-sensitive phosphatase calcineurin [80]. An important calcineurin substrate is the family of NFAT (nuclear factor of activated T cells) transcription factors [80]. NFAT family members were originally discovered in cells of the lymphoid lineage, but NFAT isoforms are also expressed in non-immune cells, with some family members expressed ubiquitously [81]. In quiescent cells, NFAT isoforms are phosphorylated and located in the cytoplasm [81,82]. Calcineurin dephosphorylates NFAT, which permits translocation to the nucleus and stimulation of gene transcription. An important gene target of calcineurin is the ion channel TRPC6 [61,74,77]. As shown in Figure 2, this pathway creates a positive feedback loop characterized by enhanced intracellular calcium levels, stimulation of calcineurin-NFAT signaling, and induction of TRPC6, which further augments intracellular calcium levels. This positive feedback pathway plays a key role in cardiovascular disease processes such as pathologic cardiac hypertrophy [77,78,83] and, more recently, this signaling pathway has been demonstrated to play a role in kidney diseases [61,84,85], including animal models of FSGS [61,74,84] and diabetic kidney disease [65,66]. Indeed, studies by Wang et al. [84] found that podocyte-specific expression of a constitutive active NFAT isoform caused glomerulosclerosis resembling FSGS.

In addition to NFAT, calcineurin has numerous substrates including transcription factors, receptors, ion channels, cytoskeletal proteins, targeting proteins, and proteins involved in apoptotic pathways [86]. Thus, TRPC6-induced calcineurin activation affects numerous downstream signaling pathways that may contribute to disease progression in CKD. For example, the podocyte protein synaptopodin associates with the actin cytoskeleton and plays a key role in maintaining the complex morphology of the glomerular podocyte, as well as inhibiting cell surface expression of TRPC6 [87]. As shown in Figure 3, Faul et al. [88] found that synaptopodin was phosphorylated by either protein kinase A (PKA) or calcium-dependent protein kinase II (CaMKII). Phosphorylation of synaptopodin provides a docking site for 14-3-3 proteins and prevents degradation of synaptopodin by the cysteine peptidase cathepsin L [88]. Dephosphorylation of the 14-3-3 docking site by calcineurin promotes synaptopodin degradation, destabilizes the actin cytoskeleton, and disrupts the integrity of the glomerular filtration barrier.

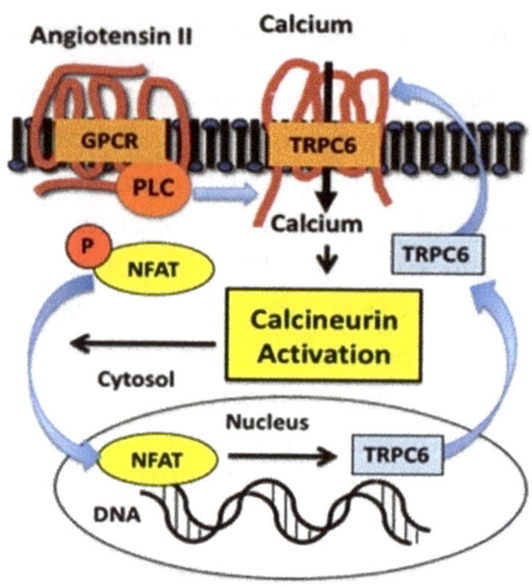

Figure 2. Positive feedback loop induced by TRPC6 activation. Stimulation of phospholipase C (PLC)-coupled receptors such as the G protein coupled receptor (GPCR) for angiotensin II activates TRPC6, which induces calcium entry into the cell, calcineurin activation, dephosphorylation of nuclear factor of activated T cells (NFAT), and translocation of NFAT to the nucleus. NFAT stimulates transcription of multiple genes including TRPC6, which further increases TRPC6 expression and enhances the calcium influx, creating a positive feedback loop.

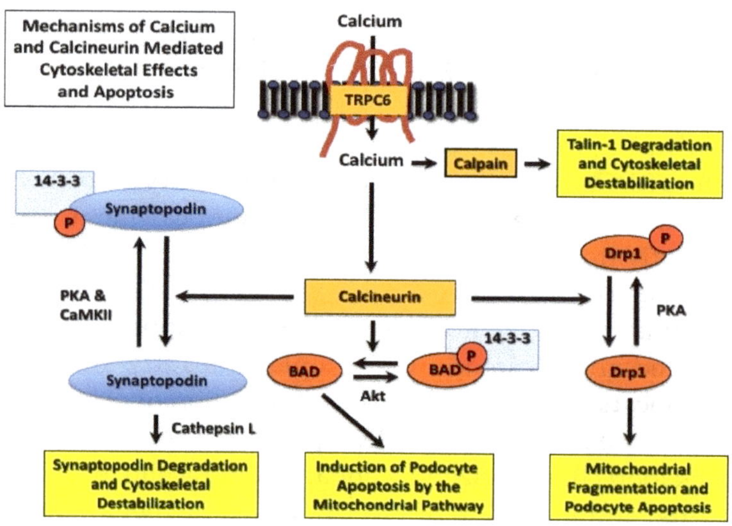

Figure 3. Mechanisms of calcium- and calcineurin-mediated podocyte injury. The podocyte protein synaptopodin is an actin associated protein that plays a role in stabilizing the podocyte cytoskeleton. Synaptopodin is phosphorylated by protein kinase A (PKA) and calcium/calmodulin-dependent protein kinase II (CaMKII), which promotes 14-3-3 binding and protects synaptopodin from degradation by cathepsin L. Calcineurin dephosphorylates synaptopodin, which permits its degradation by cathepsin L and, in turn, destabilizes the actin cytoskeleton and promotes proteinuria. Calcineurin also causes podocyte apoptosis. The mechanisms of calcineurin-induced apoptosis are incompletely understood, but both BAD (Bcl-2-associated death promoter) and Drp1 (dynamin-related protein 1) play a role in preclinical disease models. Similar to synaptopodin, BAD is phosphorylated at a 14-3-3 docking site by Akt, which inhibits its activity. Calcineurin dephosphorylates BAD and induces apoptosis by the mitochondrial pathway. Drp1 is phosphorylated and inhibited by PKA. Dephosphorylation of Drp1 by calcineurin promotes apoptosis by inducing mitochondrial fragmentation. Lastly, recent studies suggest that the calcium-activated cysteine protease calpain plays a key role in promoting podocyte injury. Calpain degrades numerous cytoskeletal proteins including the large cytoskeletal protein talin-1. Calpain-induced talin-1 degradation destabilizes the podocyte cytoskeleton and impairs glomerular filtration barrier integrity.

As discussed above, podocytes have a limited capacity for proliferation [5,6]. As a result, a decrease in podocyte number leads to collapse of the glomerular tuft, glomerulosclerosis, and disease progression [5,6,22,23]. TRPC6-induced calcium/calcineurin/NFAT signaling enhances podocyte loss by inducing podocyte apoptosis [84,89,90]. As shown in Figure 3, mechanisms of calcineurin-induced apoptosis include stimulating mitochondrial fragmentation by Drp1 (dynamin-related protein 1) [91] and activation of the apoptosis inducing Bcl-2 family member BAD (Bcl-2-associated death promoter) [92]. As shown in Figure 3, Drp1 is phosphorylated and inhibited by PKA [91], and BAD is phosphorylated by Akt, which causes sequestration of BAD by 14-3-3 proteins [92]. Dephosphorylation of both proteins by calcineurin induces apoptosis [91,92]), and both Drp1- and BAD-dependent podocyte apoptosis have been implicated in CKD progression [15,93–95].

TRPC6 activation also contributes to the pathogenesis of glomerular diseases by mechanisms that are independent of calcineurin activation. For example, calcium influx induced by TRPC6 activates the cysteine protease calpain [96], as shown in Figure 3. Recent studies suggest that TRPC6 binds calpain-1 and calpain-2, which causes membrane localization of calpain isoforms and promotes their activation [97]. Calpains have numerous downstream substrates including cytoskeletal proteins [97,98] such as the large cytoskeletal protein talin-1, which links integrins to the actin cytoskeleton [99]. Knockout of talin-1 specifically in glomerular podocytes causes severe proteinuria [99], and TRPC6-induced calcium influx increases calpain-1 activity [96]. These observations are relevant to proteinuric kidney diseases because calpain-induced cleavage of talin-1 is increased in animal models of glomerular disease, and urinary calpain activity is increased in patients with FSGS and MCD [96,99]. Moreover, calpain inhibitors attenuate proteinuria in animal models [96,99]. Taken together, these data suggest an important role for the calcium sensitive protease calpain in TRPC6-induced kidney injury.

In addition to enhancing intracellular calcium levels, TRPC family members are reported to activate the small GTPases RhoA and Rac1 [100–102], and both these Rho GTPase family members are implicated in the pathogenesis of idiopathic and hereditary glomerular diseases [103–107]. Indeed, RhoA and Rac1 play key roles in regulating cytoskeletal dynamics in podocytes, and dysregulated activity of these small GTPases in glomerular disease processes causes proteinuria [103,107]. In this regard, studies by Greka and co-workers found that Rac1 and RhoA associate with, and are activated by, TRPC5 and TRPC6, respectively [100]. Consistent with an important role for TRPC5 in glomerular diseases, additional studies by this same group suggested that inhibition of TRPC5 ameliorated glomerular injury in proteinuric rodent models [108,109], as discussed further below.

Glomerular podocytes are reported to express TRPC1, TRPC3, TRPC4, TRPC5, and TRPC6; however, only TPRC3, TRPC5, and TRPC6 have been shown to contribute to calcium entry in podocytes using electrophysiologic and pharmacologic methodologies [110]. Although TRPC5 and TRPC6 have received the most attention, accumulating evidence suggests that TRPC3 also plays a role in kidney diseases [75]. Similar to other TRPC family members, activation of TRPC3 enhances intracellular calcium levels and stimulates downstream calcium signaling cascades. An important observation was that TRPC3 is upregulated in glomerular diseases in a fashion similar to TRPC6 [61,71,73,111,112], with no change in expression of TRPC5 [61,71,73,112]. Like TRPC6, upregulation of TRPC3 occurs by calcineurin-dependent mechanisms in pathologic processes [78]. This observation may be important in glomerular diseases because increased expression of TRPC3 and TRPC6 in kidney diseases may enhance the relative contributions of these TRPC family members to elevated intracellular calcium levels. Moreover, compensatory upregulation of TRPC3 is observed in vascular smooth muscle cells of TRPC6 knockout mice, which promoted higher basal cation entry and likely contributed to enhanced vascular contractility and increased systemic blood pressure in this model [113]. Similarly, TRPC3 was upregulated in renal cortices of TRPC6 knockout rats under basal conditions [71,73]. Thus, selective blockade of TRPC6 may promote compensatory upregulation of other TRPC family members and may not be sufficient in inhibiting the calcium influx induced by TRPC activation in pathologic processes.

6. Targeting TRPC6 to Treat FSGS

Since the discovery that mutations in TRPC6 caused familial forms of FSGS, over 50 genes have been linked to inherited causes of glomerular disease [114]. However, relatively few non-syndromic, genetic causes of nephrosis had been reported in the year (2005) that mutations in *TRPC6* were linked to the development of autosomal dominant FSGS [44]. These mutations included genes encoding nephrin [115], podocin [116], CD2AP [117,118], and α-actinin-4 [119]. At the time, all these proteins were considered structural elements of either the slit diaphragm or cytoskeleton, although data were emerging to suggest that nephrin, podocin, and CD2AP formed a novel signaling complex at the SD (see above). In contrast, TRPC6 was a classical signaling molecule, an ion channel, which might play an important role in non-familial forms of glomerular disease. As a result, TRPC6 was immediately recognized as an important target for drug development.

To examine the potential therapeutic benefits of targeting TRPC6 in glomerular diseases, Winn and colleagues [111] examined the effects of infusing angiotensin II in whole-body TRPC6 knockout mice [113]. In these experiments, TRPC6-deficient mice developed less albuminuria, as well as a trend toward improved glomerular histology during the 4 week angiotensin II infusion period. Because mice treated with angiotensin II develop severe hypertension, this model evaluated both the indirect effects systemic high blood pressure on the kidney, as well as the direct effects of angiotensin II on the renal tubular, glomerular, vascular, and interstitial compartments of the kidney. Surprisingly, there was no significant effect of TRPC6 knockout on systemic blood pressure at baseline or after angiotensin II infusion using either tail cuff manometry or the "gold standard" for monitoring systemic blood pressure, radiotelemetry [111]. The lack of a difference in blood pressure at baseline was unanticipated, as previous studies had found a modest increase in systemic blood pressure in the knockout mice, as discussed above [113]; however, differences in the genetic backgrounds used in the two studies may have contributed to the differing results [111,113]. Importantly, because Winn and colleagues found that blood pressure was not affected in mice lacking TRPC6, these studies were some of the first observations to suggest that inhibition of TRPC6 had direct protective effects in the kidney.

To investigate in the role of TRPC6 in a glomerular disease process, our laboratory [61] developed a TG mouse that expressed a constitutively active Gq α-subunit specifically in podocytes (Gq mice). Gq links GPCRs such as the receptor for angiotensin II to PLC and activates TRPC6. Thus, this model caused continuous activation of TRPC6. Surprisingly, this TG mouse had no kidney phenotype at baseline, which is reminiscent of humans expressing gain-of-function mutations in TRPC6. We therefore determined if a "second hit" would induce more severe disease, as has been suggested for familial forms of FSGS due to TRPC6 mutations [59,60]. For the studies, TG animals were treated with the podocyte toxin PAN, which normally produces only mild disease in wild type mice. In Gq mice, however, treatment with PAN caused severe nephrosis, prominent tubulointerstitial disease, and glomerulosclerosis resembling the lesions observed in humans with FSGS [61], as shown in Figure 4. Similarly, Krall et al. found that podocyte-specific overexpression of wild type or activating TRPC6 mutants caused mild proteinuria and modest glomerular changes [63]. Although different genetic backgrounds were used in our studies [61] and the Krall et al. study [63], the baseline phenotypes in both studies were either normal or mild, and it would have been of interest to determine if a "second hit" augmented the phenotype in mice overexpressing the wild type and mutant forms of TRPC6 in the Krall et al. model.

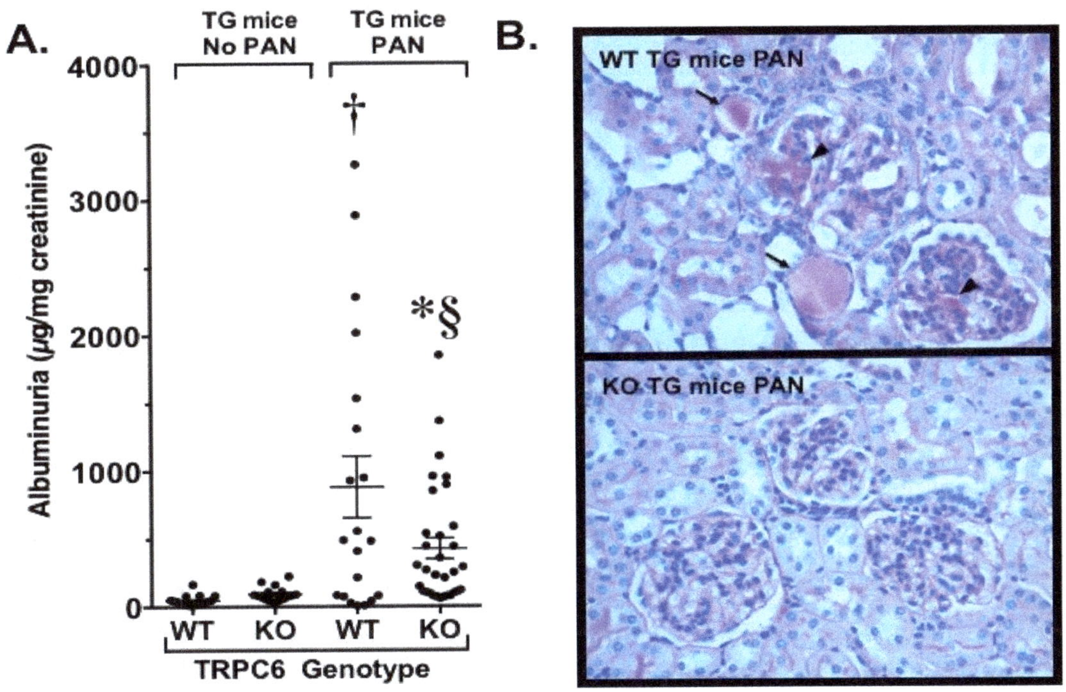

Figure 4. Effect of TRPC6 knockout (KO) in an animal model of focal segmental glomerulosclerosis (FSGS). Our lab developed a transgenic (TG) mouse model that promoted continuous activation of endogenous TRPC6 specifically in podocytes. This model had no kidney phenotype at baseline. In contrast, the podocyte toxin puromycin aminonucleoside (PAN) induced heavy proteinuria in TG mice but only mild proteinuria in non-TG animals (see text). Using this TG model, we found that whole-body knockout of TRPC6 attenuated albuminuria compared to wild type (WT) TG mice expressing TRPC6 (**A**), and reduced both segmental glomerulosclerosis (arrowheads) and tubular injury (arrows) in the knockout animals (**B**). * $p < 0.05$ vs. WT TG mice treated with PAN, † $p < 0.005$ vs. WT TG mice at baseline (no PAN), § $p < 0.005$ vs. KO TG mice at baseline (no PAN).

On the basis of our findings in Gq mice, we next crossed our TG animals with the whole body TRPC6 knockout mice and treated the animals with PAN to induce glomerular disease. As shown in Figure 4, we found that knockout of TRPC6 significantly reduced proteinuria, tubule dilation, and casts, and markedly reduced the severity of glomerulosclerosis [61]. More recently, Dryer and coworkers created a whole body TRPC6 knockout model in rats [73]. This model had an advantage in that rats are generally more susceptible to glomerular disease compared to mice, including the development of robust glomerular disease following treatment of wild type rats with PAN. Dryer and coworkers found that both wild type and knockout mice injected with PAN developed similar levels of heavy proteinuria during the early phase of the disease, but the albuminuria was significantly reduced in the knockout mice during the later, more chronic phase of the disease process. This reduction in proteinuria was associated with a significant improvement in glomerulosclerosis, tubular damage, interstitial inflammation, and fibrosis. Thus, in both our studies and the study by Dryer and coworkers, whole body knockout of TRPC6 improved the disease process in multiple kidney compartments (glomerular, tubular, and interstitial), perhaps due to beneficial effects of whole body TRPC6 knockout in multiple cell types in the kidney. These data suggest that systemic knockout of TRPC6 has beneficial effects on kidney disease in animal models of FSGS.

Pharmacologic inhibition of either TRPC6 activity or expression has also been shown to ameliorate glomerular disease in animal models of FSGS [64,120]. Although there are currently no selective TRPC6 antagonists in clinical trials, three drug classes commonly used for the treatment of FSGS [121] regulate TRPC6 expression, including angiotensin-converting enzyme inhibitors (ACEIs), angiotensin II receptor blockers (ARBs), and calcineurin inhibitors (CNIs) [61,74,77]. ACEIs and ARBs reduce podocyte TRPC6 activation and, in turn, reduce expression of TRPC6 by inhibiting angiotensin II-induced calcium influx and calcineurin activation [74]. CNIs directly inhibit NFAT-induced TRPC6 transcription, which reduces TRPC6-induced calcium currents, as discussed above. In addition to these commonly utilized FSGS therapies [121], agonists of protein kinase G (PKG) have been shown to inhibit TRPC6 activity by directly phosphorylating TRPC6 on threonine 69 (Thr69) [122–125]. PKG is stimulated by activation of either soluble-guanylyl cyclases (sGCs) or particulate-GCs (pGCs) by nitric oxide and natriuretic peptides, respectively [122,123,126]. Moreover, inhibition of TRPC6 by PKG can be potentiated by blocking dephosphorylation of Thr69 by phosphodiesterase (PDE) family members such as PDE5 and PDE9 [125,127,128]. For example, Hall et al. showed that PDE5 inhibition promoted PKG-mediated phosphorylation of Thr69 in cultured podocytes, and negatively regulated TRPC6-mediated calcium conductance [125]. In this study, calcineurin was also shown to dephosphorylate TRPC6 at Thr69, suggesting that the beneficial effects of CNIs may be due, in part, to inhibiting TRPC6 dephosphorylation [125]. In addition, PDE5 inhibition has been shown to negatively regulate TRPC6 expression through cGMP/PKG/PPARγ-mediated transcriptional repression [64]. In a study by Sonneveld et al., treatment with a PDE5 inhibitor reduced proteinuria and glomerular injury in a rat model of FSGS (Adriamycin nephrosis), as well as in a mouse model of diabetic nephropathy [64]. Taken together, these data suggest that repurposing currently approved PDE inhibitors may be useful for the treatment of glomerular diseases by inhibiting both TRPC6 expression and activity. Indeed, PDE5 inhibitors have shown promise in clinical trials for the treatment of patients with established diabetic kidney disease [129].

7. Targeting TRPC Family Members to Treat Diabetic Nephropathy

Diabetic kidney disease is the most common cause of ESKD in the United States (U.S.) and Europe, which costs the U.S. ≈20 billion annually [130]. The disease develops in ≈20–40% of patients with diabetes, and progresses to ESKD in ≈20% of patients with overt nephropathy [130]. As a result, there is much interest in developing new therapies.

Similar to FSGS, glomerular podocytes are thought to play a key role in diabetic nephropathy [22,23]. In this regard, podocyte damage and dysfunction are early features of diabetic kidney disease, eventually leading to a decrease in podocyte number and, in turn, disease progression [22,23]. In support of a role for TRPC6 in diabetic nephropathy, glomerular expression of TRPC6 is upregulated in kidneys from rodent models of diabetes [61,64–67,69], and knockdown of TRPC6 in cultured podocytes both inhibits hyperglycemia-induced apoptosis [90,131] and preserves podocin expression [69]. In addition, several studies suggest that inhibitors of TRPC6 transcription [64,65,72,77] ameliorate albuminuria and the histologic features of diabetic kidney disease in rodent models [64,66,132]. Lastly, hyperglycemia may contribute to kidney injury in diabetes by promoting NOX-dependent ROS generation [133] and, in turn, activation of TRPC6 [41,134]. In support of this possibility, knockout of NOX4 inhibits angiotensin II-stimulated calcium flux in isolated glomeruli from streptozotocin-treated rats, and attenuates diabetic kidney disease in the knockout animals [134].

On the basis of these observations, Spires et al. [112] studied the effect of whole body TRPC6 knockout in Dahl salt-sensitive rats treated with streptozotocin to induce type 1 diabetes. In this study, TRPC6 knockout had no significant effect on hyperglycemia, albuminuria, glomerular injury, interstitial fibrosis, or tubular cast formation. The authors, however, did report that diabetic rats lacking TRPC6 exhibited a reduction in urinary nephrin excretion and a subtle decrease in podocyte injury at the ultrastructural level. On the basis of these data, the authors suggested that TRPC6 inhibition had partial renoprotective effects in diabetic kidney disease.

Our laboratory also examined the effects of whole body TRPC6 knockout in Akita mice, a type 1 model of diabetes [135]. As shown in Figure 5A, we found a reduction in albuminuria early in the disease process, but this difference disappeared as the animals aged [135]. At the end of the study, diabetic TRPC6 knockout exhibited reduced tubular injury, but mesangial expansion was significantly increased (Figure 5B). The adverse effect of TRPC6 knockout on glomerular pathology was associated with insulin resistance that was, at least partially, due to decreased expression of the calcineurin-responsive gene IRS2 (insulin receptor substrate 2), which plays a critical role in insulin signaling. Given that podocytes are insulin-responsive cells [136,137], the adverse effects of TRPC6 knockout on the glomerular compartment may have been exacerbated by podocyte insulin resistance. In support of this possibility, (1) insulin signaling was impaired in TRPC6 knockout podocytes compared to wild type podocytes [135], and (2) previous studies by Welsh et al. [136] found that podocyte specific knockout of the insulin receptor caused heavy proteinuria and histopathologic features of diabetic kidney disease in the normoglycemic environment. Surprisingly, insulin resistance in knockout Akita mice was not associated with changes in blood glucose or hemoglobin A1c levels in our experiments [135]. These observations are, however, consistent with published studies suggesting that insulin sensitizers are beneficial in rodent models of diabetic kidney disease without altering glycemic control [138–140]. Taken together with the studies by Spires et al. [112], these data suggest that selective targeting of TRPC6 is unlikely to be an effective treatment strategy in diabetic kidney disease.

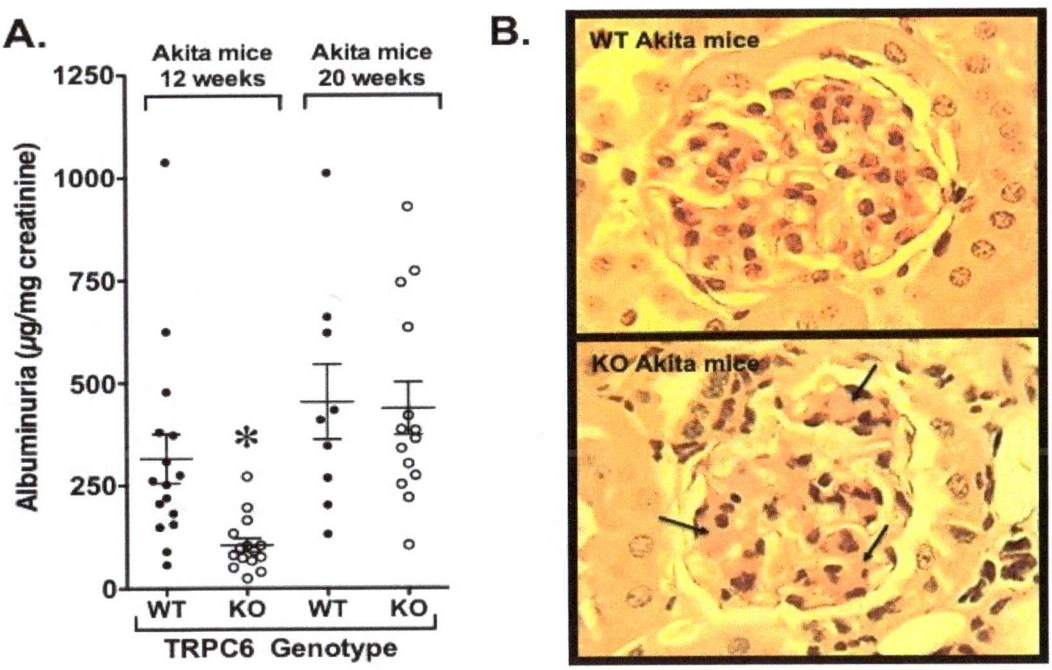

Figure 5. Effect of TRPC6 knockout in an animal model of diabetic kidney disease. Using a model of type 1 diabetes mellitus (Akita mice), we found that whole-body knockout of TRPC6 attenuated albuminuria early in the disease process (12 weeks of age), but this difference disappeared by 20 weeks of age (**A**). Histologic examination of kidneys was performed at the 20 week time point. Knockout of TRPC6 enhanced mesangial expansion (arrows) in knockout Akita mice compared to wild type (WT) Akita mice expressing TRPC6 (**B**). * $p < 0.05$ vs. WT Akita mice at 12 weeks of age.

Although selective blockade of TRPC6 was only modestly beneficial in diabetic kidney disease, it is possible that inhibition of multiple TRPC family members might be a more effective approach. Indeed, compensatory upregulation of other TRPC family members might compensate for selective inhibition of TRPC6, as discussed above. Liu et al. [141] tested this hypothesis in streptozotocin-treated mice lacking TRPC3, TRPC6, and TRPC7. Despite similar levels of hyperglycemia, knockout mice had decreased glomerular and kidney hypertrophy, reduced albuminuria, and better preserved renal cortical expression of the podocyte marker WT1 (Wilms tumor protein-1). These beneficial effects were associated with a reduction TGFβ (transforming growth factor β) signaling and markers of apoptosis in the knockout mice. Although these findings were impressive, knockout of TRPC3, TRPC6, and TRPC7 markedly reduced body weight in both vehicle-treated and streptozotocin-treated mice, which may have affected the results, as reported in another type 1 diabetic model [142]. Thus, although additional research is needed, currently available studies do not suggest an important therapeutic role for TRPC inhibition in diabetic kidney disease.

8. Targeting TRPC6 in Immune-Mediated Glomerular Diseases

In addition to direct effects in the kidney, TRPC6 may influence inflammatory responses [143]. For example, TRPC6 modulates chemotaxis, phagocytosis, cytokine release, and transendothelial migration [143–146]. To investigate the role of TRPC6 in an immune-mediated injury model, investigators have studied the effects of TRPC6 in nephrotoxic serum nephritis (NTS) [70,71]. In this model, glomerular injury was induced by injection of anti-GBM antibodies [70,71]. A recent study by Dryer and coworkers used the NTS model to examine the effects of TRPC6 knockout in rats [71]. In these studies, the investigators found that deletion of TRPC6 had no significant effect on proteinuria, renal function or tubulointerstitial inflammation and fibrosis compared to wild type animals [71]. In contrast, systemic knockout of TRPC6 significantly reduced glomerulosclerosis and attenuated the decrease in the podocyte marker podocin observed in wild type rats.

In a separate study, Kistler et al. investigated the effects of anti-GBM antiserum in wild type mice and in mice either over-expressing TRPC6 specifically in podocytes or in TRPC6 knockout mice [70]. Unexpectedly, these investigators found that podocyte-specific overexpression of TRPC6 attenuated albuminuria and FP effacement in NTS. In contrast, proteinuria was enhanced in the early stages of the disease process in TRPC6 knockout mice, and this increase in albuminuria was significantly reduced by complement depletion prior to induction of NTS. The authors attributed the beneficial effects of TRPC6 overexpression to enhanced activation of CaMKII on the basis of the following observations: (1) increased intracellular calcium levels protected podocytes from complement-mediated cellular injury [147]; (2) pharmacologic blockage of CaMKII exacerbated complement-mediated cellular injury in cultured podocytes [70]; and (3) CaMKII activation was decreased in TRPC6 knockout mice, but was increased in mice overexpressing TRPC6 specifically in podocytes [70]. In this study, the effects of TRPC6 knockout on glomerulosclerosis were not specifically evaluated, and the downstream effector pathways of CaMKII were not further explored. However, the differing effects of TRPC6 knockout in animal models of NTS, FSGS, and diabetic kidney disease suggest that targeting TRPC6 to treat glomerular disease processes is likely to be disease-specific.

9. Targeting TRPC5 in Proteinuric Kidney Diseases

As discussed above, Rho GTPase family members such as RhoA, Rac1, and Cdc42 play key roles in glomerular disease processes [107]. Excessive activation or loss of Rho GTPase family members causes proteinuria and effacement of podocyte foot processes in animal models [103,105,107,148–152]. Moreover, Rho GTPases promote podocyte loss by inducing podocyte apoptosis [152] and podocyte detachment [105]. Thus, targeting small GTPases for the treatment of glomerular disease processes is an active area of investigation.

A role for TRPC channels in regulating podocyte Rho GTPase activity was suggested by Greka and colleagues [100]. These investigators found that TRPC6 and TRPC5 were coupled to activation of RhoA and Rac1, respectively, and regulated actin cytoskeletal dynamics [100]. The authors suggested that TRPC6 promotes stress fiber formation and a contractile phenotype, which is essential for maintaining normal filtration barrier integrity [100,101]. In contrast, TRPC5 inhibited stress fiber formation and reduced podocyte contractility, which the authors suggested may play a role in adapting to hydrostatic stresses in the glomerulus [100]. In this scenario, the coupling between TRPC5 and Rac1 is of interest because Rac1 induces rapid translocation and insertion of TRPC5 into the cell membrane and increases calcium influx [153]. This creates a positive feedback loop with TRPC5, inducing Rac1 activation and, in turn, Rac1 promoting enhanced TRPC5 activity [100,101]. Greka and colleagues hypothesized that unopposed and excessive Rac1 signaling might play a role in glomerular diseases by promoting maladaptive cytoskeletal remodeling and induce proteinuria [101]. In support of this hypothesis,

TG expression of a constitutively active Rac1 construct in podocytes induces proteinuria, FP effacement, glomerulosclerosis, and excretion of podocytes expressing the transgene in urine [105,151].

To determine if TRPC5 played a pathogenetic role in proteinuric kidney diseases, Greka and coworkers [108] examined the effects of TRPC5 inhibition in animal models of proteinuria and FP effacement. In these experiments, whole body knockout of TRPC5 inhibited both albuminuria and effacement of podocyte FPs in the lipopolysaccharide (LPS) model of proteinuria. Similarly, knockout of TRPC5 inhibited FP effacement using the ex vivo, protamine sulfate (PS) model of glomerular filtration barrier disruption. The investigators then examined pharmacologic inhibition of TRPC5 using the combined TRPC4 and TRPC5 inhibitor ML204 [154]. This compound is selective for TRPC4 and TRPC5 [154], and data from this research group indicated that TRPC4 was not a major contributor to angiotensin II-induced calcium entry in podocytes [100]. On the basis of these data, the investigators suggested that examining TRPC channel activity using ML204 selectively examines the contribution of TRPC5 to podocyte biology. Indeed, the investigators found that ML204 had effects similar to TRPC5 knockout using both the LPS and PS models. On the basis of these observations, the researchers hypothesized that TRPC5 inhibition might be a useful strategy for treatment of proteinuric kidney disease.

To further investigate this hypothesis, Greka and co-workers examined the effects of ML204 in a more aggressive proteinuria model induced by TG overexpression of the human type 1 angiotensin II receptor (AT1R) specifically in podocytes in rats (AT1R TG rats) [155]. In these studies, ML204 inhibited albuminuria and podocyte loss, and improved glomerular histology in the AT1R TG model, even when treatment began in rats after the onset of disease [109]. To more selectively examine the role of TRPC5 in the disease process, the investigators developed a specific TRPC5 inhibitor (AC1903) based on the structures of published TRPC5 inhibitors including the TRPC4/5 inhibitor ML204 [154,156]. In these studies, AC1903 suppressed proteinuria, reduced podocyte loss, and improved glomerular histology in the in AT1R TG rats [109]. Similar beneficial effects of AC1903 were also observed in Dahl salt-sensitive rats, which are a model of hypertension-induced glomerulosclerosis. Thus, the data support a role for TRPC5 in the pathogenesis of proteinuric kidney diseases, provided that the doses of the pharmacologic agents maintained selectivity for TRPC5 in vivo.

Despite these promising findings, the role of TRPC5 in glomerular disease processes is controversial. Reiser and colleagues [157] studied the effects of overexpressing either wild type TRPC5 or a dominant-negative TRPC5 using a promoter that expressed the TG TRPC5 constructs ubiquitously [158]. The investigators found that both TG and non-TG mice exhibited similar levels of proteinuria as the mice aged, as well as after treatment with LPS. Furthermore, injection of the TRPC5 activator englerin-A did not cause proteinuria in non-TG mice or in TG animals, and treatment with ML204 did not inhibit LPS-induced albuminuria in any of the groups. The authors suggested that TRPC5 does not cause or exacerbate glomerular injury. However, interpretation of this study is complicated. First, primary podocyte cultures from animals overexpressing wild type TRPC5 demonstrated higher calcium responses to carbachol compared to podocytes overexpressing the dominant negative construct; however, no comparison of calcium responses was made with primary podocytes from non-TG mice. As a result, it is not known if the TG mice exhibited significantly altered calcium responses compared to non-TG animals. In addition, although the dose englerin-A used in these studies was biologically active in other model systems [159–161], the treatment regimen may not have been of sufficient strength or duration to cause adverse renal effects. Lastly, the dosage of ML204 used in the studies by Reiser and colleagues [157] was ≈10-fold lower than the dosage used in the studies by Greka and coworkers [108,109]. Thus, the dosage may have been too low to be effective in the studies by Reiser and colleagues [157] or, alternatively, the dosage used by Greka and coworkers [108,109] may have had beneficial effects due to blockade of other TRPC family members.

On the basis of these publications, further studies will be necessary to elucidate the role of TRPC5 in kidney diseases. In this regard, TRPC6 is the major TRPC family member linked to GPCR-coupled calcium entry in podocytes under basal conditions [41,43,162]. In disease states, however, other TRPC family members may play a role in disease pathogenesis. For example, active TRPC5 channels are difficult to detect prior to disease onset in the AT1R TG rat described above [109]. In contrast, with the onset of disease, functional TRPC5 channels are readily detected, and their activity may increase further as the disease progresses [109]. The mechanism(s) of enhanced TRPC5 activity in this model was not further investigated in this published study, but changes in the level of TRPC5 expression in the kidney have not been observed in animal models of glomerular disease [61,71,73,111,112]. However, the level of channel activity is also modulated by the number of functional channels that traffic to the cell surface [163]. This observation is directly relevant to TRPC5 channels, because cell surface expression of TRPC5 may be regulated by some of the same stimuli that activate TRPC6, including mechanical stimuli and oxidative stress [31,32,38,39]. In this scenario, both TRPC5 and TRPC6 might traffic to the cell surface in a coordinated fashion in disease states and, in turn, contribute calcium entry and podocyte injury in proteinuric kidney diseases.

10. Targeting TRPC Family Members in Other Acquired Kidney Diseases

In addition to podocytes, TRPC6 is expressed in multiple cell types in the kidney [35]. Recent studies suggest an important role for the TRPC family members TRPC3 and TRPC6 in fibroblast proliferation, as well as in fibroblast to myofibroblast transformation [75,164]. These cell types play a critical role in wound healing and are the key cellular mediators of fibrosis in renal and extrarenal tissues [75,76,164]. Saliba et al. found that selective pharmacologic blockade of TRPC3 using Pyr3 [165] inhibited fibroblast proliferation, myofibroblast transformation, and production of extracellular matrix proteins in primary renal fibroblasts [75]. In vivo, treatment with Pyr3 inhibited fibroblast activation, attenuated both interstitial fibrosis and inflammatory cell infiltration, and decreased total renal tissue collagen content in obstructed kidneys of both Wistar rats and wild type mice undergoing unilateral ureteral obstruction (UUO) [75]. Pharmacologic blockade of TRPC3 also inhibited upregulation of TRPC3 in obstructed kidneys, and the beneficial histologic effects of TRPC3 inhibition were recapitulated in TRPC3 knockout mice.

In a separate study, Wu et al. found that TRPC6 knockout provided partial protection from renal fibrosis in mice subjected to UUO, and a comparable beneficial effect was observed in obstructed kidneys following treatment with the non-selective TRPC inhibitor BTP2 [76]. Moreover, a similar beneficial effect was observed by another group in a mouse UUO model using the selective TRPC6 inhibitor BI-749327 [166]. In the Wu et al. study, the authors also examined the effects of soluble klotho in the UUO model on the basis of the following observations: (1) the investigators had previously demonstrated that soluble klotho inhibits TRPC6 exocytosis and TRPC6 currents in the heart [167], and (2) treatment with soluble klotho inhibits renal fibrosis in obstructed kidneys [168]. However, soluble klotho provided no additional protection in TRPC6 knockout mice, suggesting that the beneficial effects of klotho in UUO were mediated by inhibition of TRPC6. Lastly, both TRPC3 and TRPC6 mRNA were potently upregulated in interstitial fibroblasts of obstructed kidneys [76], but combined TRPC3 and TRPC6 knockout in UUO provided no additional protection from renal fibrosis compared to TRPC6 knockout mice. Given that either TRPC3 or TRPC6 knockout attenuated fibrosis in UUO, it is of interest that combined TRPC3 and TRPC6 knockout was not additive in the Wu et al. study [76]. We can only speculate on the mechanisms of this effect; however, TRPC1, TRPC3, and TRPC6 co-immunoprecipitate in freshly isolated renal fibroblasts, suggesting that these TRPC family members form a macromolecular complex in these cells [75]. Moreover, TRPC6 has been shown to form heterodimers with TRPC3 in other cell types [35,169]. These results suggest that TRPC6 and TRPC3 are components of the same signaling pathways, perhaps by forming heterodimers or macromolecular complexes with other TRPC family members.

11. Conclusions

In summary, the discovery that gain-of-function mutations in TRPC6 caused familial forms of FSGS generated significant interest in targeting TRPC6, and perhaps other TRPC family members, to treat glomerular disease processes. Since that time, preclinical studies have examined the role of TRPC channels in diverse animal models of kidney disease. Additional studies have suggested that TRPC6 is a component of a novel signaling complex at the SD that likely plays a key role in podocyte biology. Interpretation of available studies is, however, limited by differing results between disease models, as well as generalizability of preclinical results to human disease processes. Although we acknowledge the limitations of preclinical models, these model systems have significantly advanced our understanding of both normal physiology and pathophysiologic processes. Moreover, preclinical models will continue to play an important role in developing molecular-targeted therapies for human disease. In this regard, a major limitation of current model systems is the lack of inducible, cell-specific TRPC knockout models. Conditional knockout models would enhance our ability to discern the biologic role of TRPC family members in organs and tissues composed of multiple, diverse cell types such as the kidney. The study of glomerular biology is also limited by current cell culture systems, which cannot recapitulate the multicellular environment and hydrostatic pressures of the glomerulus. Recent progress in cell culture systems may circumvent some of these limitations. For example, newly developed microfluidic devices are able to support the growth of multicellular culture systems, which closely simulate the natural tissue–tissue interface of the glomerulus [170]. It is likely that the development of both new animal models and innovative cell culture technologies will facilitate the study of glomerular biology. Given the need for new therapies to treat kidney diseases, the development of these new technologies provides an opportunity to better understand normal physiology and pathophysiologic processes, as well as to test new therapeutic strategies.

Acknowledgments: We thank William Eisner for his technical assistance with our animal studies.

References

1. Sarnak, M.J.; Levey, A.S.; Schoolwerth, A.C.; Coresh, J.; Culleton, B.; Hamm, L.L.; McCullough, P.A.; Kasiske, B.L.; Kelepouris, E.; Klag, M.J.; et al. Kidney disease as a risk factor for development of cardiovascular disease: A statement from the American Heart Association Councils on Kidney in Cardiovascular Disease, High Blood Pressure Research, Clinical Cardiology, and Epidemiology and Prevention. *Circulation* **2003**, *108*, 2154–2169. [CrossRef] [PubMed]
2. Greenberg, A.; Cheung, A.K. *Primer on Kidney Diseases*, 4th ed.; Elsevier Saunders: Philadelphia, PA, USA, 2005; p. 608.
3. Foley, R.N.; Collins, A.J. The USRDS: What you need to know about what it can and can't tell us about ESRD. *Clin. J. Am. Soc. Nephrol.* **2013**, *8*, 845–851. [CrossRef] [PubMed]
4. Go, A.S.; Chertow, G.M.; Fan, D.; McCulloch, C.E.; Hsu, C.Y. Chronic kidney disease and the risks of death, cardiovascular events, and hospitalization. *N. Engl. J. Med.* **2004**, *351*, 1296–1305. [CrossRef] [PubMed]
5. Kriz, W.; Gretz, N.; Lemley, K.V. Progression of glomerular diseases: Is the podocyte the culprit? *Kidney Int.* **1998**, *54*, 687–697. [CrossRef]
6. Pavenstadt, H.; Kriz, W.; Kretzler, M. Cell biology of the glomerular podocyte. *Physiol. Rev.* **2003**, *83*, 253–307. [CrossRef]
7. Martin, C.E.; Jones, N. Nephrin Signaling in the Podocyte: An Updated View of Signal Regulation at the Slit Diaphragm and Beyond. *Front. Endocrinol. (Lausanne)* **2018**, *9*, 302. [CrossRef]
8. Neal, C.R. Podocytes ... What's Under Yours? (Podocytes and Foot Processes and How They Change in Nephropathy). *Front. Endocrinol. (Lausanne)* **2015**, *6*, 9. [CrossRef]
9. Schwarz, K.; Simons, M.; Reiser, J.; Saleem, M.A.; Faul, C.; Kriz, W.; Shaw, A.S.; Holzman, L.B.; Mundel, P. Podocin, a raft-associated component of the glomerular slit diaphragm, interacts with CD2AP and nephrin. *J. Clin. Investig.* **2001**, *108*, 1621–1629. [CrossRef]

10. Harita, Y.; Kurihara, H.; Kosako, H.; Tezuka, T.; Sekine, T.; Igarashi, T.; Ohsawa, I.; Ohta, S.; Hattori, S. Phosphorylation of Nephrin Triggers Ca^{2+} Signaling by Recruitment and Activation of Phospholipase C-{gamma}1. *J. Biol. Chem.* **2009**, *284*, 8951–8962. [CrossRef]
11. Jones, N.; Blasutig, I.M.; Eremina, V.; Ruston, J.M.; Bladt, F.; Li, H.; Huang, H.; Larose, L.; Li, S.S.; Takano, T.; et al. Nck adaptor proteins link nephrin to the actin cytoskeleton of kidney podocytes. *Nature* **2006**, *440*, 818–823. [CrossRef]
12. Li, H.; Lemay, S.; Aoudjit, L.; Kawachi, H.; Takano, T. SRC-family kinase Fyn phosphorylates the cytoplasmic domain of nephrin and modulates its interaction with podocin. *J. Am. Soc. Nephrol.* **2004**, *15*, 3006–3015. [CrossRef] [PubMed]
13. Verma, R.; Wharram, B.; Kovari, I.; Kunkel, R.; Nihalani, D.; Wary, K.K.; Wiggins, R.C.; Killen, P.; Holzman, L.B. Fyn binds to and phosphorylates the kidney slit diaphragm component Nephrin. *J. Biol. Chem.* **2003**, *278*, 20716–20723. [CrossRef] [PubMed]
14. Huber, T.B.; Kottgen, M.; Schilling, B.; Walz, G.; Benzing, T. Interaction with podocin facilitates nephrin signaling. *J. Biol. Chem.* **2001**, *276*, 41543–41546. [CrossRef] [PubMed]
15. Huber, T.B.; Hartleben, B.; Kim, J.; Schmidts, M.; Schermer, B.; Keil, A.; Egger, L.; Lecha, R.L.; Borner, C.; Pavenstadt, H.; et al. Nephrin and CD2AP associate with phosphoinositide 3-OH kinase and stimulate AKT-dependent signaling. *Mol. Cell. Biol.* **2003**, *23*, 4917–4928. [CrossRef]
16. Pollak, M.R.; Quaggin, S.E.; Hoenig, M.P.; Dworkin, L.D. The glomerulus: The sphere of influence. *Clin. J. Am. Soc. Nephrol.* **2014**, *9*, 1461–1469. [CrossRef]
17. Kriz, W.; Lemley, K.V. A potential role for mechanical forces in the detachment of podocytes and the progression of CKD. *J. Am. Soc. Nephrol.* **2015**, *26*, 258–269. [CrossRef]
18. Kriz, W.; Lemley, K.V. Potential relevance of shear stress for slit diaphragm and podocyte function. *Kidney Int.* **2017**, *91*, 1283–1286. [CrossRef]
19. Lin, J.S.; Jeon, J.S.; Fan, Q.; Wong, H.N.; Palmer, M.B.; Holzman, L.B. ARF6 mediates nephrin tyrosine phosphorylation-induced podocyte cellular dynamics. *PLoS ONE* **2017**, *12*, e0184575. [CrossRef]
20. George, B.; Verma, R.; Soofi, A.A.; Garg, P.; Zhang, J.; Park, T.J.; Giardino, L.; Ryzhova, L.; Johnstone, D.B.; Wong, H.; et al. Crk1/2-dependent signaling is necessary for podocyte foot process spreading in mouse models of glomerular disease. *J. Clin. Investig.* **2012**, *122*, 674–692. [CrossRef]
21. Verma, R.; Venkatareddy, M.; Kalinowski, A.; Patel, S.R.; Garg, P. Integrin Ligation Results in Nephrin Tyrosine Phosphorylation In Vitro. *PLoS ONE* **2016**, *11*, e0148906. [CrossRef]
22. Wiggins, R.C. The spectrum of podocytopathies: A unifying view of glomerular diseases. *Kidney Int.* **2007**, *71*, 1205–1214. [CrossRef] [PubMed]
23. Wolf, G.; Chen, S.; Ziyadeh, F.N. From the periphery of the glomerular capillary wall toward the center of disease: Podocyte injury comes of age in diabetic nephropathy. *Diabetes* **2005**, *54*, 1626–1634. [CrossRef] [PubMed]
24. Kim, Y.H.; Goyal, M.; Kurnit, D.; Wharram, B.; Wiggins, J.; Holzman, L.; Kershaw, D.; Wiggins, R. Podocyte depletion and glomerulosclerosis have a direct relationship in the PAN-treated rat. *Kidney Int.* **2001**, *60*, 957–968. [CrossRef] [PubMed]
25. Wharram, B.L.; Goyal, M.; Wiggins, J.E.; Sanden, S.K.; Hussain, S.; Filipiak, W.E.; Saunders, T.L.; Dysko, R.C.; Kohno, K.; Holzman, L.B.; et al. Podocyte depletion causes glomerulosclerosis: Diphtheria toxin-induced podocyte depletion in rats expressing human diphtheria toxin receptor transgene. *J. Am. Soc. Nephrol.* **2005**, *16*, 2941–2952. [CrossRef] [PubMed]
26. Gees, M.; Colsoul, B.; Nilius, B. The role of transient receptor potential cation channels in Ca2+ signaling. *Cold Spring Harb. Perspect. Biol.* **2010**, *2*, a003962. [CrossRef]
27. Nilius, B.; Owsianik, G.; Voets, T.; Peters, J.A. Transient receptor potential cation channels in disease. *Physiol. Rev.* **2007**, *87*, 165–217. [CrossRef]
28. Nishizuka, Y. Intracellular signaling by hydrolysis of phospholipids and activation of protein kinase C. *Science* **1992**, *258*, 607–614. [CrossRef]
29. Maroto, R.; Raso, A.; Wood, T.G.; Kurosky, A.; Martinac, B.; Hamill, O.P. TRPC1 forms the stretch-activated cation channel in vertebrate cells. *Nat. Cell Biol.* **2005**, *7*, 179–185. [CrossRef]
30. Spassova, M.A.; Hewavitharana, T.; Xu, W.; Soboloff, J.; Gill, D.L. A common mechanism underlies stretch activation and receptor activation of TRPC6 channels. *Proc. Natl. Acad. Sci. USA* **2006**, *103*, 16586–16591. [CrossRef]

31. Gomis, A.; Soriano, S.; Belmonte, C.; Viana, F. Hypoosmotic- and pressure-induced membrane stretch activate TRPC5 channels. *J. Physiol.* **2008**, *586*, 5633–5649. [CrossRef]
32. Shen, B.; Wong, C.O.; Lau, O.C.; Woo, T.; Bai, S.; Huang, Y.; Yao, X. Plasma membrane mechanical stress activates TRPC5 channels. *PLoS ONE* **2015**, *10*, e0122227. [CrossRef] [PubMed]
33. Yamaguchi, Y.; Iribe, G.; Nishida, M.; Naruse, K. Role of TRPC3 and TRPC6 channels in the myocardial response to stretch: Linking physiology and pathophysiology. *Prog. Biophys. Mol. Biol.* **2017**, *130*, 264–272. [CrossRef] [PubMed]
34. Wilson, C.; Dryer, S.E. A mutation in TRPC6 channels abolishes their activation by hypoosmotic stretch but does not affect activation by diacylglycerol or G protein signaling cascades. *Am. J. Physiol. Ren. Physiol.* **2014**, *306*, F1018–F1025. [CrossRef] [PubMed]
35. Dryer, S.E.; Roshanravan, H.; Kim, E.Y. TRPC channels: Regulation, dysregulation and contributions to chronic kidney disease. *Biochim. Biophys. Acta Mol. Basis. Dis.* **2019**, *1865*, 1041–1066. [CrossRef] [PubMed]
36. Anderson, M.; Kim, E.Y.; Hagmann, H.; Benzing, T.; Dryer, S.E. Opposing effects of podocin on the gating of podocyte TRPC6 channels evoked by membrane stretch or diacylglycerol. *Am. J. Physiol. Cell Physiol.* **2013**, *305*, C276–C289. [CrossRef] [PubMed]
37. Nikolaev, Y.A.; Cox, C.D.; Ridone, P.; Rohde, P.R.; Cordero-Morales, J.F.; Vasquez, V.; Laver, D.R.; Martinac, B. Mammalian TRP ion channels are insensitive to membrane stretch. *J. Cell. Sci.* **2019**. [CrossRef]
38. Yoshida, T.; Inoue, R.; Morii, T.; Takahashi, N.; Yamamoto, S.; Hara, Y.; Tominaga, M.; Shimizu, S.; Sato, Y.; Mori, Y. Nitric oxide activates TRP channels by cysteine S-nitrosylation. *Nat. Chem. Biol.* **2006**, *2*, 596–607. [CrossRef]
39. Yamamoto, S.; Takahashi, N.; Mori, Y. Chemical physiology of oxidative stress-activated TRPM2 and TRPC5 channels. *Prog. Biophys. Mol. Biol.* **2010**, *103*, 18–27. [CrossRef]
40. Ding, Y.; Winters, A.; Ding, M.; Graham, S.; Akopova, I.; Muallem, S.; Wang, Y.; Hong, J.H.; Gryczynski, Z.; Yang, S.H.; et al. Reactive oxygen species-mediated TRPC6 protein activation in vascular myocytes, a mechanism for vasoconstrictor-regulated vascular tone. *J. Biol. Chem.* **2011**, *286*, 31799–31809. [CrossRef]
41. Anderson, M.; Roshanravan, H.; Khine, J.; Dryer, S.E. Angiotensin II activation of TRPC6 channels in rat podocytes requires generation of reactive oxygen species. *J. Cell. Physiol.* **2014**, *229*, 434–442. [CrossRef]
42. Kim, E.Y.; Anderson, M.; Wilson, C.; Hagmann, H.; Benzing, T.; Dryer, S.E. NOX2 interacts with podocyte TRPC6 channels and contributes to their activation by diacylglycerol: Essential role of podocin in formation of this complex. *Am. J. Physiol. Cell Physiol.* **2013**, *305*, C960–C971. [CrossRef] [PubMed]
43. Roshanravan, H.; Dryer, S.E. ATP acting through P2Y receptors causes activation of podocyte TRPC6 channels: Role of podocin and reactive oxygen species. *Am. J. Physiol. Ren. Physiol.* **2014**, *306*, F1088–F1097. [CrossRef] [PubMed]
44. Winn, M.P.; Conlon, P.J.; Lynn, K.L.; Farrington, M.K.; Creazzo, T.; Hawkins, A.F.; Daskalakis, N.; Kwan, S.Y.; Ebersviller, S.; Burchette, J.L.; et al. A mutation in the TRPC6 cation channel causes familial focal segmental glomerulosclerosis. *Science* **2005**, *308*, 1801–1804. [CrossRef] [PubMed]
45. Reiser, J.; Polu, K.R.; Moller, C.C.; Kenlan, P.; Altintas, M.M.; Wei, C.; Faul, C.; Herbert, S.; Villegas, I.; Avila-Casado, C.; et al. TRPC6 is a glomerular slit diaphragm-associated channel required for normal renal function. *Nat. Genet.* **2005**, *37*, 739–744. [CrossRef]
46. Huber, T.B.; Schermer, B.; Muller, R.U.; Hohne, M.; Bartram, M.; Calixto, A.; Hagmann, H.; Reinhardt, C.; Koos, F.; Kunzelmann, K.; et al. Podocin and MEC-2 bind cholesterol to regulate the activity of associated ion channels. *Proc. Natl. Acad. Sci. USA* **2006**, *103*, 17079–17086. [CrossRef]
47. Faul, C.; Asanuma, K.; Yanagida-Asanuma, E.; Kim, K.; Mundel, P. Actin up: Regulation of podocyte structure and function by components of the actin cytoskeleton. *Trends Cell Biol.* **2007**, *17*, 428–437. [CrossRef]
48. Drenckhahn, D.; Franke, R.P. Ultrastructural organization of contractile and cytoskeletal proteins in glomerular podocytes of chicken, rat, and man. *Lab. Investig.* **1988**, *59*, 673–682.
49. Riehle, M.; Buscher, A.K.; Gohlke, B.O.; Kassmann, M.; Kolatsi-Joannou, M.; Brasen, J.H.; Nagel, M.; Becker, J.U.; Winyard, P.; Hoyer, P.F.; et al. TRPC6 G757D Loss-of-Function Mutation Associates with FSGS. *J. Am. Soc. Nephrol.* **2016**, *27*, 2771–2783. [CrossRef]
50. Santin, S.; Ars, E.; Rossetti, S.; Salido, E.; Silva, I.; Garcia-Maset, R.; Gimenez, I.; Ruiz, P.; Mendizabal, S.; Luciano Nieto, J.; et al. TRPC6 mutational analysis in a large cohort of patients with focal segmental glomerulosclerosis. *Nephrol. Dial. Transplant.* **2009**, *24*, 3089–3096. [CrossRef]

51. Mir, S.; Yavascan, O.; Berdeli, A.; Sozeri, B. TRPC6 gene variants in Turkish children with steroid-resistant nephrotic syndrome. *Nephrol. Dial. Transplant.* **2012**, *27*, 205–209. [CrossRef]
52. Buscher, A.K.; Kranz, B.; Buscher, R.; Hildebrandt, F.; Dworniczak, B.; Pennekamp, P.; Kuwertz-Broking, E.; Wingen, A.M.; John, U.; Kemper, M.; et al. Immunosuppression and renal outcome in congenital and pediatric steroid-resistant nephrotic syndrome. *Clin. J. Am. Soc. Nephrol.* **2010**, *5*, 2075–2084. [CrossRef] [PubMed]
53. Gigante, M.; Caridi, G.; Montemurno, E.; Soccio, M.; d'Apolito, M.; Cerullo, G.; Aucella, F.; Schirinzi, A.; Emma, F.; Massella, L.; et al. TRPC6 mutations in children with steroid-resistant nephrotic syndrome and atypical phenotype. *Clin. J. Am. Soc. Nephrol.* **2011**, *6*, 1626–1634. [CrossRef] [PubMed]
54. Heeringa, S.F.; Moller, C.C.; Du, J.; Yue, L.; Hinkes, B.; Chernin, G.; Vlangos, C.N.; Hoyer, P.F.; Reiser, J.; Hildebrandt, F. A novel TRPC6 mutation that causes childhood FSGS. *PLoS ONE* **2009**, *4*, e7771. [CrossRef] [PubMed]
55. Zhu, B.; Chen, N.; Wang, Z.H.; Pan, X.X.; Ren, H.; Zhang, W.; Wang, W.M. Identification and functional analysis of a novel TRPC6 mutation associated with late onset familial focal segmental glomerulosclerosis in Chinese patients. *Mutat. Res.* **2009**, *664*, 84–90. [CrossRef] [PubMed]
56. Hofstra, J.M.; Lainez, S.; van Kuijk, W.H.; Schoots, J.; Baltissen, M.P.; Hoefsloot, L.H.; Knoers, N.V.; Berden, J.H.; Bindels, R.J.; van der Vlag, J.; et al. New TRPC6 gain-of-function mutation in a non-consanguineous Dutch family with late-onset focal segmental glomerulosclerosis. *Nephrol. Dial. Transplant.* **2013**, *28*, 1830–1838. [CrossRef]
57. Buscher, A.K.; Konrad, M.; Nagel, M.; Witzke, O.; Kribben, A.; Hoyer, P.F.; Weber, S. Mutations in podocyte genes are a rare cause of primary FSGS associated with ESRD in adult patients. *Clin. Nephrol.* **2012**, *78*, 47–53. [CrossRef]
58. Winn, M.P.; Conlon, P.J.; Lynn, K.L.; Howell, D.N.; Slotterbeck, B.D.; Smith, A.H.; Graham, F.L.; Bembe, M.; Quarles, L.D.; Pericak-Vance, M.A.; et al. Linkage of a gene causing familial focal segmental glomerulosclerosis to chromosome 11 and further evidence of genetic heterogeneity. *Genomics* **1999**, *58*, 113–120. [CrossRef]
59. Moller, C.C.; Flesche, J.; Reiser, J. Sensitizing the Slit Diaphragm with TRPC6 ion channels. *J. Am. Soc. Nephrol.* **2009**, *20*, 950–953. [CrossRef]
60. El Hindi, S.; Reiser, J. TRPC channel modulation in podocytes-inching toward novel treatments for glomerular disease. *Pediatr. Nephrol.* **2011**, *26*, 1057–1064. [CrossRef]
61. Wang, L.; Jirka, G.; Rosenberg, P.B.; Buckley, A.F.; Gomez, J.A.; Fields, T.A.; Winn, M.P.; Spurney, R.F. Gq signaling causes glomerular injury by activating TRPC6. *J. Clin. Investig.* **2015**, *125*, 1913–1926. [CrossRef]
62. Moller, C.C.; Wei, C.; Altintas, M.M.; Li, J.; Greka, A.; Ohse, T.; Pippin, J.W.; Rastaldi, M.P.; Wawersik, S.; Schiavi, S.; et al. Induction of TRPC6 channel in acquired forms of proteinuric kidney disease. *J. Am. Soc. Nephrol.* **2007**, *18*, 29–36. [CrossRef] [PubMed]
63. Krall, P.; Canales, C.P.; Kairath, P.; Carmona-Mora, P.; Molina, J.; Carpio, J.D.; Ruiz, P.; Mezzano, S.A.; Li, J.; Wei, C.; et al. Podocyte-specific overexpression of wild type or mutant trpc6 in mice is sufficient to cause glomerular disease. *PLoS ONE* **2010**, *5*, e12859. [CrossRef] [PubMed]
64. Sonneveld, R.; Hoenderop, J.G.; Isidori, A.M.; Henique, C.; Dijkman, H.B.; Berden, J.H.; Tharaux, P.L.; van der Vlag, J.; Nijenhuis, T. Sildenafil Prevents Podocyte Injury via PPAR-gamma-Mediated TRPC6 Inhibition. *J. Am. Soc. Nephrol.* **2016**. [CrossRef]
65. Sonneveld, R.; van der Vlag, J.; Baltissen, M.P.; Verkaart, S.A.; Wetzels, J.F.; Berden, J.H.; Hoenderop, J.G.; Nijenhuis, T. Glucose specifically regulates TRPC6 expression in the podocyte in an AngII-dependent manner. *Am. J. Pathol.* **2014**, *184*, 1715–1726. [CrossRef]
66. Ma, R.; Liu, L.; Jiang, W.; Yu, Y.; Song, H. FK506 ameliorates podocyte injury in type 2 diabetic nephropathy by down-regulating TRPC6 and NFAT expression. *Int. J. Clin. Exp. Pathol.* **2015**, *8*, 14063–14074.
67. Ilatovskaya, D.V.; Levchenko, V.; Lowing, A.; Shuyskiy, L.S.; Palygin, O.; Staruschenko, A. Podocyte injury in diabetic nephropathy: Implications of angiotensin II-dependent activation of TRPC channels. *Sci. Rep.* **2015**, *5*, 17637. [CrossRef]
68. Ma, R.; Xu, Y.; Zhou, H.; Zhang, D.; Yao, D.; Song, L.; Liu, Y. Participation of the AngII/TRPC6/NFAT axis in the pathogenesis of podocyte injury in rats with type 2 diabetes. *Mol. Med. Rep.* **2019**, *19*, 2421–2430. [CrossRef]

69. Lu, X.Y.; Liu, B.C.; Cao, Y.Z.; Song, C.; Su, H.; Chen, G.; Klein, J.D.; Zhang, H.X.; Wang, L.; Ma, H.P. High glucose reduces the expression of podocin in cultured human podocytes by stimulating TRPC6. *Am. J. Physiol. Ren. Physiol.* **2019**. [CrossRef]
70. Kistler, A.D.; Singh, G.; Altintas, M.M.; Yu, H.; Fernandez, I.C.; Gu, C.; Wilson, C.; Srivastava, S.K.; Dietrich, A.; Walz, K.; et al. Transient receptor potential channel 6 (TRPC6) protects podocytes during complement-mediated glomerular disease. *J. Biol. Chem.* **2013**, *288*, 36598–36609. [CrossRef]
71. Kim, E.Y.; Shotorbani, P.Y.; Dryer, S.E. TRPC6 inactivation does not affect loss of renal function in nephrotoxic serum glomerulonephritis in rats, but reduces severity of glomerular lesions. *Biochem. Biophys. Rep.* **2019**, *17*, 139–150. [CrossRef]
72. Sonneveld, R.; Ferre, S.; Hoenderop, J.G.; Dijkman, H.B.; Berden, J.H.; Bindels, R.J.; Wetzels, J.F.; van der Vlag, J.; Nijenhuis, T. Vitamin D down-regulates TRPC6 expression in podocyte injury and proteinuric glomerular disease. *Am. J. Pathol.* **2013**, *182*, 1196–1204. [CrossRef] [PubMed]
73. Kim, E.Y.; Yazdizadeh Shotorbani, P.; Dryer, S.E. Trpc6 inactivation confers protection in a model of severe nephrosis in rats. *J. Mol. Med. (Berl.)* **2018**, *96*, 631–644. [CrossRef] [PubMed]
74. Nijenhuis, T.; Sloan, A.J.; Hoenderop, J.G.; Flesche, J.; van Goor, H.; Kistler, A.D.; Bakker, M.; Bindels, R.J.; de Boer, R.A.; Moller, C.C.; et al. Angiotensin II contributes to podocyte injury by increasing TRPC6 expression via an NFAT-mediated positive feedback signaling pathway. *Am. J. Pathol.* **2011**, *179*, 1719–1732. [CrossRef] [PubMed]
75. Saliba, Y.; Karam, R.; Smayra, V.; Aftimos, G.; Abramowitz, J.; Birnbaumer, L.; Fares, N. Evidence of a Role for Fibroblast Transient Receptor Potential Canonical 3 Ca^{2+} Channel in Renal Fibrosis. *J. Am. Soc. Nephrol.* **2015**, *26*, 1855–1876. [CrossRef]
76. Wu, Y.L.; Xie, J.; An, S.W.; Oliver, N.; Barrezueta, N.X.; Lin, M.H.; Birnbaumer, L.; Huang, C.L. Inhibition of TRPC6 channels ameliorates renal fibrosis and contributes to renal protection by soluble klotho. *Kidney Int.* **2017**, *91*, 830–841. [CrossRef]
77. Kuwahara, K.; Wang, Y.; McAnally, J.; Richardson, J.A.; Bassel-Duby, R.; Hill, J.A.; Olson, E.N. TRPC6 fulfills a calcineurin signaling circuit during pathologic cardiac remodeling. *J. Clin. Investig.* **2006**, *116*, 3114–3126. [CrossRef]
78. Bush, E.W.; Hood, D.B.; Papst, P.J.; Chapo, J.A.; Minobe, W.; Bristow, M.R.; Olson, E.N.; McKinsey, T.A. Canonical transient receptor potential channels promote cardiomyocyte hypertrophy through activation of calcineurin signaling. *J. Biol. Chem.* **2006**, *281*, 33487–33496. [CrossRef]
79. Onohara, N.; Nishida, M.; Inoue, R.; Kobayashi, H.; Sumimoto, H.; Sato, Y.; Mori, Y.; Nagao, T.; Kurose, H. TRPC3 and TRPC6 are essential for angiotensin II-induced cardiac hypertrophy. *EMBO J.* **2006**, *25*, 5305–5316. [CrossRef]
80. Hogan, P.G.; Chen, L.; Nardone, J.; Rao, A. Transcriptional regulation by calcium, calcineurin, and NFAT. *Genes. Dev.* **2003**, *17*, 2205–2232. [CrossRef]
81. Johnson, S.A.; Spurney, R.F. Twenty years after ACEIs and ARBs: Emerging treatment strategies for diabetic nephropathy. *Am. J. Physiol. Ren. Physiol.* **2015**, *309*, F807–F820. [CrossRef]
82. Horsley, V.; Pavlath, G.K. NFAT: Ubiquitous regulator of cell differentiation and adaptation. *J. Cell Biol.* **2002**, *156*, 771–774. [CrossRef] [PubMed]
83. Wilkins, B.J.; Dai, Y.S.; Bueno, O.F.; Parsons, S.A.; Xu, J.; Plank, D.M.; Jones, F.; Kimball, T.R.; Molkentin, J.D. Calcineurin/NFAT coupling participates in pathological, but not physiological, cardiac hypertrophy. *Circ. Res.* **2004**, *94*, 110–118. [CrossRef] [PubMed]
84. Wang, Y.; Jarad, G.; Tripathi, P.; Pan, M.; Cunningham, J.; Martin, D.R.; Liapis, H.; Miner, J.H.; Chen, F. Activation of NFAT signaling in podocytes causes glomerulosclerosis. *J. Am. Soc. Nephrol.* **2010**, *21*, 1657–1666. [CrossRef] [PubMed]
85. Schlondorff, J.; Del Camino, D.; Carrasquillo, R.; Lacey, V.; Pollak, M.R. TRPC6 mutations associated with focal segmental glomerulosclerosis cause constitutive activation of NFAT-dependent transcription. *Am. J. Physiol. Cell Physiol.* **2009**, *296*, C558–C569. [CrossRef]
86. Li, H.; Rao, A.; Hogan, P.G. Interaction of calcineurin with substrates and targeting proteins. *Trends Cell Biol.* **2011**, *21*, 91–103. [CrossRef]
87. Yu, H.; Kistler, A.; Faridi, M.H.; Meyer, J.O.; Tryniszewska, B.; Mehta, D.; Yue, L.; Dryer, S.; Reiser, J. Synaptopodin Limits TRPC6 Podocyte Surface Expression and Attenuates Proteinuria. *J. Am. Soc. Nephrol.* **2016**, *27*, 3308–3319. [CrossRef]

88. Faul, C.; Donnelly, M.; Merscher-Gomez, S.; Chang, Y.H.; Franz, S.; Delfgaauw, J.; Chang, J.M.; Choi, H.Y.; Campbell, K.N.; Kim, K.; et al. The actin cytoskeleton of kidney podocytes is a direct target of the antiproteinuric effect of cyclosporine A. *Nat. Med.* **2008**, *14*, 931–938. [CrossRef]
89. Wang, L.; Chang, J.H.; Paik, S.Y.; Tang, Y.; Eisner, W.; Spurney, R.F. Calcineurin (CN) activation promotes apoptosis of glomerular podocytes both in vitro and in vivo. *Mol. Endocrinol.* **2011**, *25*, 1376–1386. [CrossRef]
90. Liu, B.C.; Song, X.; Lu, X.Y.; Li, D.T.; Eaton, D.C.; Shen, B.Z.; Li, X.Q.; Ma, H.P. High glucose induces podocyte apoptosis by stimulating TRPC6 via elevation of reactive oxygen species. *Biochim. Biophys. Acta* **2013**, *1833*, 1434–1442. [CrossRef]
91. Cribbs, J.T.; Strack, S. Reversible phosphorylation of Drp1 by cyclic AMP-dependent protein kinase and calcineurin regulates mitochondrial fission and cell death. *EMBO Rep.* **2007**, *8*, 939–944. [CrossRef]
92. Shibasaki, F.; Hallin, U.; Uchino, H. Calcineurin as a multifunctional regulator. *J. Biochem.* **2002**, *131*, 1–15. [CrossRef] [PubMed]
93. Wang, W.; Wang, Y.; Long, J.; Wang, J.; Haudek, S.B.; Overbeek, P.; Chang, B.H.; Schumacker, P.T.; Danesh, F.R. Mitochondrial fission triggered by hyperglycemia is mediated by ROCK1 activation in podocytes and endothelial cells. *Cell Metab.* **2012**, *15*, 186–200. [CrossRef] [PubMed]
94. Yu, S.Y.; Qi, R. Role of bad in podocyte apoptosis induced by puromycin aminonucleoside. *Transplant. Proc.* **2013**, *45*, 569–573. [CrossRef] [PubMed]
95. Sanz, A.B.; Santamaria, B.; Ruiz-Ortega, M.; Egido, J.; Ortiz, A. Mechanisms of renal apoptosis in health and disease. *J. Am. Soc. Nephrol.* **2008**, *19*, 1634–1642. [CrossRef] [PubMed]
96. Verheijden, K.A.T.; Sonneveld, R.; Bakker-van Bebber, M.; Wetzels, J.F.M.; van der Vlag, J.; Nijenhuis, T. The Calcium-Dependent Protease Calpain-1 Links TRPC6 Activity to Podocyte Injury. *J. Am. Soc. Nephrol.* **2018**, *29*, 2099–2109. [CrossRef]
97. Farmer, L.K.; Rollason, R.; Whitcomb, D.J.; Ni, L.; Goodliff, A.; Lay, A.C.; Birnbaumer, L.; Heesom, K.J.; Xu, S.Z.; Saleem, M.A.; et al. TRPC6 Binds to and Activates Calpain, Independent of Its Channel Activity, and Regulates Podocyte Cytoskeleton, Cell Adhesion, and Motility. *J. Am. Soc. Nephrol.* **2019**, *30*, 1910–1924. [CrossRef]
98. Chan, S.L.; Mattson, M.P. Caspase and calpain substrates: Roles in synaptic plasticity and cell death. *J. Neurosci. Res.* **1999**, *58*, 167–190. [CrossRef]
99. Tian, X.; Kim, J.J.; Monkley, S.M.; Gotoh, N.; Nandez, R.; Soda, K.; Inoue, K.; Balkin, D.M.; Hassan, H.; Son, S.H.; et al. Podocyte-associated talin1 is critical for glomerular filtration barrier maintenance. *J. Clin. Investig.* **2014**, *124*, 1098–1113. [CrossRef]
100. Tian, D.; Jacobo, S.M.; Billing, D.; Rozkalne, A.; Gage, S.D.; Anagnostou, T.; Pavenstadt, H.; Hsu, H.H.; Schlondorff, J.; Ramos, A.; et al. Antagonistic regulation of actin dynamics and cell motility by TRPC5 and TRPC6 channels. *Sci. Signal.* **2010**, *3*, ra77. [CrossRef]
101. Greka, A.; Mundel, P. Balancing calcium signals through TRPC5 and TRPC6 in podocytes. *J. Am. Soc. Nephrol.* **2011**, *22*, 1969–1980. [CrossRef]
102. Jiang, L.; Ding, J.; Tsai, H.; Li, L.; Feng, Q.; Miao, J.; Fan, Q. Over-expressing transient receptor potential cation channel 6 in podocytes induces cytoskeleton rearrangement through increases of intracellular Ca^{2+} and RhoA activation. *Exp. Biol. Med. (Maywood)* **2011**, *236*, 184–193. [CrossRef] [PubMed]
103. Hall, G.; Spurney, R.F. Losing their footing: Rac1 signaling causes podocyte detachment and FSGS. *Kidney Int.* **2017**, *92*, 283–285. [CrossRef] [PubMed]
104. Gupta, I.R.; Baldwin, C.; Auguste, D.; Ha, K.C.; El Andalousi, J.; Fahiminiya, S.; Bitzan, M.; Bernard, C.; Akbari, M.R.; Narod, S.A.; et al. ARHGDIA: A novel gene implicated in nephrotic syndrome. *J. Med. Genet.* **2013**, *50*, 330–338. [CrossRef] [PubMed]
105. Robins, R.; Baldwin, C.; Aoudjit, L.; Cote, J.F.; Gupta, I.R.; Takano, T. Rac1 activation in podocytes induces the spectrum of nephrotic syndrome. *Kidney Int.* **2017**, *92*, 349–364. [CrossRef] [PubMed]
106. Akilesh, S.; Suleiman, H.; Yu, H.; Stander, M.C.; Lavin, P.; Gbadegesin, R.; Antignac, C.; Pollak, M.; Kopp, J.B.; Winn, M.P.; et al. Arhgap24 inactivates Rac1 in mouse podocytes, and a mutant form is associated with familial focal segmental glomerulosclerosis. *J. Clin. Investig.* **2011**, *121*, 4127–4137. [CrossRef] [PubMed]
107. Mouawad, F.; Tsui, H.; Takano, T. Role of Rho-GTPases and their regulatory proteins in glomerular podocyte function. *Can. J. Physiol. Pharmacol.* **2013**, *91*, 773–782. [CrossRef]

108. Schaldecker, T.; Kim, S.; Tarabanis, C.; Tian, D.; Hakroush, S.; Castonguay, P.; Ahn, W.; Wallentin, H.; Heid, H.; Hopkins, C.R.; et al. Inhibition of the TRPC5 ion channel protects the kidney filter. *J. Clin. Investig.* **2013**, *123*, 5298–5309. [CrossRef]
109. Zhou, Y.; Castonguay, P.; Sidhom, E.H.; Clark, A.R.; Dvela-Levitt, M.; Kim, S.; Sieber, J.; Wieder, N.; Jung, J.Y.; Andreeva, S.; et al. A small-molecule inhibitor of TRPC5 ion channels suppresses progressive kidney disease in animal models. *Science* **2017**, *358*, 1332–1336. [CrossRef]
110. Ilatovskaya, D.V.; Staruschenko, A. TRPC6 channel as an emerging determinant of the podocyte injury susceptibility in kidney diseases. *Am. J. Physiol. Ren. Physiol.* **2015**, *309*, F393–F397. [CrossRef]
111. Eckel, J.; Lavin, P.J.; Finch, E.A.; Mukerji, N.; Burch, J.; Gbadegesin, R.; Wu, G.; Bowling, B.; Byrd, A.; Hall, G.; et al. TRPC6 enhances angiotensin II-induced albuminuria. *J. Am. Soc. Nephrol.* **2011**, *22*, 526–535. [CrossRef]
112. Spires, D.; Ilatovskaya, D.V.; Levchenko, V.; North, P.E.; Geurts, A.M.; Palygin, O.; Staruschenko, A. Protective role of Trpc6 knockout in the progression of diabetic kidney disease. *Am. J. Physiol. Ren. Physiol.* **2018**, *315*, F1091–F1097. [CrossRef] [PubMed]
113. Dietrich, A.; Mederos, Y.S.M.; Gollasch, M.; Gross, V.; Storch, U.; Dubrovska, G.; Obst, M.; Yildirim, E.; Salanova, B.; Kalwa, H.; et al. Increased vascular smooth muscle contractility in TRPC6-/- mice. *Mol. Cell. Biol.* **2005**, *25*, 6980–6989. [CrossRef] [PubMed]
114. Bullich, G.; Domingo-Gallego, A.; Vargas, I.; Ruiz, P.; Lorente-Grandoso, L.; Furlano, M.; Fraga, G.; Madrid, A.; Ariceta, G.; Borregan, M.; et al. A kidney-disease gene panel allows a comprehensive genetic diagnosis of cystic and glomerular inherited kidney diseases. *Kidney Int.* **2018**, *94*, 363–371. [CrossRef] [PubMed]
115. Kestila, M.; Lenkkeri, U.; Mannikko, M.; Lamerdin, J.; McCready, P.; Putaala, H.; Ruotsalainen, V.; Morita, T.; Nissinen, M.; Herva, R.; et al. Positionally cloned gene for a novel glomerular protein–nephrin–is mutated in congenital nephrotic syndrome. *Mol. Cell* **1998**, *1*, 575–582. [CrossRef]
116. Boute, N.; Gribouval, O.; Roselli, S.; Benessy, F.; Lee, H.; Fuchshuber, A.; Dahan, K.; Gubler, M.C.; Niaudet, P.; Antignac, C. NPHS2, encoding the glomerular protein podocin, is mutated in autosomal recessive steroid-resistant nephrotic syndrome. *Nat. Genet.* **2000**, *24*, 349–354. [CrossRef]
117. Shih, N.Y.; Li, J.; Karpitskii, V.; Nguyen, A.; Dustin, M.L.; Kanagawa, O.; Miner, J.H.; Shaw, A.S. Congenital nephrotic syndrome in mice lacking CD2-associated protein. *Science* **1999**, *286*, 312–315. [CrossRef]
118. Kim, J.M.; Wu, H.; Green, G.; Winkler, C.A.; Kopp, J.B.; Miner, J.H.; Unanue, E.R.; Shaw, A.S. CD2-associated protein haploinsufficiency is linked to glomerular disease susceptibility. *Science* **2003**, *300*, 1298–1300. [CrossRef]
119. Kaplan, J.M.; Kim, S.H.; North, K.N.; Rennke, H.; Correia, L.A.; Tong, H.Q.; Mathis, B.J.; Rodriguez-Perez, J.C.; Allen, P.G.; Beggs, A.H.; et al. Mutations in ACTN4, encoding alpha-actinin-4, cause familial focal segmental glomerulosclerosis. *Nat. Genet.* **2000**, *24*, 251–256. [CrossRef]
120. Staffel, J.; Valletta, D.; Federlein, A.; Ehm, K.; Volkmann, R.; Fuchsl, A.M.; Witzgall, R.; Kuhn, M.; Schweda, F. Natriuretic Peptide Receptor Guanylyl Cyclase-A in Podocytes is Renoprotective but Dispensable for Physiologic Renal Function. *J. Am. Soc. Nephrol.* **2017**, *28*, 260–277. [CrossRef]
121. Korbet, S.M. Treatment of primary FSGS in adults. *J. Am. Soc. Nephrol.* **2012**, *23*, 1769–1776. [CrossRef]
122. Takahashi, S.; Lin, H.; Geshi, N.; Mori, Y.; Kawarabayashi, Y.; Takami, N.; Mori, M.X.; Honda, A.; Inoue, R. Nitric oxide-cGMP-protein kinase G pathway negatively regulates vascular transient receptor potential channel TRPC6. *J. Physiol.* **2008**, *586*, 4209–4223. [CrossRef] [PubMed]
123. Kinoshita, H.; Kuwahara, K.; Nishida, M.; Jian, Z.; Rong, X.; Kiyonaka, S.; Kuwabara, Y.; Kurose, H.; Inoue, R.; Mori, Y.; et al. Inhibition of TRPC6 channel activity contributes to the antihypertrophic effects of natriuretic peptides-guanylyl cyclase-A signaling in the heart. *Circ. Res.* **2010**, *106*, 1849–1860. [CrossRef] [PubMed]
124. Nishida, M.; Watanabe, K.; Sato, Y.; Nakaya, M.; Kitajima, N.; Ide, T.; Inoue, R.; Kurose, H. Phosphorylation of TRPC6 channels at Thr69 is required for anti-hypertrophic effects of phosphodiesterase 5 inhibition. *J. Biol. Chem.* **2010**, *285*, 13244–13253. [CrossRef] [PubMed]
125. Hall, G.; Rowell, J.; Farinelli, F.; Gbadegesin, R.A.; Lavin, P.; Wu, G.; Homstad, A.; Malone, A.; Lindsey, T.; Jiang, R.; et al. Phosphodiesterase 5 inhibition ameliorates angiontensin II-induced podocyte dysmotility via the protein kinase G-mediated downregulation of TRPC6 activity. *Am. J. Physiol. Ren. Physiol.* **2014**, *306*, F1442–F1450. [CrossRef] [PubMed]
126. Francis, S.H.; Busch, J.L.; Corbin, J.D.; Sibley, D. cGMP-dependent protein kinases and cGMP phosphodiesterases in nitric oxide and cGMP action. *Pharmacol. Rev.* **2010**, *62*, 525–563. [CrossRef] [PubMed]

127. Takimoto, E.; Champion, H.C.; Li, M.; Belardi, D.; Ren, S.; Rodriguez, E.R.; Bedja, D.; Gabrielson, K.L.; Wang, Y.; Kass, D.A. Chronic inhibition of cyclic GMP phosphodiesterase 5A prevents and reverses cardiac hypertrophy. *Nat. Med.* **2005**, *11*, 214–222. [CrossRef] [PubMed]
128. Lee, D.I.; Zhu, G.; Sasaki, T.; Cho, G.S.; Hamdani, N.; Holewinski, R.; Jo, S.H.; Danner, T.; Zhang, M.; Rainer, P.P.; et al. Phosphodiesterase 9A controls nitric-oxide-independent cGMP and hypertrophic heart disease. *Nature* **2015**, *519*, 472–476. [CrossRef]
129. Scheele, W.; Diamond, S.; Gale, J.; Clerin, V.; Tamimi, N.; Le, V.; Walley, R.; Grover-Paez, F.; Perros-Huguet, C.; Rolph, T.; et al. Phosphodiesterase Type 5 Inhibition Reduces Albuminuria in Subjects with Overt Diabetic Nephropathy. *J. Am. Soc. Nephrol.* **2016**. [CrossRef]
130. Molitch, M.E.; DeFronzo, R.A.; Franz, M.J.; Keane, W.F.; Mogensen, C.E.; Parving, H.H.; Steffes, M.W. Nephropathy in diabetes. *Diabetes Care* **2004**, *27*, S79–S83.
131. Yang, H.; Zhao, B.; Liao, C.; Zhang, R.; Meng, K.; Xu, J.; Jiao, J. High glucose-induced apoptosis in cultured podocytes involves TRPC6-dependent calcium entry via the RhoA/ROCK pathway. *Biochem. Biophys. Res. Commun.* **2013**, *434*, 394–400. [CrossRef]
132. Zhang, X.; Song, Z.; Guo, Y.; Zhou, M. The novel role of TRPC6 in vitamin D ameliorating podocyte injury in STZ-induced diabetic rats. *Mol. Cell. Biochem.* **2015**, *399*, 155–165. [CrossRef] [PubMed]
133. Susztak, K.; Raff, A.C.; Schiffer, M.; Bottinger, E.P. Glucose-induced reactive oxygen species cause apoptosis of podocytes and podocyte depletion at the onset of diabetic nephropathy. *Diabetes* **2006**, *55*, 225–233. [CrossRef] [PubMed]
134. Ilatovskaya, D.V.; Blass, G.; Palygin, O.; Levchenko, V.; Pavlov, T.S.; Grzybowski, M.N.; Winsor, K.; Shuyskiy, L.S.; Geurts, A.M.; Cowley, A.W., Jr.; et al. A NOX4/TRPC6 Pathway in Podocyte Calcium Regulation and Renal Damage in Diabetic Kidney Disease. *J. Am. Soc. Nephrol.* **2018**, *29*, 1917–1927. [CrossRef] [PubMed]
135. Wang, L.; Chang, J.H.; Buckley, A.F.; Spurney, R.F. Knockout of TRPC6 promotes insulin resistance and exacerbates glomerular injury in Akita mice. *Kidney Int.* **2019**, *95*, 321–332. [CrossRef]
136. Welsh, G.I.; Hale, L.J.; Eremina, V.; Jeansson, M.; Maezawa, Y.; Lennon, R.; Pons, D.A.; Owen, R.J.; Satchell, S.C.; Miles, M.J.; et al. Insulin signaling to the glomerular podocyte is critical for normal kidney function. *Cell Metab.* **2010**, *12*, 329–340. [CrossRef]
137. Coward, R.J.; Welsh, G.I.; Yang, J.; Tasman, C.; Lennon, R.; Koziell, A.; Satchell, S.; Holman, G.D.; Kerjaschki, D.; Tavare, J.M.; et al. The human glomerular podocyte is a novel target for insulin action. *Diabetes* **2005**, *54*, 3095–3102. [CrossRef]
138. Isshiki, K.; Haneda, M.; Koya, D.; Maeda, S.; Sugimoto, T.; Kikkawa, R. Thiazolidinedione compounds ameliorate glomerular dysfunction independent of their insulin-sensitizing action in diabetic rats. *Diabetes* **2000**, *49*, 1022–1032. [CrossRef]
139. Nicholas, S.B.; Kawano, Y.; Wakino, S.; Collins, A.R.; Hsueh, W.A. Expression and function of peroxisome proliferator-activated receptor-gamma in mesangial cells. *Hypertension* **2001**, *37*, 722–727. [CrossRef]
140. Zhang, H.; Saha, J.; Byun, J.; Schin, M.; Lorenz, M.; Kennedy, R.T.; Kretzler, M.; Feldman, E.L.; Pennathur, S.; Brosius, F.C., 3rd. Rosiglitazone reduces renal and plasma markers of oxidative injury and reverses urinary metabolite abnormalities in the amelioration of diabetic nephropathy. *Am. J. Physiol. Ren. Physiol.* **2008**, *295*, F1071–F1081. [CrossRef]
141. Liu, B.; He, X.; Li, S.; Xu, B.; Birnbaumer, L.; Liao, Y. Deletion of diacylglycerol-responsive TRPC genes attenuates diabetic nephropathy by inhibiting activation of the TGFbeta1 signaling pathway. *Am. J. Transl. Res.* **2017**, *9*, 5619–5630.
142. Chen, N.Y.; Chen, W.Y.; Bellush, L.; Yang, C.W.; Striker, L.J.; Striker, G.E.; Kopchick, J.J. Effects of streptozotocin treatment in growth hormone (GH) and GH antagonist transgenic mice. *Endocrinology* **1995**, *136*, 660–667. [CrossRef] [PubMed]
143. Ramirez, G.A.; Coletto, L.A.; Sciorati, C.; Bozzolo, E.P.; Manunta, P.; Rovere-Querini, P.; Manfredi, A.A. Ion Channels and Transporters in Inflammation: Special Focus on TRP Channels and TRPC6. *Cells* **2018**, *7*, 70. [CrossRef] [PubMed]
144. Weber, E.W.; Han, F.; Tauseef, M.; Birnbaumer, L.; Mehta, D.; Muller, W.A. TRPC6 is the endothelial calcium channel that regulates leukocyte transendothelial migration during the inflammatory response. *J. Exp. Med.* **2015**, *212*, 1883–1899. [CrossRef] [PubMed]

145. Riazanski, V.; Gabdoulkhakova, A.G.; Boynton, L.S.; Eguchi, R.R.; Deriy, L.V.; Hogarth, D.K.; Loaec, N.; Oumata, N.; Galons, H.; Brown, M.E.; et al. TRPC6 channel translocation into phagosomal membrane augments phagosomal function. *Proc. Natl. Acad. Sci. USA* **2015**, *112*, E6486–E6495. [CrossRef]
146. Lindemann, O.; Umlauf, D.; Frank, S.; Schimmelpfennig, S.; Bertrand, J.; Pap, T.; Hanley, P.J.; Fabian, A.; Dietrich, A.; Schwab, A. TRPC6 regulates CXCR2-mediated chemotaxis of murine neutrophils. *J. Immunol.* **2013**, *190*, 5496–5505. [CrossRef]
147. Cybulsky, A.V.; Bonventre, J.V.; Quigg, R.J.; Lieberthal, W.; Salant, D.J. Cytosolic calcium and protein kinase C reduce complement-mediated glomerular epithelial injury. *Kidney Int.* **1990**, *38*, 803–811. [CrossRef]
148. Zhu, L.; Jiang, R.; Aoudjit, L.; Jones, N.; Takano, T. Activation of RhoA in podocytes induces focal segmental glomerulosclerosis. *J. Am. Soc. Nephrol.* **2011**, *22*, 1621–1630. [CrossRef]
149. Scott, R.P.; Hawley, S.P.; Ruston, J.; Du, J.; Brakebusch, C.; Jones, N.; Pawson, T. Podocyte-specific loss of Cdc42 leads to congenital nephropathy. *J. Am. Soc. Nephrol.* **2012**, *23*, 1149–1154. [CrossRef]
150. Blattner, S.M.; Hodgin, J.B.; Nishio, M.; Wylie, S.A.; Saha, J.; Soofi, A.A.; Vining, C.; Randolph, A.; Herbach, N.; Wanke, R.; et al. Divergent functions of the Rho GTPases Rac1 and Cdc42 in podocyte injury. *Kidney Int.* **2013**, *84*, 920–930. [CrossRef]
151. Yu, H.; Suleiman, H.; Kim, A.H.; Miner, J.H.; Dani, A.; Shaw, A.S.; Akilesh, S. Rac1 activation in podocytes induces rapid foot process effacement and proteinuria. *Mol. Cell. Biol.* **2013**, *33*, 4755–4764. [CrossRef]
152. Wang, L.; Ellis, M.J.; Gomez, J.A.; Eisner, W.; Fennell, W.; Howell, D.N.; Ruiz, P.; Fields, T.A.; Spurney, R.F. Mechanisms of the proteinuria induced by Rho GTPases. *Kidney Int.* **2012**, *81*, 1075–1085. [CrossRef] [PubMed]
153. Bezzerides, V.J.; Ramsey, I.S.; Kotecha, S.; Greka, A.; Clapham, D.E. Rapid vesicular translocation and insertion of TRP channels. *Nat. Cell Biol.* **2004**, *6*, 709–720. [CrossRef] [PubMed]
154. Miller, M.; Shi, J.; Zhu, Y.; Kustov, M.; Tian, J.B.; Stevens, A.; Wu, M.; Xu, J.; Long, S.; Yang, P.; et al. Identification of ML204, a novel potent antagonist that selectively modulates native TRPC4/C5 ion channels. *J. Biol. Chem.* **2011**, *286*, 33436–33446. [CrossRef]
155. Hoffmann, S.; Podlich, D.; Hahnel, B.; Kriz, W.; Gretz, N. Angiotensin II type 1 receptor overexpression in podocytes induces glomerulosclerosis in transgenic rats. *J. Am. Soc. Nephrol.* **2004**, *15*, 1475–1487. [CrossRef] [PubMed]
156. Richter, J.M.; Schaefer, M.; Hill, K. Clemizole hydrochloride is a novel and potent inhibitor of transient receptor potential channel TRPC5. *Mol. Pharmacol.* **2014**, *86*, 514–521. [CrossRef] [PubMed]
157. Wang, X.; Dande, R.R.; Yu, H.; Samelko, B.; Miller, R.E.; Altintas, M.M.; Reiser, J. TRPC5 Does Not Cause or Aggravate Glomerular Disease. *J. Am. Soc. Nephrol.* **2018**, *29*, 409–415. [CrossRef] [PubMed]
158. Niwa, H.; Yamamura, K.; Miyazaki, J. Efficient selection for high-expression transfectants with a novel eukaryotic vector. *Gene* **1991**, *108*, 193–199.
159. Cheung, S.Y.; Henrot, M.; Al-Saad, M.; Baumann, M.; Muller, H.; Unger, A.; Rubaiy, H.N.; Mathar, I.; Dinkel, K.; Nussbaumer, P.; et al. TRPC4/TRPC5 channels mediate adverse reaction to the cancer cell cytotoxic agent (-)-Englerin A. *Oncotarget* **2018**, *9*, 29634–29643. [CrossRef]
160. Sourbier, C.; Scroggins, B.T.; Ratnayake, R.; Prince, T.L.; Lee, S.; Lee, M.J.; Nagy, P.L.; Lee, Y.H.; Trepel, J.B.; Beutler, J.A.; et al. Englerin A stimulates PKCtheta to inhibit insulin signaling and to simultaneously activate HSF1: Pharmacologically induced synthetic lethality. *Cancer Cell* **2013**, *23*, 228–237. [CrossRef]
161. Carson, C.; Raman, P.; Tullai, J.; Xu, L.; Henault, M.; Thomas, E.; Yeola, S.; Lao, J.; McPate, M.; Verkuyl, J.M.; et al. Englerin A Agonizes the TRPC4/C5 Cation Channels to Inhibit Tumor Cell Line Proliferation. *PLoS ONE* **2015**, *10*, e0127498. [CrossRef]
162. Ilatovskaya, D.V.; Palygin, O.; Chubinskiy-Nadezhdin, V.; Negulyaev, Y.A.; Ma, R.; Birnbaumer, L.; Staruschenko, A. Angiotensin II has acute effects on TRPC6 channels in podocytes of freshly isolated glomeruli. *Kidney Int.* **2014**, *86*, 506–514. [CrossRef] [PubMed]
163. Subramanyam, P.; Colecraft, H.M. Ion channel engineering: Perspectives and strategies. *J. Mol. Biol.* **2015**, *427*, 190–204. [CrossRef] [PubMed]
164. Davis, J.; Burr, A.R.; Davis, G.F.; Birnbaumer, L.; Molkentin, J.D. A TRPC6-dependent pathway for myofibroblast transdifferentiation and wound healing in vivo. *Dev. Cell* **2012**, *23*, 705–715. [CrossRef] [PubMed]

165. Kiyonaka, S.; Kato, K.; Nishida, M.; Mio, K.; Numaga, T.; Sawaguchi, Y.; Yoshida, T.; Wakamori, M.; Mori, E.; Numata, T.; et al. Selective and direct inhibition of TRPC3 channels underlies biological activities of a pyrazole compound. *Proc. Natl. Acad. Sci. USA* **2009**, *106*, 5400–5405. [CrossRef] [PubMed]
166. Lin, B.L.; Matera, D.; Doerner, J.F.; Zheng, N.; Del Camino, D.; Mishra, S.; Bian, H.; Zeveleva, S.; Zhen, X.; Blair, N.T.; et al. In vivo selective inhibition of TRPC6 by antagonist BI 749327 ameliorates fibrosis and dysfunction in cardiac and renal disease. *Proc. Natl. Acad. Sci. USA* **2019**, *116*, 10156–10161. [CrossRef] [PubMed]
167. Xie, J.; Cha, S.K.; An, S.W.; Kuro, O.M.; Birnbaumer, L.; Huang, C.L. Cardioprotection by Klotho through downregulation of TRPC6 channels in the mouse heart. *Nat. Commun.* **2012**, *3*, 1238. [CrossRef]
168. Doi, S.; Zou, Y.; Togao, O.; Pastor, J.V.; John, G.B.; Wang, L.; Shiizaki, K.; Gotschall, R.; Schiavi, S.; Yorioka, N.; et al. Klotho inhibits transforming growth factor-beta1 (TGF-beta1) signaling and suppresses renal fibrosis and cancer metastasis in mice. *J. Biol. Chem.* **2011**, *286*, 8655–8665. [CrossRef]
169. Eder, P.; Molkentin, J.D. TRPC channels as effectors of cardiac hypertrophy. *Circ. Res.* **2011**, *108*, 265–272. [CrossRef]
170. Musah, S.; Mammoto, A.; Ferrante, T.C.; Jeanty, S.S.F.; Hirano-Kobayashi, M.; Mammoto, T.; Roberts, K.; Chung, S.; Novak, R.; Ingram, M.; et al. Mature induced-pluripotent-stem-cell-derived human podocytes reconstitute kidney glomerular-capillary-wall function on a chip. *Nat. Biomed. Eng.* **2017**, *1*, 69. [CrossRef]

3

Urinary Excretion of N^1-methyl-2-pyridone-5-carboxamide and N^1-methylnicotinamide in Renal Transplant Recipients and Donors

Carolien P. J. Deen [1,2,3,*], Anna van der Veen [2], António W. Gomes-Neto [1,4], Johanna M. Geleijnse [5], Karin J. Borgonjen-van den Berg [5], M. Rebecca Heiner-Fokkema [2], Ido P. Kema [2] and Stephan J. L. Bakker [1,3,4]

1 Department of Internal Medicine, University of Groningen, University Medical Center Groningen, 9713 GZ Groningen, The Netherlands; a.w.gomes.neto@umcg.nl (A.W.G.-N.); s.j.l.bakker@umcg.nl (S.J.L.B.)
2 Department of Laboratory Medicine, University of Groningen, University Medical Center Groningen, 9713 GZ Groningen, The Netherlands; a.van.der.veen03@umcg.nl (A.v.d.V.); m.r.heiner@umcg.nl (M.R.H.-F.); i.p.kema@umcg.nl (I.P.K.)
3 TiFN, 6709 PA Wageningen, The Netherlands
4 TransplantLines Food and Nutrition Biobank and Cohort Study, University of Groningen, University Medical Center Groningen, 9713 GZ Groningen, The Netherlands
5 Division of Human Nutrition and Health, Wageningen University, 6708 PB Wageningen, The Netherlands; marianne.geleijnse@wur.nl (J.M.G.); karin.borgonjen@wur.nl (K.J.B.-v.d.B.)
* Correspondence: c.p.j.deen@umcg.nl

Abstract: N^1-methylnicotinamide (N^1-MN) and N^1-methyl-2-pyridone-5-carboxamide (2Py) are successive end products of NAD^+ catabolism. N^1-MN excretion in 24-h urine is the established biomarker of niacin nutritional status, and recently shown to be reduced in renal transplant recipients (RTR). However, it is unclear whether 2Py excretion is increased in this population, and, if so, whether a shift in excretion of N^1-MN to 2Py can be attributed to kidney function. Hence, we assessed the 24-h urinary excretion of 2Py and N^1-MN in RTR and kidney donors before and after kidney donation, and investigated associations of the urinary ratio of 2Py to N^1-MN (2Py/N^1-MN) with kidney function, and independent determinants of urinary 2Py/N^1-MN in RTR. The urinary excretion of 2Py and N^1-MN was measured in a cross-sectional cohort of 660 RTR and 275 healthy kidney donors with liquid chromatography-tandem mass spectrometry (LC-MS/MS). Linear regression analyses were used to investigate associations and determinants of urinary 2Py/N^1-MN. Median 2Py excretion was 178.1 (130.3–242.8) μmol/day in RTR, compared to 155.6 (119.6–217.6) μmol/day in kidney donors ($p < 0.001$). In kidney donors, urinary 2Py/N^1-MN increased significantly after kidney donation (4.0 ± 1.4 to 5.2 ± 1.5, respectively; $p < 0.001$). Smoking, alcohol consumption, diabetes, high-density lipoprotein (HDL), high-sensitivity C-reactive protein (hs-CRP) and estimated glomerular filtration rate (eGFR) were identified as independent determinants of urinary 2Py/N^1-MN in RTR. In conclusion, the 24-h urinary excretion of 2Py is higher in RTR than in kidney donors, and urinary 2Py/N^1-MN increases after kidney donation. As our data furthermore reveal strong associations of urinary 2Py/N^1-MN with kidney function, interpretation of both N^1-MN and 2Py excretion may be recommended for assessment of niacin nutritional status in conditions of impaired kidney function.

Keywords: N^1-methyl-2-pyridone-5-carboxamide; N^1-methylnicotinamide; urinary excretion; renal transplantation; kidney function; biomarker; niacin status; tryptophan; vitamin B_3

1. Introduction

Niacin, or vitamin B_3, is the precursor of the nicotinamide nucleotide coenzyme NAD^+. An adequate niacin status is vital to provide reducing equivalents for energy metabolism, and substrates of NAD^+ consuming enzymes, including adenosine diphosphate (ADP)-ribosyl transferases and deacetylases, that transfer ADP-ribose moieties from NAD^+ and $NADP^+$ [1,2].

Niacin nutritional status is most commonly assessed by the 24-h urinary excretion of N^1-methylnicotinamide (N^1-MN) as a breakdown product of NAD^+, and recommended as such by authorities, including the WHO and the European Food Safety Authority (EFSA) [3,4]. However, N^1-methyl-2-pyridone-5-carboxamide (2Py) is the end product of NAD^+ catabolism, after aldehyde oxidase (AOX1)-dependent oxidation of N^1-MN (Figure 1) [5,6]. Although the 24-h urinary excretion of N^1-MN has shown the most sensitive response to oral test doses of niacin equivalents [3,7], excretion of 2Py, whether or not combined with that of N^1-MN, has also been implicated for the assessment of niacin status [8–11].

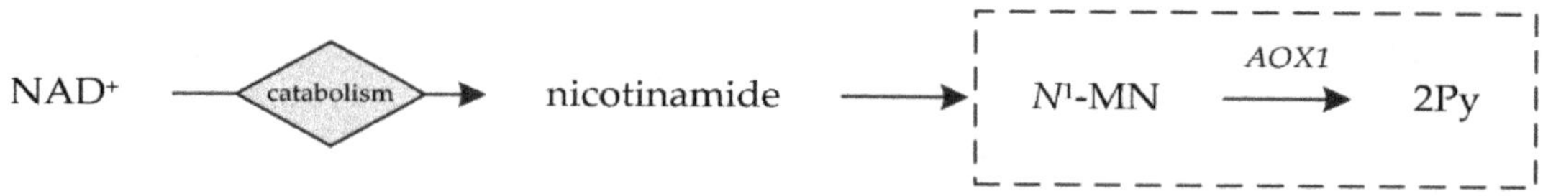

Figure 1. Schematic overview of NAD^+ catabolism. 2Py is the end product of NAD^+ catabolism after AOX1-dependent oxidation of N^1-MN, framed by the dotted line. AOX1, aldehyde oxidase; N^1-MN, N^1-methylnicotinamide; 2Py, N^1-methyl-2-pyridone-5-carboxamide.

In a recent study, we found that N^1-MN excretion is lower in renal transplant recipients (RTR) than in healthy controls [12]. As this discrepancy could not be explained by lower dietary intake of niacin equivalents, enhanced enzymatic conversion of N^1-MN to 2Py by AOX1 might be present in this population due to the suggested contribution of AOX1 to N^1-MN clearance with lower kidney function [13,14]. It is unclear whether 2Py excretion is increased in RTR, and if so, whether a shift in excretion of N^1-MN to 2Py can be attributed to kidney function.

Hence, to evaluate the applicability of N^1-MN excretion as a biomarker of niacin nutritional status in conditions of impaired kidney function, we measured the 24-h urinary excretion of 2Py and N^1-MN in RTR and kidney donors before and after kidney donation, allowing us to (1) compare the 24-h urinary excretion of 2Py in RTR and kidney donors, (2) investigate the effect of kidney donation on the excretion of 2Py and N^1-MN in kidney donors, (3) assess whether the urinary ratio of 2Py to N^1-MN (2Py/N^1-MN) is associated with kidney function, and (4) identify determinants of urinary 2Py/N^1-MN in RTR.

2. Materials and Methods

2.1. Study Population

This cross-sectional study was based on a well-characterized, single-center cohort of 707 RTR (aged ≥18 years) who visited the outpatient clinic of the University Medical Center Groningen, Groningen, the Netherlands, between 2008 and 2011, with a functioning graft for at least 1 year and no history of alcohol and/or drug abuse [15–17]. As a control group, 367 healthy kidney donors were included who participated in a screening program before kidney donation, and of whom biomaterial was collected before and, after declared eligible, 3 months after kidney donation. Exclusion of subjects with missing biomaterial or niacin supplementation use left 660 RTR and 275 kidney donors, of which 85 underwent donor nephrectomy during the inclusion period, eligible for statistical analyses. Signed informed consent was obtained from all participating subjects and the study protocol was approved by the institutional review board (METc 2008/186) adhering to the Declaration of Helsinki. This study included the same cohort of 660 RTR and 275 kidney donors for data collection as reported previously [12].

2.2. Data Collection and Measurements

Participants were instructed to collect a 24-h urine sample on the day before their morning visit to the outpatient clinic, and to fast overnight for 8 to 12 h. Urine samples were collected under oil, and chlorhexidine was added as an antiseptic agent. Fasting blood samples were drawn after completion of the urine collection. Laboratory measurements were performed directly with spectrophotometric-based routine clinical laboratory methods (Roche Diagnostics, Rotkreuz, Switzerland). Body composition and hemodynamic parameters were measured according to a previously described, strict protocol [15]. Diabetes was diagnosed if fasting plasma glucose was ≥7.0 mmol/L or antidiabetic medication was used. Proteinuria was diagnosed if total urinary protein excretion was ≥0.5 g/day as measured by a biuret reaction-based assay (MEGA AU510; Merck Diagnostica, Darmstadt, Germany).

Dietary intake was assessed with a validated semi-quantitative food frequency questionnaire (FFQ) [18,19]. The self-administered questionnaire was filled out at home and inquired about 177 food items over the last month. During the outpatient clinic visit, the FFQ was checked for completeness by a trained researcher and inconsistent answers were verified with the participant. The FFQ was validated for RTR as previously reported [16]. Dietary data were converted into daily nutrient intake using the Dutch Food Composition Table of 2006 [20]. Intake of niacin equivalents was calculated by adding up niacin and one-sixtieth of tryptophan intake. Subjects who were using niacin supplementation were excluded. Smoking behavior was assessed with a separate questionnaire [21]. Data on medication and vitamin supplements use, and medical history were obtained from medical records [21].

The estimated glomerular filtration rate (eGFR) was calculated by the combined creatinine and cystatin C-based Chronic Kidney Disease Epidemiology Collaboration equation [22], which has shown to be the most accurate equation in RTR [23]. The glomerular filtration rate (GFR) was measured by infusion of ^{125}I-Iothalamate as described previously [24].

2.3. Assessment of 2Py and N^1-MN Excretion

Measurement of 2Py and N^1-MN concentrations was performed with a validated liquid chromatography (Luna HILIC column; Phenomenex, Torrance, CA, USA) isotope dilution-tandem mass spectrometry (Quattro Premier; Waters, Milford, MA, USA) (LC-MS/MS) method, as described previously [25], with the addition of N^1-methyl-2-pyridone-5-carboxamide-d_3 in acetonitrile as an internal standard. The 24-h urinary excretion of 2Py and N^1-MN (μmol/day) was obtained by multiplying concentrations (μmol/L) by total urine volume calculated from weight (L/day).

2.4. Statistical Analysis

Data are presented as the mean ± SD, median (IQR) and absolute number (percentage) for normally distributed, skewed and nominal data, respectively. Assumptions for normality were checked by visual judgments of the corresponding frequency distribution and Q-Q plot.

Baseline characteristics of RTR and the total cohort of kidney donors were compared by means of *t*, Mann–Whitney, and Chi-Square tests, of which age, sex, body surface area, N^1-MN excretion and eGFR have been reported previously [12]. Crude associations of 2Py and N^1-MN excretion with intake of niacin equivalents were investigated with linear regression analyses. Characteristics of kidney donors before and after kidney donation were compared by means of paired samples *t* and Wilcoxon signed rank tests.

Linear regression analyses were used to investigate associations of urinary 2Py/N^1-MN with kidney function in RTR and kidney donors, with additional adjustments for age and sex. Effect modification between either age or sex and kidney function with urinary 2Py/N^1-MN was assessed by including the corresponding cross product term in the linear regression model.

Linear regression analyses were furthermore employed to investigate cross-sectional associations of urinary 2Py/N^1-MN with baseline variables in RTR. Variables were 2-base log-transformed when assumptions of normality and homogeneity of variance of the residuals, based on visual judgement of

P-P and scatter plots, respectively, were not met. Multivariable linear regression analyses were used to identify determinants of urinary 2Py/N^1-MN, by entering terms with p-value <0.1 in univariable analysis, and eliminating the least significant term stepwise until the remaining terms contributed significantly to the model.

For all statistical analyses, a two-sided p-value of less than 0.05 was considered to indicate statistical significance and SPSS Statistics version 23.0 (IBM, Armonk, NY, USA) was used as software.

3. Results

3.1. Excretion of 2Py in Kidney Donors and RTR

The total cohort consisted of 660 stable RTR (57% male; mean age 53.0 ± 12.7 years), included at a median time of 5.6 (2.0–12.0) years after transplantation, and 275 healthy kidney donors (41% male; mean age 53.3 ± 10.7 years) (Table 1). Differences in the 24-h urinary excretion of 2Py and N^1-MN and kidney function are shown in Table 1. 2Py excretion was higher in RTR than in kidney donors (178.1 (130.3–242.8) versus 155.6 (119.6–217.6) µmol/day, respectively; $p < 0.001$), while N^1-MN excretion was lower in RTR than in kidney donors (22.0 (15.8–31.8) versus 41.4 (31.6–57.2) µmol/day, respectively; $p < 0.001$). Kidney function was significantly lower in RTR than in kidney donors (eGFR: 45.8 ± 18.7 versus 91.0 ± 14.2 mL/min/1.73 m^2, respectively; $p < 0.001$ and GFR: 52.4 ± 17.4 versus 82.3 ± 29.7 mL/min/1.73 m^2, respectively; $p < 0.001$). Urinary 2Py/N^1-MN was significantly higher in RTR than in kidney donors (8.7 ± 3.8 versus 4.0 ± 1.4, respectively; $p < 0.001$), while the sum of 2Py and N^1-MN excretion was similar (198.3 (155.9–269.4) versus 203.7 (149.4–274.7) µmol/day, respectively; $p = 0.98$). The urinary fraction of 2Py was higher in RTR than in kidney donors (89.1% (86.4%–91.3%) versus 79.0% (75.6%–82.1%), respectively; $p < 0.001$), and that of N^1-MN was lower (10.9% (8.7%–13.6%) versus 21.0% (17.9%–24.4%), respectively; $p < 0.001$). The 24-h urinary excretion of 2Py, N^1-MN and the sum of 2Py and N^1-MN, but not urinary 2Py/N^1-MN, were directly associated with intake of niacin equivalents (Table S1).

3.2. Excretion of 2Py and N^1-MN before and after Kidney Donation in Kidney Donors

The 24-h urinary excretion of 2Py and N^1-MN and kidney function in 85 kidney donors before and after kidney donation are shown in Table 1 and Figure 2. At a median time of 1.64 (1.61–1.87) months after kidney donation, 2Py excretion did not change significantly (152.8 (124.4–215.1) to 161.7 (116.6–227.8) µmol/day, respectively; $p = 0.31$), while N^1-MN decreased (40.9 (31.0–58.2) to 32.5 (23.4–44.0) µmol/day, respectively; $p < 0.001$). Kidney function decreased significantly after kidney donation (eGFR: 92.8 ± 13.9 to 60.1 ± 12.1 mL/min/1.73 m^2, respectively; $p < 0.001$ and GFR: 103.7 ± 16.7 to 65.3 ± 10.4 mL/min/1.73 m^2, respectively; $p < 0.001$). Urinary 2Py/N^1-MN increased after kidney donation (4.0 ± 1.4 to 5.2 ± 1.5, respectively; $p < 0.001$), while the sum of 2Py and N^1-MN excretion did not change (198.3 (162.3–270.8) to 189.7 (141.9–271.6) µmol/day, respectively; $p = 0.90$). The urinary fraction of 2Py increased after kidney donation (78.3% (75.5%–81.8%) to 83.5% (80.0%–86.0%), respectively; $p < 0.001$), and that of N^1-MN decreased (21.7% (18.2%–24.5%) to 16.5% (14.0%–20.0%), respectively; $p < 0.001$).

3.3. Associations of Urinary 2Py/N^1-MN with Kidney Function

Urinary 2Py/N^1-MN was associated with kidney function in RTR (eGFR: $\beta = -0.40$; $p < 0.001$ and GFR: $\beta = -0.39$; $p < 0.001$) and the total cohort of kidney donors (eGFR: $\beta = -0.17$; $p = 0.03$ and GFR: $\beta = -0.20$; $p = 0.003$), but not in the pre- (eGFR: $\beta = -0.01$; $p = 0.94$ and GFR: $\beta = -0.02$; $p = 0.89$) and post-donation subgroups of kidney donors (eGFR: $\beta = -0.11$; $p = 0.42$ and GFR: $\beta = 0.15$; $p = 0.27$), with adjustment for age and sex (Table 2). No significant interaction between either age or sex with kidney function was found in the association with urinary 2Py/N^1-MN in RTR and kidney donors.

Table 1. Excretion of 2Py and N^1-MN and kidney function in RTR and kidney donors before and after kidney donation [1].

Variable	RTR $n = 660$	Kidney Donors $n = 275$	Population Difference	Kidney Donors $n = 85$		Paired Difference
	Total Cohort	Total Cohort	p-Value [2]	Pre-Donation	Post-Donation	p-Value [3]
Age, years	53.0 ± 12.7	53.3 ± 10.7	0.68	52.2 ± 10.5	52.6 ± 10.4	<0.001
Male, n (%)	379 (57)	112 (41)	0.001	43 (51)	43 (51)	-
Body surface area, m^2	1.9 ± 0.2	1.9 ± 0.2	0.90	2.0 ± 0.2	1.9 ± 0.2	0.01
BMI, kg/m^2	26.6 ± 4.8	25.9 ± 3.4	0.01	26.0 ± 3.4	25.7 ± 3.2	0.03
Urinary excretion						
2Py, µmol/day	178.1 (130.3–242.8)	155.6 (119.6–217.6)	0.001	152.8 (124.4–215.1)	161.7 (116.6–227.8)	0.31
N^1-MN, µmol/day	22.0 (15.8–31.8)	41.4 (31.6–57.2)	<0.001	40.9 (31.0–58.2)	32.5 (23.4–44.0)	<0.001
2Py/N^1-MN	8.7 ± 3.8	4.0 ± 1.4	<0.001	4.0 ± 1.4	5.2 ± 1.5	<0.001
Sum of 2Py and N^1-MN, µmol/day	198.3 (155.9–269.4)	203.7 (149.4–274.7)	0.98	198.3 (162.3–270.8)	189.7 (141.9–271.6)	0.90
2Py fraction, % [4]	89.1 (86.4–91.3)	79.0 (75.6–82.1)	<0.001	78.3 (75.5–81.8)	83.5 (80.0–86.0)	<0.001
N^1-MN fraction, % [4]	10.9 (8.7–13.6)	21.0 (17.9–24.4)	<0.001	21.7 (18.2–24.5)	16.5 (14.0–20.0)	<0.001
Kidney function						
eGFR, mL/min/1.73 m^2	45.8 ± 18.7	91.0 ± 14.2	<0.001	92.8 ± 13.9	60.1 ± 12.1	<0.001
GFR, mL/min/1.73 m^2	52.4 ± 17.4	82.3 ± 29.7	<0.001	103.7 ± 16.7	65.3 ± 10.4	<0.001

[1] Data are presented as mean ± SD, median (IQR) and absolute number (percentage) for normally distributed, skewed and nominal data, respectively. [2] p-value for difference between RTR and the total cohort of kidney donors was tested by t and Mann–Whitney tests for normally and skewed distributed continuous variables, respectively. [3] p-value for difference between kidney donors before and after kidney donation was tested by paired samples t and Wilcoxon signed rank tests for normally and skewed distributed continuous variables, respectively. [4] The urinary fraction of 2Py or N^1-MN (percentage) was calculated by dividing 2Py or N^1-MN excretion by the sum of 2Py and N^1-MN excretion, respectively, and multiplying by 100. BMI, body mass index; eGFR, estimated glomerular filtration rate; GFR, glomerular filtration rate; N^1-MN, N^1-methylnicotinamide; RTR, renal transplant recipients; 2Py, N^1-methyl-2-pyridone-5-carboxamide; 2Py/N^1-MN, ratio of 2Py to N^1-MN.

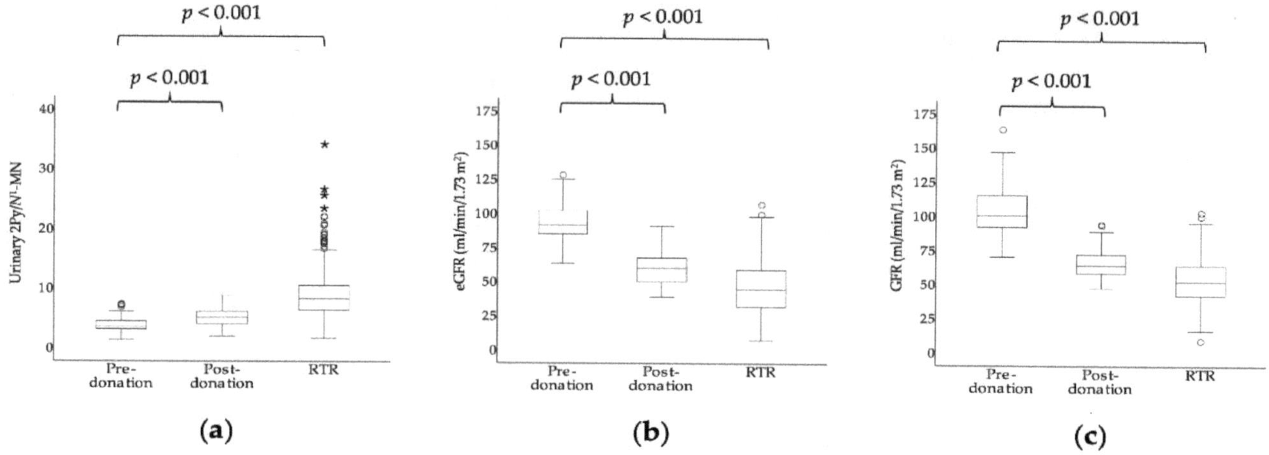

Figure 2. Box plots of (**a**) urinary 2Py/N^1-MN, (**b**) eGFR and (**c**) GFR in kidney donors before ($n = 85$) and after kidney donation ($n = 85$) and RTR ($n = 660$), respectively. Boxes, bars and whiskers represent IQRs, medians and values <1.5 × IQR, respectively, whereas outliers (1.5–3 × IQR) are indicated by circles and extreme outliers (>3 × IQR) by asterisks. p-value for difference between kidney donors before and after kidney donation was tested by paired samples t and Wilcoxon signed rank tests for normally and skewed distributed continuous variables, respectively. p-value for difference between RTR and kidney donors before donation was tested by t and Mann–Whitney tests for normally and skewed distributed continuous variables, respectively. eGFR, estimated glomerular filtration rate; GFR, glomerular filtration rate; N^1-MN, N^1-methylnicotinamide; RTR, renal transplant recipients; 2Py, N^1-methyl-2-pyridone-5-carboxamide; 2Py/N^1-MN, ratio of 2Py to N^1-MN.

Table 2. Associations of urinary 2Py/N^1-MN with kidney function in RTR and kidney donors before and after kidney donation [1].

Variable	RTR	Kidney Donors		
		Total Cohort	Pre-Donation	Post-Donation
	$n = 660$	$n = 275$	$n = 85$	$n = 85$
eGFR, mL/min/1.73 m^2				
Standardized β	−0.40	−0.17	−0.01	−0.11
p-value	<0.001	0.03	0.94	0.42
GFR, mL/min/1.73 m^2				
Standardized β	−0.39	−0.20	−0.02	0.15
p-value	<0.001	0.003	0.89	0.27

[1] Linear regression analyses were performed to investigate associations of urinary 2Py/N^1-MN with kidney function, with adjustment for age and sex. eGFR, estimated glomerular filtration rate; GFR, glomerular filtration rate; N^1-MN, N^1-methylnicotinamide; RTR, renal transplant recipients; 2Py, N^1-methyl-2-pyridone-5-carboxamide; 2Py/N^1-MN, ratio of 2Py to N^1-MN.

3.4. Characteristics and Associations with Urinary 2Py/N^1-MN in RTR

Characteristics of the RTR cohort are shown in Table 3. Urinary 2Py/N^1-MN was positively associated with body surface area, body mass index (BMI), glucose homeostasis parameters, triglycerides, mean arterial pressure, high-sensitivity C-reactive protein (hs-CRP), proteinuria, and use of antidiabetics, antihypertensives, acetylsalicylic acid, proton pump inhibitors and tacrolimus. Inverse associations were found between urinary 2Py/N^1-MN and smoking, alcohol consumption, energy intake, vitamin B_6 intake, high-density lipoprotein (HDL) and eGFR.

Table 3. Associations of urinary 2Py/N^1-MN with characteristics in 660 RTR [1,2].

Variable	Value	Standardized β	p-Value
Urinary 2Py/N^1-MN	8.7 ± 3.8	-	-
2Py excretion, μmol/day	178.1 (130.3–242.8)	-	-
N^1-MN excretion, μmol/day	22.0 (15.8–31.8)	-	-
Age, years	53.0 ± 12.7	0.03	0.09
Male, n (%)	379 (57)	−0.004	0.92
Body surface area, m^2	1.9 ± 0.22	0.11	0.006
BMI, kg/m^2	26.6 ± 4.8	0.17	<0.001
Creatinine excretion, mmol/day	11.7 ± 3.4	−0.05	0.22
Time since transplantation, years	5.6 (2.0–12.0)	−0.07	0.07
Lifestyle			
Current smoker, n (%)	78 (13)	−0.10	0.02
Alcohol consumption, g/day	3.1 (0.0–11.9)	−0.15	<0.001
Nutrition			
Energy intake, kcal/day	2182 ± 642	−0.09	0.03
Niacin equivalents intake, mg/day	35.6 ± 9.2	−0.06	0.14
Vitamin B_6 intake, mg/day	1.8 ± 0.5	−0.09	0.03
Glucose homeostasis			
Glucose, mmol/L	5.3 (4.8–6.0)	0.15	<0.001
HbA1c, %	5.8 (5.5–6.2)	0.12	0.002
Diabetes, n (%)	152 (23)	0.16	<0.001
Lipid homeostasis			
Total cholesterol, mmol/L	5.1 ± 1.1	0.03	0.38
LDL, mmol/L	3.0 ± 0.9	0.07	0.10
HDL, mmol/L	1.3 (1.1–1.7)	−0.20	<0.001
Triglycerides, mmol/L	1.7 (1.2–2.3)	0.17	<0.001
Hemodynamic			
Systolic blood pressure, mmHg	135.8 ± 17.3	0.07	0.08
Diastolic blood pressure, mmHg	82.5 ± 11.0	0.08	0.05
Mean arterial pressure, mmHg	107.0 ± 15.0	0.10	0.02
Inflammation			
Hs-CRP, mg/L	1.6 (0.7–4.6)	0.19	<0.001
Kidney function			
eGFR, mL/min/1.73 m^2	45.8 ± 18.7	−0.40	<0.001
Proteinuria, n (%)	132 (20)	0.08	0.04
Nonimmunosuppressive medication			
Antidiabetic, n (%)	96 (15)	0.14	<0.001
Statin, n (%)	349 (53)	0.06	0.15
Antihypertensive, n (%)	581 (88)	0.09	0.02
Acetylsalicylic acid, n (%)	127 (19)	0.09	0.03
Proton pump inhibitor, n (%)	326 (49)	0.08	0.04
Immunosuppressive medication			
Prednisolon dose, mg/day	3.0 (2.0–3.0)	0.07	0.07
Proliferation inhibitor, n (%)	548 (83)	−0.02	0.71
Tacrolimus, n (%)	120 (18)	0.11	0.007
Cyclosporine, n (%)	253 (38)	−0.01	0.72

[1] Data are presented as mean ± SD, median (IQR) and absolute number (percentage) for normally distributed, skewed and nominal data, respectively. [2] Linear regression analyses were performed to investigate associations of urinary 2Py/N^1-MN with baseline variables, of which standardized β and p-value are presented. BMI, body mass index; eGFR, estimated glomerular filtration rate; HbA1c, hemoglobin A1c; HDL, high-density lipoprotein; hs-CRP, high-sensitivity C-reactive protein; LDL, low-density lipoprotein; N^1-MN, N^1-methylnicotinamide; RTR, renal transplant recipients; 2Py, N^1-methyl-2-pyridone-5-carboxamide; 2Py/N^1-MN, ratio of 2Py to N^1-MN.

3.5. Determinants of Urinary 2Py/N^1-MN in RTR

Stepwise multivariable linear regression analyses with backward elimination revealed smoking, alcohol consumption, diabetes, HDL, hs-CRP and eGFR as independent determinants of urinary 2Py/N^1-MN in RTR (Table 4). In the final model, urinary 2Py/N^1-MN was positively associated with diabetes ($\beta = 0.10$; $p = 0.01$) and hs-CRP ($\beta = 0.10$; $p = 0.009$), and inversely associated with smoking ($\beta = -0.13$; $p = 0.001$), alcohol consumption ($\beta = -0.12$; $p = 0.002$), HDL ($\beta = -0.12$; $p = 0.002$) and eGFR ($\beta = -0.38$; $p < 0.001$).

Table 4. Independent determinants of urinary 2Py/N^1-MN in RTR.

Variable	Univariable		Multivariable [1]	
	Standardized β	*p*-Value	Standardized β	*p*-Value
Age, years	0.03	0.09	-	-
Male, *n* (%)	−0.004	0.92	-	-
BMI, kg/m^2	0.17	<0.001	-	-
Time since transplantation, years	−0.07	0.07	-	-
Lifestyle				
Current smoker, *n* (%)	−0.10	0.02	−0.13	0.001
Alcohol consumption, g/day	−0.15	<0.001	−0.12	0.002
Nutrition				
Energy intake, kcal/day	−0.09	0.03	-	-
Niacin equivalents intake, mg/day	−0.06	0.14	-	-
Vitamin B_6 intake, mg/day	−0.09	0.03	-	-
Glucose homeostasis				
Diabetes, *n* (%)	0.16	<0.001	0.10	0.01
Lipid homeostasis				
LDL, mmol/L	0.07	0.10	-	-
HDL, mmol/L	−0.20	<0.001	−0.12	0.002
Hemodynamic				
Mean arterial pressure, mmHg	0.10	0.02	-	-
Inflammation				
Hs-CRP, mg/L	0.19	<0.001	0.10	0.009
Kidney function				
eGFR, mL/min/1.73 m^2	−0.40	<0.001	−0.38	<0.001
Proteinuria, *n* (%)	0.08	0.04	-	-
Nonimmunosuppressive medication				
Antihypertensive, *n* (%)	0.09	0.02	-	-
Acetylsalicylic acid, *n* (%)	0.09	0.03	-	-
Proton pump inhibitor, *n* (%)	0.08	0.04	-	-
Immunosuppressive medication				
Prednisolon dose, mg/day	0.07	0.07	-	-
Tacrolimus, *n* (%)	0.11	0.007	-	-
R^2	0.28		0.26	
Adjusted R^2	0.25		0.25	

[1] Stepwise multivariable linear regression with backward elimination was performed to identify determinants of urinary 2Py/N^1-MN, of which standardized β and *p*-value are presented. BMI, body mass index; eGFR, estimated glomerular filtration rate; HDL, high-density lipoprotein; hs-CRP, high-sensitivity C-reactive protein; LDL, low-density lipoprotein; N^1-MN, N^1-methylnicotinamide; RTR, renal transplant recipients; 2Py, N^1-methyl-2-pyridone-5-carboxamide; 2Py/N^1-MN, ratio of 2Py to N^1-MN.

4. Discussion

This study aimed to investigate the 24-h urinary excretion of both 2Py and N^1-MN as major catabolic products of NAD^+ with regard to kidney function. We assessed 2Py and N^1-MN excretion in RTR and healthy kidney donors as a model of renal disease, and in kidney donors before and after unilateral nephrectomy as a model of isolated renal function impairment. In RTR, 2Py excretion was significantly higher compared to that in kidney donors. Urinary 2Py/N^1-MN increased significantly in kidney donors after donation. In both RTR and kidney donors, urinary 2Py/N^1-MN was associated with kidney function. Kidney function was furthermore revealed as the strongest determinant of urinary 2Py/N^1-MN in RTR.

NAD^+ is formed either de novo from tryptophan via the kynurenine pathway, or via salvage pathways from preformed nicotinamide, nicotinic acid and nicotinamide riboside [26], commonly known as niacin, or vitamin B_3. NAD^+ catabolism proceeds via nicotinamide and its downstream metabolites N^1-MN and 2Py, respectively (Figure 1), and these products are found in both plasma and urine [27]. N^1-MN itself exhibits anti-inflammatory properties, and is produced by muscle in response to hypoxia and depletion of energy stores, besides its primary production in the liver [28]. Whereas nicotinamide is reabsorbed by renal tubules and only small amounts appear in urine, N^1-MN and 2Py account for 20%–35% and 45%–60%, respectively, of all urinary NAD^+ metabolites [29]. The WHO and the EFSA recommend the 24-h urinary excretion of N^1-MN for laboratory assessment of niacin nutritional status accordingly [3,4]. In a previous study, we found that N^1-MN excretion is clearly reduced in RTR compared to healthy kidney donors [12]. The fact that this is paralleled by a significant elevation of 2Py excretion in the present study, raises speculation that enhanced enzymatic conversion of N^1-MN to 2Py by AOX1 may be present in RTR. Furthermore, the opposing shifts of 2Py and N^1-MN excretion in kidney donors after donation, may imply a putative isolated effect of renal function impairment on urinary 2Py/N^1-MN.

Regarding kidney function, urinary 2Py/N^1-MN was positively associated with kidney function in both RTR and the total cohort of kidney donors. Renal clearance of N^1-MN is affected by lower kidney function [13,14], being freely filtered at the glomerulus and tubular secreted, with negligible and saturable tubular reabsorption [30,31]. 2Py has previously been classified as a uremic retention product by the European Uremic Toxin Working Group [32,33], though specific mechanisms of its renal clearance have yet not been characterized. Whereas plasma concentrations of 2Py are reported to increase progressively with chronic kidney disease stages [34], those of N^1-MN are suggested to be less sensitive to kidney function because of the contribution of AOX1 to N^1-MN clearance [13,14]. In view of this, we can speculate upon slower excretion of N^1-MN, hence prolonged exposure to 2Py-forming AOX1 that is related to kidney function, rather than retention of 2Py primarily. This speculation is supported by the fact that kidney function appeared to have only a minor effect on the daily excretion of the sum of 2Py and N^1-MN in all groups. The presence of a significant association of urinary 2Py/N^1-MN with kidney function in the total cohort of kidney donors, but not in the pre- and post-donation subgroups, is most likely due to smaller effect sizes in the latter subgroups of kidney donors being declared eligible after pre-donation screening.

The identification of eGFR as the strongest independent determinant of urinary 2Py/N^1-MN in RTR further supports the notion of an isolated effect of kidney function. Other identified determinant factors include those that are known to affect the enzymatic activity of the aforementioned 2Py-forming AOX1 and most likely contribute as such. In fact, urinary 2Py/N^1-MN has been used as an index to estimate in vivo AOX1 levels and activity [35], being regulated by a wide variety of endogenous and exogenous factors [36]. Smoking and alcohol consumption are well-known factors [37,38] that showed an inverse association with urinary 2Py/N^1-MN in RTR. Diabetes and inflammatory mediators [37], including hs-CRP [39,40], have also been implicated in AOX1 activity, as well as HDL-cholesterol-levels via interaction of AOX1 with the ATP-binding cassette transporter A1 (ABCA1) which is a regulator of HDL metabolism [41,42]. Surprisingly, medication use did not appear to affect urinary 2Py/N^1-MN in RTR, despite the significant function of AOX1 in metabolizing xenobiotics. Importantly, the fact that urinary 2Py/N^1-MN has multiple determinants in addition to eGFR, precludes its use as a biomarker of kidney function.

Excessive poly (ADP-ribose) polymerase (PARP) activation induced by stressors such as inflammation, oxidative stress and DNA damage that are predominant in RTR [43,44], has also been implicated in higher production of 2Py from NAD^+ degradation [45,46]. One would, however, expect that this would be reflected by an overall increase of NAD^+ catabolites, which is opposed by the two-fold reduction of N^1-MN excretion in our RTR population.

In general, higher urinary output of NAD^+ metabolites indicates higher niacin nutritional status, being excreted after the pool of pyridine nucleotide coenzymes is filled [47]. Acute stress may alter this output, but not steady state conditions, in which elimination and production rates are equal [48]. However, the ratio of metabolites is subject to factors that affect not only the activity of 2Py-forming AOX1, but according to our data also kidney function. In a previous study, we found N^1-MN excretion to be lower in RTR independent of dietary intake of niacin equivalents, as well as to be positively associated with kidney function [12]. According to the present study, the latter association remains when taking into account 2Py excretion, by means of urinary 2Py/N^1-MN. Therefore, although urinary excretion of N^1-MN is the most common and recommended index [3,4], our findings suggest that this index might be of limited value in conditions of kidney function impairment and future studies may confirm whether 2Py excretion should at least be additionally interpreted for evaluation of niacin nutritional status.

The speculative presence of slower excretion, hence prolonged exposure of N^1-MN to 2Py-forming AOX1 with kidney function impairment has not been confirmed in previous studies. In fact, this speculation indicates straight substrate conversion kinetics, which is unlikely to fully account for the previously reported, increased serum concentrations of 2Py in patients with chronic renal failure [46]. More specifically, Rutkowski et al. suggested high serum concentrations of 2Py in chronic renal failure to be a result of kidney function impairment, based on the fact that serum concentrations of 2Py were approximately 20-fold higher in patients with advanced renal failure than in healthy subjects (15.5 ± 5.8 μmol/L versus 0.83 ± 0.18 μmol/L), with only a transient drop after dialysis, and a permanent reduction after kidney transplantation [46]. Accordingly, given its accumulation, along with a deterioration of kidney function, and its toxic properties due to significant inhibition of PARP activity, 2Py has been identified as a uremic toxin [32,45,46]. As we only measured urinary excretion of 2Py, it cannot be ruled out whether increased urinary excretion of 2Py is solely the consequence of increased serum concentrations of 2Py, due to decreased renal clearance, rather than conversion kinetics of N^1-MN to 2Py by AOX1, and future studies are warranted to address this matter.

Strengths of this study include the large sample size of a specific patient group and the availability of healthy kidney donors before donation as a control group, and after donation as a model of isolated renal function impairment. Moreover, the extensive characterization of RTR allowed us to control for other factors that could affect 2Py/N^1-MN in 24-h urine, and to comprehensively identify determinants of urinary 2Py/N^1-MN. The ratio of metabolites in 24-h urine provides a measure to demonstrate changes in metabolism related to renal function, while being the least sensitive to 24-h urine collection errors. Limitations of this study are its observational nature, which prohibits causal inferences, as well as final conclusions on underlying mechanisms of increased urinary 2Py/N^1-MN in RTR and kidney donors after kidney donation, and associations with kidney function. Therefore, it remains to be determined whether the association of urinary 2Py/N^1-MN with kidney function is a causal relation. The observational design of this study did neither allow us to rule out increased serum concentrations of 2Py due to decreased renal clearance, or higher production of 2Py from NAD^+ degradation due to PARP activation by means of an experimental design. Conclusions are yet additionally supported by the presence of direct associations of the 24-h urinary excretion of 2Py, N^1-MN, and the sum of 2Py and N^1-MN, but not urinary 2Py/N^1-MN, with niacin nutritional intake (Table S1). Future studies are strongly encouraged to elaborate on serum concentrations of 2Py and N^1-MN along with their urinary excretion. The present study is confined to the urinary excretion of the major NAD^+

metabolites, comprising the most common and recommended indices of niacin nutritional status according to existing literature and authorities, including the WHO and the EFSA [3,4], respectively. Other indices, including serum or erythrocyte concentrations of niacin and its metabolites [49], are considered inferior as urinary concentrations have shown the most sensitive response to oral test doses of niacin equivalents [3,7]. Given the aforementioned limitations, this study should be conceived as a descriptive report that precludes final conclusions on the applicability of N^1-MN excretion as a biomarker of niacin nutritional status in conditions of impaired kidney function. Finally, although niacin deficiency is considered to be uncommon in the developed world, it might be prevalent in subpopulations, including RTR [12]. Still, it should be emphasized that assessment of niacin nutritional status might not be feasible in the developing world given the costs.

5. Conclusions

The 24-h urinary excretion of 2Py is higher in RTR than in kidney donors, and urinary 2Py/N^1-MN clearly increases after kidney donation. Urinary 2Py/N^1-MN is associated with kidney function in both RTR and kidney donors, and kidney function is identified as the strongest determinant of urinary 2Py/N^1-MN in RTR. Therefore, interpretation of both N^1-MN and 2Py excretion, rather than N^1-MN alone, may be recommended for assessment of niacin nutritional status in conditions of impaired kidney function.

Author Contributions: Conceptualization, I.P.K. and S.J.L.B.; Formal Analysis, C.P.J.D. and S.J.L.B.; Investigation, C.P.J.D. and A.v.d.V.; Resources, J.M.G. and K.J.B.-v.d.B.; Data Curation, A.W.G.-N and S.J.L.B.; Writing—Original Draft Preparation, C.P.J.D.; Writing—Review & Editing, A.v.d.V., A.W.G.-N., K.J.B.-v.d.B, M.R.H.-F. and S.J.L.B.; Supervision, M.R.H.-F., S.J.L.B.; Funding Acquisition, S.J.L.B. All authors have read and agreed to the published version of the manuscript.

Acknowledgments: Supported by FrieslandCampina and Danone Nutricia Research. The cohort on which the study was based is registered at clinicaltrials.gov as "TransplantLines Food and Nutrition Biobank and Cohort Study (TxL-FN)" with number NCT02811835.

References

1. Bogan, K.L.; Brenner, C. Nicotinic acid, nicotinamide, and nicotinamide riboside: A molecular evaluation of NAD+ precursor vitamins in human nutrition. *Annu. Rev. Nutr.* **2008**, *28*, 115–130. [CrossRef]
2. Soldi, L.R.; Maltos, A.L.; da Cunha, D.F.; Portari, G.V. Correlation Between First Morning Single Void and 24-Hour Urines: The Reliability to Quantify Niacin Status. *Med. Sci. Monit. Basic Res.* **2018**, *24*, 206–209. [CrossRef] [PubMed]
3. EFSA NDA Panel. Scientific Opinion on Dietary Reference Values for niacin. *EFSA J.* **2014**, *12*, 3759. [CrossRef]
4. World Health Organization and United Nations High Commissions for Refugees. Pellagra and Its Prevention and Control in Major Emergencies; WHO/NHD/00.10.2000. Available online: http://apps.who.int/iris/bitstream/handle/10665/66704/WHO_NHD_00.10.pdf?sequence=1&isAllowed=y (accessed on 26 March 2018).
5. Menon, R.M.; Gonzalez, M.A.; Adams, M.H.; Tolbert, D.S.; Leu, J.H.; Cefali, E.A. Effect of the rate of niacin administration on the plasma and urine pharmacokinetics of niacin and its metabolites. *J. Clin. Pharmacol.* **2007**, *47*, 681–688. [CrossRef] [PubMed]
6. Pissios, P. Nicotinamide N-Methyltransferase: More Than a Vitamin B3 Clearance Enzyme. *Trends Endocrinol. Metab.* **2017**, *28*, 340–353. [CrossRef]

7. Jacob, R.A.; Swendseid, M.E.; McKee, R.W.; Fu, C.S.; Clemens, R.A. Biochemical markers for assessment of niacin status in young men: Urinary and blood levels of niacin metabolites. *J. Nutr.* **1989**, *119*, 591–598. [CrossRef]
8. Delange, D.J.; Joubert, C.P. Assessment of Nicotinic Acid Status of Population Groups. *Am. J. Clin. Nutr.* **1964**, *15*, 169–174. [CrossRef]
9. Hegyi, J.; Schwartz, R.A.; Hegyi, V. Pellagra: Dermatitis, dementia, and diarrhea. *Int. J. Dermatol.* **2004**, *43*, 1–5. [CrossRef]
10. Strohm, D.; Bechthold, A.; Isik, N.; Leschik-Bonnet, E.; Heseker, H. Revised reference values for the intake of thiamin (vitamin B1), riboflavin (vitamin B2), and niacin. *NFS J.* **2016**, *3*, 20–24. [CrossRef]
11. Shibata, K.; Matsuo, H. Correlation between niacin equivalent intake and urinary excretion of its metabolites, N′-methylnicotinamide, N′-methyl-2-pyridone-5-carboxamide, and N′-methyl-4-pyridone-3-carboxamide, in humans consuming a self-selected food. *Am. J. Clin. Nutr.* **1989**, *50*, 114–119. [CrossRef]
12. Deen, C.P.J.; van der Veen, A.; van Faassen, M.; Minovic, I.; Gomes-Neto, A.W.; Geleijnse, J.M.; Borgonjen-van den Berg, K.J.; Kema, I.P.; Bakker, S.J.L. Urinary Excretion of N(1)-Methylnicotinamide, as a Biomarker of Niacin Status, and Mortality in Renal Transplant Recipients. *J. Clin. Med.* **2019**, *8*, 1948. [CrossRef]
13. Maiza, A.; Waldek, S.; Ballardie, F.W.; Daley-Yates, P.T. Estimation of renal tubular secretion in man, in health and disease, using endogenous N-1-methylnicotinamide. *Nephron* **1992**, *60*, 12–16. [CrossRef] [PubMed]
14. Muller, F.; Sharma, A.; Konig, J.; Fromm, M.F. Biomarkers for In Vivo Assessment of Transporter Function. *Pharmacol. Rev.* **2018**, *70*, 246–277. [CrossRef]
15. van den Berg, E.; Engberink, M.F.; Brink, E.J.; van Baak, M.A.; Joosten, M.M.; Gans, R.O.; Navis, G.; Bakker, S.J. Dietary acid load and metabolic acidosis in renal transplant recipients. *Clin. J. Am. Soc. Nephrol.* **2012**, *7*, 1811–1818. [CrossRef] [PubMed]
16. van den Berg, E.; Engberink, M.F.; Brink, E.J.; van Baak, M.A.; Gans, R.O.; Navis, G.; Bakker, S.J. Dietary protein, blood pressure and renal function in renal transplant recipients. *Br. J. Nutr.* **2013**, *109*, 1463–1470. [CrossRef] [PubMed]
17. van den Berg, E.; Pasch, A.; Westendorp, W.H.; Navis, G.; Brink, E.J.; Gans, R.O.; van Goor, H.; Bakker, S.J. Urinary sulfur metabolites associate with a favorable cardiovascular risk profile and survival benefit in renal transplant recipients. *J. Am. Soc. Nephrol.* **2014**, *25*, 1303–1312. [CrossRef] [PubMed]
18. Siebelink, E.; Geelen, A.; de Vries, J.H. Self-reported energy intake by FFQ compared with actual energy intake to maintain body weight in 516 adults. *Br. J. Nutr.* **2011**, *106*, 274–281. [CrossRef]
19. Streppel, M.T.; de Vries, J.H.; Meijboom, S.; Beekman, M.; de Craen, A.J.; Slagboom, P.E.; Feskens, E.J. Relative validity of the food frequency questionnaire used to assess dietary intake in the Leiden Longevity Study. *Nutr. J.* **2013**, *12*, 75. [CrossRef]
20. Dutch Nutrient Databank. *NEVO Table 2006*; Voorlichtingsbureau Voor de Voeding: The Hague, The Netherlands, 2006.
21. Eisenga, M.F.; Kieneker, L.M.; Soedamah-Muthu, S.S.; van den Berg, E.; Deetman, P.E.; Navis, G.J.; Gans, R.O.; Gaillard, C.A.; Bakker, S.J.; Joosten, M.M. Urinary potassium excretion, renal ammoniagenesis, and risk of graft failure and mortality in renal transplant recipients. *Am. J. Clin. Nutr.* **2016**, *104*, 1703–1711. [CrossRef]
22. Inker, L.A.; Schmid, C.H.; Tighiouart, H.; Eckfeldt, J.H.; Feldman, H.I.; Greene, T.; Kusek, J.W.; Manzi, J.; Van Lente, F.; Zhang, Y.L.; et al. Estimating glomerular filtration rate from serum creatinine and cystatin C. *N. Engl. J. Med.* **2012**, *367*, 20–29. [CrossRef]
23. Salvador, C.L.; Hartmann, A.; Asberg, A.; Bergan, S.; Rowe, A.D.; Morkrid, L. Estimating Glomerular Filtration Rate in Kidney Transplant Recipients: Comparing a Novel Equation with Commonly Used Equations in this Population. *Transplant. Direct* **2017**, *3*, e332. [CrossRef] [PubMed]
24. Apperloo, A.J.; de Zeeuw, D.; Donker, A.J.; de Jong, P.E. Precision of glomerular filtration rate determinations for long-term slope calculations is improved by simultaneous infusion of 125I-iothalamate and 131I-hippuran. *J. Am. Soc. Nephrol.* **1996**, *7*, 567–572. [PubMed]
25. Bouma, G.; van Faassen, M.; Kats-Ugurlu, G.; de Vries, E.G.; Kema, I.P.; Walenkamp, A.M. Niacin (Vitamin B3) Supplementation in Patients with Serotonin-Producing Neuroendocrine Tumor. *Neuroendocrinology* **2016**, *103*, 489–494. [CrossRef] [PubMed]
26. Kennedy, B.E.; Sharif, T.; Martell, E.; Dai, C.; Kim, Y.; Lee, P.W.; Gujar, S.A. NAD(+) salvage pathway in cancer metabolism and therapy. *Pharmacol. Res.* **2016**, *114*, 274–283. [CrossRef]

27. Badawy, A.A. Kynurenine Pathway of Tryptophan Metabolism: Regulatory and Functional Aspects. *Int. J. Tryptophan Res.* **2017**, *10*, 1–20. [CrossRef]

28. Wozniacka, A.; Wieczorkowska, M.; Gebicki, J.; Sysa-Jedrzejowska, A. Topical application of 1-methylnicotinamide in the treatment of rosacea: A pilot study. *Clin. Exp. Dermatol.* **2005**, *30*, 632–635. [CrossRef]

29. Kremer, J.I.; Gompel, K.; Bakuradze, T.; Eisenbrand, G.; Richling, E. Urinary Excretion of Niacin Metabolites in Humans after Coffee Consumption. *Mol. Nutr. Food Res.* **2018**, *62*, e1700735. [CrossRef]

30. Nasseri, K.; Daley-Yates, P.T. A comparison of N-1-methylnicotinamide clearance with 5 other markers of renal function in models of acute and chronic renal failure. *Toxicol. Lett.* **1990**, *53*, 243–245. [CrossRef]

31. Weber, W.; Toussaint, S.; Looby, M.; Nitz, M.; Kewitz, H. System analysis in multiple dose kinetics: Evidence for saturable tubular reabsorption of the organic cation N1-methylnicotinamide in humans. *J. Pharm. Biopharm.* **1991**, *19*, 553–574. [CrossRef]

32. Duranton, F.; Cohen, G.; De Smet, R.; Rodriguez, M.; Jankowski, J.; Vanholder, R.; Argiles, A.; European Uremic Toxin Work Group. Normal and pathologic concentrations of uremic toxins. *J. Am. Soc. Nephrol.* **2012**, *23*, 1258–1270. [CrossRef]

33. Vanholder, R.; Van Laecke, S.; Glorieux, G. What is new in uremic toxicity? *Pediatr. Nephrol.* **2008**, *23*, 1211–1221. [CrossRef] [PubMed]

34. Lenglet, A.; Liabeuf, S.; Bodeau, S.; Louvet, L.; Mary, A.; Boullier, A.; Lemaire-Hurtel, A.S.; Jonet, A.; Sonnet, P.; Kamel, S.; et al. N-methyl-2-pyridone-5-carboxamide (2PY)-Major Metabolite of Nicotinamide: An Update on an Old Uremic Toxin. *Toxins* **2016**, *8*, 339. [CrossRef] [PubMed]

35. Tayama, Y.; Sugihara, K.; Sanoh, S.; Miyake, K.; Kitamura, S.; Ohta, S. Developmental changes of aldehyde oxidase activity and protein expression in human liver cytosol. *Drug Metab. Pharm.* **2012**, *27*, 543–547. [CrossRef] [PubMed]

36. Garattini, E.; Terao, M. The role of aldehyde oxidase in drug metabolism. *Expert Opin. Drug Metab. Toxicol.* **2012**, *8*, 487–503. [CrossRef] [PubMed]

37. Pryde, D.C.; Dalvie, D.; Hu, Q.; Jones, P.; Obach, R.S.; Tran, T.D. Aldehyde oxidase: An enzyme of emerging importance in drug discovery. *J. Med. Chem.* **2010**, *53*, 8441–8460. [CrossRef]

38. Chen, C.H.; Ferreira, J.C.; Gross, E.R.; Mochly-Rosen, D. Targeting aldehyde dehydrogenase 2: New therapeutic opportunities. *Physiol. Rev.* **2014**, *94*, 1–34. [CrossRef]

39. Xu, F.; Chen, Y.G.; Xue, L.; Li, R.J.; Zhang, H.; Bian, Y.; Zhang, C.; Lv, R.J.; Feng, J.B.; Zhang, Y. Role of aldehyde dehydrogenase 2 Glu504lys polymorphism in acute coronary syndrome. *J. Cell Mol. Med.* **2011**, *15*, 1955–1962. [CrossRef]

40. Pan, C.; Xing, J.H.; Zhang, C.; Zhang, Y.M.; Zhang, L.T.; Wei, S.J.; Zhang, M.X.; Wang, X.P.; Yuan, Q.H.; Xue, L.; et al. Aldehyde dehydrogenase 2 inhibits inflammatory response and regulates atherosclerotic plaque. *Oncotarget* **2016**, *7*, 35562–35576. [CrossRef]

41. Graessler, J.; Fischer, S. The dual substrate specificity of aldehyde oxidase 1 for retinal and acetaldehyde and its role in ABCA1 mediated efflux. *Horm. Metab. Res.* **2007**, *39*, 775–776. [CrossRef]

42. Sigruener, A.; Buechler, C.; Orso, E.; Hartmann, A.; Wild, P.J.; Terracciano, L.; Roncalli, M.; Bornstein, S.R.; Schmitz, G. Human aldehyde oxidase 1 interacts with ATP-binding cassette transporter-1 and modulates its activity in hepatocytes. *Horm. Metab. Res.* **2007**, *39*, 781–789. [CrossRef]

43. Chini, C.C.S.; Tarrago, M.G.; Chini, E.N. NAD and the aging process: Role in life, death and everything in between. *Mol. Cell Endocrinol.* **2017**, *455*, 62–74. [CrossRef] [PubMed]

44. Canto, C.; Menzies, K.J.; Auwerx, J. NAD(+) Metabolism and the Control of Energy Homeostasis: A Balancing Act between Mitochondria and the Nucleus. *Cell Metab.* **2015**, *22*, 31–53. [CrossRef] [PubMed]

45. Slominska, E.M.; Smolenski, R.T.; Szolkiewicz, M.; Leaver, N.; Rutkowski, B.; Simmonds, H.A.; Swierczynski, J. Accumulation of plasma N-methyl-2-pyridone-5-carboxamide in patients with chronic renal failure. *Mol. Cell Biochem.* **2002**, *231*, 83–88. [CrossRef] [PubMed]

46. Rutkowski, B.; Slominska, E.; Szolkiewicz, M.; Smolenski, R.T.; Striley, C.; Rutkowski, P.; Swierczynski, J. N-methyl-2-pyridone-5-carboxamide: A novel uremic toxin? *Kidney Int.* **2003**, *63*, S19–S21. [CrossRef]

47. Okamoto, H.; Ishikawa, A.; Yoshitake, Y.; Kodama, N.; Nishimuta, M.; Fukuwatari, T.; Shibata, K. Diurnal variations in human urinary excretion of nicotinamide catabolites: Effects of stress on the metabolism of nicotinamide. *Am. J. Clin. Nutr.* **2003**, *77*, 406–410. [CrossRef]
48. Orlando, R.; Floreani, M.; Napoli, E.; Padrini, R.; Palatini, P. Renal clearance of N(1)-methylnicotinamide: A sensitive marker of the severity of liver dysfunction in cirrhosis. *Nephron* **2000**, *84*, 32–39. [CrossRef]
49. Fu, C.S.; Swendseid, M.E.; Jacob, R.A.; McKee, R.W. Biochemical markers for assessment of niacin status in young men: Levels of erythrocyte niacin coenzymes and plasma tryptophan. *J. Nutr.* **1989**, *119*, 1949–1955. [CrossRef]

4

Changes in Serum Creatinine Levels and Natural Evolution of Acute Kidney Injury with Conservative Management of Hemodynamically Significant Patent Ductus Arteriosus in Extremely Preterm Infants at 23–26 Weeks of Gestation

Eun Seop Seo †, Se In Sung †, So Yoon Ahn, Yun Sil Chang and Won Soon Park *

Department of Pediatrics, Samsung Medical Center, Sungkyunkwan University School of Medicine, 06351 Seoul, Korea; eunseop720@gmail.com (E.S.S.); sein.sung@samsung.com (S.I.S.); soyoon.ahn@samsung.com (S.Y.A.); yschang@skku.edu (Y.S.C.)

* Correspondence: wonspark@skku.edu

† These authors equally contributed to the manuscript.

Abstract: Changes in kidney function in extremely preterm infants (EPT) with conservatively managed hemodynamically significant (HS) patent ductus arteriosus (PDA) are not known well. We aimed to present the postnatal course in serum creatinine levels (sCr), prevalence of acute kidney injury (AKI), then relevance between AKI and adverse outcomes in EPT with conservatively managed HS PDA. By review of medical records, we analyzed the postnatal course of sCr and prevalence of stage 3 AKI defined by the modified Kidney Disease Improving Global Outcome (KDIGO) in EPT at gestational age of 23 to 26 weeks with conservatively treated HS PDA. We investigated if the presence and/or prolonged duration of stage 3 AKI elevated the risk of adverse outcomes. The results showed that, neither factor was associated with adverse outcomes. While the average PDA closure date was at postnatal day (P) 41 and 53, sCr peaked at P 10 and 14 and the cumulative prevalence of stage 3 AKI was 57% and 72% in the EPT of 25–26 and 23–24 weeks' gestation, respectively. The high prevalence of stage 3 AKI without adverse outcomes in EPT with conservatively managed HS PDA suggests that it might reflect renal immaturity rather than pathologic conditions.

Keywords: acute kidney injury; patent ductus arteriosus; conservative management

1. Introduction

Assessing kidney function is crucial for meticulous fluid, electrolyte, and nutritional support, and the adjustment of medication dosage in extremely preterm infants (EPT) [1–4]. Serum creatinine level (sCr) is a commonly used in evaluating renal function and could also be applied in assessment of glomerular filtration rate (GFR) in neonates and infants [4–7]. However, the use of sCr for renal function assessment in preterm infants is problematic as their sCr at birth reflects maternal levels [8,9], and sCr is quite variable according to gestational age (GA), birth weight, and chronological age [4,7,10,11]. Limited data are available on how sCr is affected by gestational age and birth weight and how this value changes over time, especially in the peri-viable EPT [5,7,10,12–14]. Despite these limitations, all the three current available acute kidney injury (AKI) definitions use change in sCr to classify the stage of AKI in the newborn infants [5,15,16].

AKI in premature infants are known to be related to increased mortality [11,17–21] and morbidities, which includes bronchopulmonary dysplasia (BPD) [2,22,23] and intraventricular hemorrhage (IVH) [24]. However, these associations have not been well reported and elucidated in EPT, although

EPT are at high risk for acute AKI because of low GFR resulting from under-developed kidney systems, exhibiting incomplete nephrogenesis and low nephron number [25,26]. Meanwhile, hemodynamically significant (HS) patent ductus arteriosus (PDA) could promote developing AKI by decreasing renal perfusion in the preterm infants in recent studies [16,17,27–29]. However, growing evidences support that the conservative management of HS PDA could be safe and feasible without increased mortality and/or morbidities [30–33]. Furthermore, the risks of developing AKI and the ensuing adverse outcomes with the conservative management of HS PDA have not yet been delineated. Therefore, we conducted this investigation to provide the natural postnatal course of changes in sCr, and the prevalence of AKI in EPT at gestation of 23–26 weeks with HS PDA exclusively managed with a conservative approach [31,32]. We also examined if the presence or persistence of AKI stage 3 adversely affected the risk of adverse events by comparing mortality and morbidities between EPT with and without AKI stage 3.

2. Experimental Section

2.1. Study Sample

The Samsung Medical Center (SMC) Institutional Review Board approved our investigation and waived the need for consent on October 10, 2019 (No. SMC 2015-10-156). We reviewed medical charts of 97 EPT at gestation of 23–26 weeks admitted to our Neonatal Intensive Care Unit (NICU) from January 2011 to June 2014 presenting with HS PDA, and treated exclusively by a conservative approach [31,32]. We stratified the extremely preterm infants into 23–24 ($n = 50$) and 25–26 ($n = 47$) weeks' gestation, and analyzed rates of mortality and morbidities, such as necrotizing enterocolitis (NEC), BPD, and intraventricular hemorrhage (IVH) in accordance with the presence/absence of and duration of AKI stage 3 [5,16,18].

2.2. AKI

AKI events occurring during the 6-week postnatal period were detected by the neonatal modified KIDGO sCr criteria [5,16,18] (Table 1). Measuring a chemistry panel including sCr q 1–3 days is usual at our NICU if the infant's condition is critical during the first few weeks of life, and increasing the interval up to q 1–2 weeks, if the infant's condition has become stabilized. Although we did not adopt urine amount criteria to classify stage, we calculated urine output from flow sheets, and reported the incidence of oliguria (<0.5 mL/kg/day) at each stage of AKI.

Table 1. The maximum AKI stage within a first month after birth according to neonatal acute kidney injury KDIGO classification.

Stage	Serum Creatinine	GA 23–24 Weeks $n = 50$	GA 25–26 Weeks $n = 47$	Total $n = 97$	Total with Oliguria (<0.5 mL/kg/day) $n = 97$
0	No change in SCr or rise < 0.3 mg/DL	4 (8%)	3 (6%)	7(7%)	1(1%)
1	SCr rise ≥ 0.3 mg/dL within 48 h or SCr rise ≥ 1.5–1.9 × reference SCr [a] within 7 days	2 (4%)	5 (11%)	7(7%)	1(1%)
2	SCr rise ≥ 2.0–2.9 × reference SCr [a]	7 (14%)	11 (23%)	18(19%)	1(1%)
3	SCr rise ≥ 3 × reference SCr [a] or SCr ≥ 2.5 mg/dL [b] or receipt of dialysis	36 (72%)	27 (57%)	63(66%)	18(19%)

[a] Reference SCr will be considered as the lowest prior SCr value. [b] SCr value of 2.5 mg/dL corresponds to GFR less than 10 mL/min/1.73 m^2. AKI, acute kidney injury; SCr, serum creatinine; KDIGO, Kidney Disease Improving Global Outcomes.

2.3. HS PDA

We defined HS PDA as more than 2 mm in ductal diameter plus predominant left to right flow on echocardiography initially performed at average postnatal day 7; requiring ventilator support accompanying signs and symptoms consistent with symptomatic PDA, such as hypotension with mean airway pressure below GA; grade ≥ 2 cardiac murmur; pulse pressure widening (>30 mmHg); or need for increased respiratory support [31,32]. We deferred until postnatal day 7 as spontaneous ductal closures could occur even in EPT for the first postnatal week [17,34]. Follow-up echocardiography was conducted regularly at 2–4 weeks intervals until PDA closure. During the study period, 50/54 (93%) and 47/74 (64%) in the EPT of 23–26 weeks of gestation were diagnosed with HS PDA, respectively.

2.4. Fluid Therapy

We managed all EPT with HS PDA with non-interventional conservative management without any pharmacologic and/or surgical intervention. We judiciously restricted the fluid intake starting with the first-day mean fluid volume around 67 mL/kg/day, and maintaining mean fluid intake around 107–115 mL/kg/day from days 7 to 28 for the first two months of life [31,32]. We individualized and adjusted the target fluid volume for each EPT q 24 h after assessment of volume status by body weight, serum sodium level, urine output and specific gravity, or cardiomegaly. In this present study, we could obtain judicious fluid restriction in EPT through meticulous NICU care including better room care delivery, minimal handling, and high humidification [35,36].

2.5. Data Collection and Definition

We analyzed clinical characteristics, which included sex, birth weight, GA, Apgar score at 1-min and 5-min, mode of delivery, chorioamnionitis, use of inotropic drugs, antenatal steroid use, and oliguria. We determined GA using the last menstrual period of mother and modified Ballard score. We confirmed chorioamnionitis using placental pathology. We reported oliguria when urine amount is less than 0.5 mL/kg for a day.

We analyzed adverse outcomes including ≥ moderate BPD [37], cystic periventricular leukomalacia, IVH (grade ≥ 3) [38], NEC (Bell's stage ≥ 2b) [39], retinopathy of prematurity (ROP) (stage ≥ 3) [40], and mortality.

To present the time course of sCr and AKI by gestational age, cumulative incidence rates of AKI in EPT at gestational age of 23–24 and 25–26 weeks were evaluated. We measured the adjusted odds ratios (ORs) of mortality and morbidities by the presence and/or persistence (per increase of week) of AKI stage 3 using multivariate regression analyses.

2.6. Statistical Analyses

We analyzed the categorical variables by χ^2 tests and Fisher's exact test. For continuous variables, we analyzed data through Student's *t*-tests and Mann–Whitney *U* tests. We also did multivariable analyses by binary logistic regression to measure adjusted ORs and 95% CI of the association between the duration of stage 3 AKI and adverse outcomes including mortality within the entire cohort. We considered a p value less than 0.05 as statistically significant. We used SPSS version 21 (SPSS Inc., Chicago, IL, USA) in all data analyses.

3. Results

3.1. Natural Course of sCr

For the time course of sCr, the initial increase in sCr peaked at postnatal day (P) 10 and postnatal week 2 in EPT at 25–26 and 23–24 weeks of gestation, respectively (Figure 1A). The peak sCr showed a higher tendency without statistical significance in EPT at gestation of 23–24 weeks than in those at 25–26 weeks. After this, sCr gradually declined until postnatal week 9 in both subgroups and reached sCr at birth at postnatal week 6 and 7 in EPT at 25–26 and 23–24 weeks' gestation, respectively. In EPT of 25–26 weeks' gestation without HS PDA, sCr showed a similar time course without statistical significance with the EPT of 25–26 weeks' gestation with HS PDA (Supplementary Figure S1).

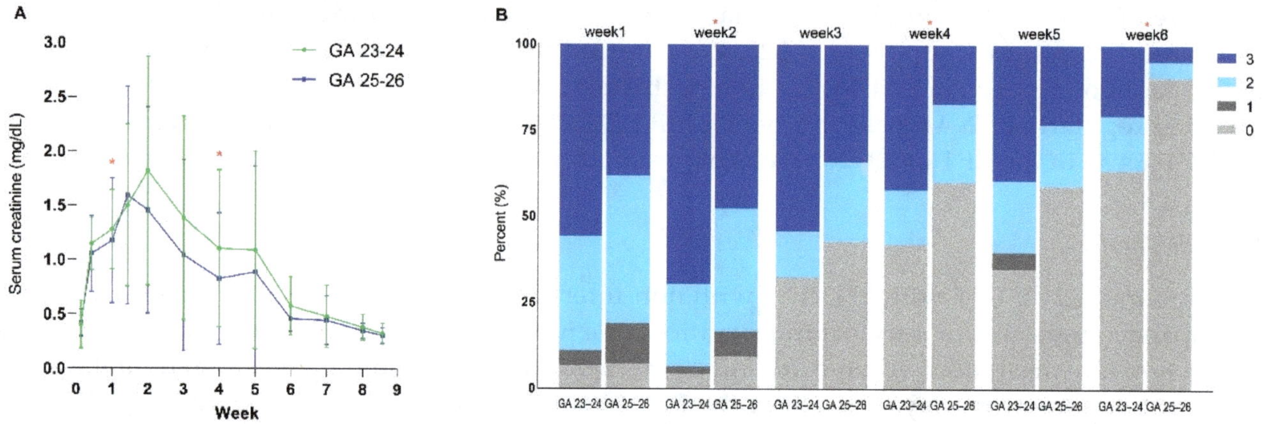

Figure 1. Time course of the mean serum creatinine levels within different gestational groups and prevalence of acute kidney injury (AKI) by stage in a week interval. (**A**) Serum creatinine profile for the 6 weeks of life in accordance to different gestational age groups; (**B**) Prevalence of AKI by stage in a week interval. * $p < 0.05$ in comparison between infants at 23–24 and those at 25–26 weeks of gestation.

3.2. *AKI Prevalence*

Table 1 demonstrates the cumulative AKI stage within the first six postnatal weeks according to neonatal KDIGO classification stratified by gestational age group. While only 6% and 8% were at AKI stage 0 in EPT at 25–26 and 23–24 weeks of gestation, respectively, the prevalence of AKI stage 3 tended to be higher (72%) in EPT at gestation of 23–24 weeks than in EPT of 25–26 weeks (57%) without statistical significance.

For the time course of the prevalence of AKI by stage in a week interval, postnatal increase in the prevalence of AKI stage 3 peaked at postnatal week 2 in both groups, and afterwards prevalence gradually declined till postnatal week 6 (Figure 1B). The prevalence of AKI stage 3 at postnatal week 2 and 6 in EPT at gestation of 23–24 weeks was higher significantly than that in EPT at gestation of 25–26 weeks.

3.3. *Clinical Characteristics According to AKI Stage*

Demographic and clinical characteristics in each study group in accordance with AKI stages are described in Table 2. In EPT with AKI stage 3, total GA was significantly lower, and male gender in EPT at gestation of 25–26 weeks had higher GA than in EPT with AKI 0–2. While total oliguria and oliguria in EPT at 25–26 weeks of gestation with AKI stage 3 were higher compared with those with AKI stage 0–2 significantly, no differences were observed in other clinical variables between AKI stage 3 and stage 0–2 groups.

3.4. *Adverse Outcomes According to AKI Stage*

While sepsis in EPT at 25–26 weeks of gestation with AKI stage 3 was slightly higher than infants with AKI stage 0–2, no significant differences were found in other adverse outcomes, including mortality and BPD, between the AKI stage 3 and stage 0–2 groups (Table 3).

Table 2. Demographics and clinical characteristics of EPT in period II: Stage 0–2 AKI vs. stage 3 AKI.

Clinical Characteristics	Total (n = 97)					
	GA 23–24 Weeks (n = 50)		GA 25–26 Weeks (n = 47)		Total (n = 97)	
	AKI 0–2 (n = 13)	AKI 3 (n = 36)	AKI 0–2 (n = 18)	AKI 3 (n = 27)	AKI 0–2 (n = 31)	AKI 3 (n = 63)
Gestational age (weeks)	23.9 ± 0.4	23.6 ± 0.5	25.6 ± 0.5 †	25.3 ± 0.4 †	24.8 ± 1.0	24.3 ± 1.0 *
Birth weight, mean (SD), g	684 ± 90	636 ± 79	743 ± 145	829 ± 140 †	718 ± 127	719 ± 145
Male, n (%)	6(46)	19(53)	7(39)	19(70) *	13(42)	38(60)
Apgar score at 1-min	3.9 ± 0.7	4.2 ± 1.3	4.4 ± 1.8	4.7 ± 1.4	4.2 ± 1.4	4.4 ± 1.4
Apgar score at 5-min	6.9 ± 1.1	6.5 ± 1.4	6.8 ± 1.4	6.9 ± 1.5	6.8 ± 1.3	6.7 ± 1.5
Cesarean delivery, n (%)	8 (62)	2 6(72)	16 (89)	24 (89)	24 (78)	50 (79)
Hypertension in pregnancy, n (%)	0	0	1 (6)	0	1 (3)	0
Chorioamnionitis, n (%)	6 (46)	25 (69)	9 (50)	15 (56)	15 (48)	40 (62)
Use of inotropic drugs, n (%)	3 (23)	8 (22)	4 (22)	1 (4)	7 (44)	9 (56)
Antenatal steroid use, n (%)	12 (92)	27 (75)	13 (72)	24 (89)	25 (81)	51 (81)
Oliguria, n (%)	1 (8)	9 (25)	1 (6)	9 (33) *	2 (7)	18 (29) *

* $p < 0.05$ compared with Stage 0–2 AKI. † $p < 0.05$ compared with infants at 23–24 weeks of gestation.

Table 3. Adverse outcomes of infants in period II: stage 0–2 AKI vs. stage 3 AKI.

Adverse Outcomes	Total (n = 97)					
	GA 23–24 Weeks (n = 50)		GA 25–26 Weeks (n = 47)		Total (n = 97)	
	AKI 0–2 (n = 13)	AKI 3 (n = 36)	AKI 0–2 (n = 18)	AKI 3 (n = 27)	AKI 0–2 (n = 31)	AKI 3 (n = 63)
Mortality, n (%)	1 (8)	7 (19)	1 (6)	1 (4)	2 (7)	8 (13)
Length of stay	111 ± 14	120 ± 64	130 ± 68	110 ± 59	122 ± 53	116 ± 62
NEC (Stage ≥ 2b), n (%)	0	5 (14)	2 (11)	3 (11)	2 (7)	8 (13)
ROP (requiring laser operation), n (%)	3 (23)	10 (28)	5 (28)	7 (26)	8 (26)	17 (27)
Blood culture-proven sepsis, n (%)	3 (23)	13 (36)	1 (6)	10 (37) *	4 (13)	23 (37) *
Cystic PVL, n (%)	3 (23)	7 (20)	3 (17)	2 (7)	6 (19)	9 (15)
IVH (Grade ≥ 3), n (%)	1 (8)	8 (22)	1 (6)	2 (7)	2 (7)	10 (16)
BPD (≥moderate BPD), n (%)	5 (39)	15 (47)	6 (33)	8 (30)	11 (36)	23 (39)
Survival without BPD, n (%)	1 (0)	0	1 (6)	3 (11)	2 (7)	3 (5)

* $p < 0.05$ compared with Stage 0–2 AKI.

3.5. *Adjusted ORs for Risk of Adverse Outcomes by AKI Stage 3*

The adjusted ORs for the risk of unfavorable outcomes were not increased in AKI stage 3 in multivariate analyses (Table 4). In addition, the adjusted ORs for outcomes were not elevated by prolonged duration (per week) of AKI stage 3 (Table 5).

Table 4. Adjusted ORs * for risk of adverse outcomes by presence of Stage 3 AKI.

Outcomes	Adjusted OR (95% CI)	p Value
Mortality	0.965 (0.140–6.661)	0.971
BPD (more than moderate BPD)	1.441 (0.507–4.095)	0.493
Survival without BPD	0.314 (0.018–5.559)	0.430
IVH (Grade ≥ 3), n (%)	1.923 (0.360–10.269)	0.444
Cystic PVL	0.460 (0.116–1.819)	0.268
ROP (requiring laser operation), n (%)	1.538 (0.480–4.926)	0.469
NEC (Stage ≥ 2b), n (%)	3.610 (0.439–29.654)	0.232
Blood culture-proven sepsis	3.556 (0.965–13.101)	0.057

OR, odds ratio; AKI, acute kidney injury; CI, confidence interval; BPD, bronchopulmonary dysplasia; IVH, intraventricular hemorrhage; PVL, periventricular. leukomalacia; ROP, retinopathy of prematurity; NEC, necrotizing enterocolitis. * adjusted for birth weight, gestational age, small for gestational age, antenatal steroid use, 1-min and 5-min Apgar scores, hypertension in pregnancy, chorioamnionitis.

Table 5. Adjusted ORs * for risk of adverse outcomes by duration (per week) of stage 3 AKI.

Outcomes	Adjusted OR (95% CI)	p Value
Mortality	1.040 (0.602–1.797)	0.887
BPD (more than moderate BPD)	1.043 (0.745–1.459)	0.808
Survival without BPD	0.332 (0.083–1.329)	0.119
IVH (Grade ≥ 3), n (%)	1.164 (0.074–1.823)	0.508
Cystic PVL	0.709 (0.437–1.150)	0.163
ROP (requiring laser operation), n (%)	1.000 (0.693–1.441)	0.998
NEC (Stage ≥ 2b), n (%)	1.325 (0.748–2.346)	0.335
Blood culture-proven sepsis	1.170 (0.820–1.665)	0.382

OR, odds ratio; AKI, acute kidney injury; CI, confidence interval; BPD, bronchopulmonary dysplasia; IVH, intraventricular hemorrhage; PVL, periventricular. leukomalacia; ROP, retinopathy of prematurity; NEC, necrotizing enterocolitis. * adjusted for birth weight, gestational age, small for gestational age, antenatal steroid use, 1-min and 5-min Apgar scores, hypertension in pregnancy, chorioamnionitis.

4. Discussion

This present study is the first human study demonstrating the natural postnatal evolution of sCr and the prevalence of AKI in the peri-viable EPT at gestation of 23–26 weeks with HS PDA who received exclusive conservative management. In this present study, while sCr at birth was about the same between the study groups, representing maternal levels [8,9], the peak sCr and the peak prevalence of AKI stage 3 during the first two postnatal weeks were higher in EPT at gestation of 23–24 weeks than in EPT of 25–26 weeks. These findings suggest that very low initial GFR and tubular immaturity, and its slow improvement, might be inversely related to GA in these peri-viable EPT [7,11,14,27,41]. Furthermore, as HS PDA closed averagely at postnatal day 41 and 53 in EPT of 25–26 and 23–24 weeks' gestation, respectively [31,32], our data suggests that renal immaturity inversely related to GA, rather than HS PDA induced renal hypo-perfusion [17,27–29], are primarily responsible for the initial postnatal rise in sCr and the peak prevalence of AKI stage 3 during the first two postnatal weeks [42].

sCr after peak declined rapidly, and reached a birth sCr at postnatal week 6 and 7, compatible with corrected GA of 31–32 weeks in EPT at 25–26 and 23–24 weeks of gestation, respectively, and after then, sCr approached a stable plateau in both GA subgroups, indicating a steady state between endogenous Cr production and excretion [13,27,41]. In the preterm infant, the GFR is lower until the full nephrogenesis is finished by 34–35 weeks of gestation [43–46]. Overall, our data suggest that despite its inverse relationship with GA, the postnatal renal maturation and the ensuing logarithmic increase in GFR are accelerated by 2–3 weeks in these peri-viable EPT [47].

Although AKI in premature infants has been known to be related to raised mortality [11,17–21] and morbidity rates, including BPD [2,22,23] and IVH [24], evidence supporting their direct causal relationships are lacking. In contrast, while sepsis rate was more elevated in AKI stage 3 than in stage 0–2, only in EPT at gestation of 25–26 but not of 23–24 weeks, neither the presence nor the prolonged duration of AKI stage 3 was associated with elevated mortality or any morbidities rates including BPD and IVH. The reasons for our results, which are contradictory to other studies showing increased mortality and/or morbidities [2,11,17–24], are difficult to explain. Few data are available for the peri-viable EPT of 23–24 week's gestation, and actively treated with pharmacologic agents for HS PDA could be cofounders in other studies. A further controlled study with a homogeneous patient population and same clinical management policy might be necessary to clarify these contradictory findings.

Fluid therapy and drug dosing in premature infants need to be adjusted according to renal function, i.e., GFR [3,4,45,46]. Considering our results, which showed greater and delayed peak of sCr and very high prevalence of AKI stage 3 at the first two postnatal weeks in these peri-viable EPT with HS PDA, judicious fluid restriction might be prerequisite for the success of non-interventional treatment for HS PDA [2,48,49]. In our prior studies [31,32], fluid volume of 67 mL/kg/day at day of birth, and raising up to ≤115 mL/kg/day for the first month was accomplished without restricting caloric support or elevating the risk of renal dysfunctions and electrolyte imbalance. Acute fluid overload in the newborn infants was associated with adverse outcomes, including mortality [50] and morbidities [2,48]. Furthermore, the extent of volume overload in critical adult patients also correlated with worse clinical course [51–53]. In contrast, fluid restriction was associated with reduced mortality [54] and morbidities, such as PDA and NEC [55]. Overall, these findings suggest that judicious fluid restriction might be essential for the success of the non-interventional conservative treatment of HS PDA in EPT [45].

Heterogeneous time intervals and variable number of follow-up sCr measurements for review could be limitations of this retrospective uncontrolled observational single center study. The absence of long-term outcome assessments including growth and neurodevelopment might be another limitation of this study. However, a relatively large sample size (n = 50) of the peri-viable EPT at gestation of 23–24 weeks with HS PDA exclusively managed with a conservative treatment, as well as less variation in clinical management policies, might be a strength of this single-center study.

5. Conclusions

In conclusion, the study findings suggest that AKI observed in EPT with conservatively managed HS PDA is not a pathological entity and might reflect a physiological postnatal developmental process of the immature renal system.

Author Contributions: Conceptualization, E.S.S., S.I.S. and W.S.P.; methodology, Y.S.C. and W.S.P.; software, E.S.S.; validation, S.Y.A.; formal analysis, E.S.S. and S.I.S.; resources, S.I.S. and W.S.P., data curation, E.S.S. and S.Y.A.; writing—original draft preparation, E.S.S. and S.I.S.; writing—review and editing, Y.S.C. and W.S.S.; visualization, E.S.S.; supervision, Y.S.C. and W.S.P.; project administration, E.S.S. and S.I.S. All authors have read and agree to the published version of the manuscript.

References

1. Aviles, D.H.; Fildes, R.D.; Jose, P.A. Evaluation of renal function. *Clin. Perinatol.* **1992**, *19*, 69–84. [CrossRef]
2. Rocha, G.; Ribeiro, O.; Guimaraes, H. Fluid and electrolyte balance during the first week of life and risk of bronchopulmonary dysplasia in the preterm neonate. *Clinics* **2010**, *65*, 663–674. [CrossRef] [PubMed]
3. Aperia, A.; Broberger, O.; Elinder, G.; Herin, P.; Zetterstrom, R. Postnatal development of renal function in pre-term and full-term infants. *Acta Paediatr. Scand.* **1981**, *70*, 183–187. [CrossRef] [PubMed]
4. Falcao, M.C.; Okay, Y.; Ramos, J.L. Relationship between plasma creatinine concentration and glomerular filtration in preterm newborn infants. *Rev. Hosp. Clin. Fac. Med. Sao Paulo* **1999**, *54*, 121–126. [CrossRef] [PubMed]
5. Chowdhary, V.; Vajpeyajula, R.; Jain, M.; Maqsood, S.; Raina, R.; Kumar, D.; Mhanna, M.J. Comparison of different definitions of acute kidney injury in extremely low birth weight infants. *Clin. Exp. Nephrol.* **2018**, *22*, 117–125. [CrossRef] [PubMed]
6. Raaijmakers, A.; Ortibus, E.; van Tienoven, T.P.; Vanhole, C.; Levtchenko, E.; Allegaert, K. Neonatal creatinemia trends as biomarker of subsequent cognitive outcome in extremely low birth weight neonates. *Early Hum. Dev.* **2015**, *91*, 367–372. [CrossRef]
7. Gallini, F.; Maggio, L.; Romagnoli, C.; Marrocco, G.; Tortorolo, G. Progression of renal function in preterm neonates with gestational age < or = 32 weeks. *Pediatr. Nephrol.* **2000**, *15*, 119–124. [CrossRef]
8. Lao, T.T.; Loong, E.P.; Chin, R.K.; Lam, Y.M. Renal function in the newborn. Newborn creatinine related to birth weight, maturity and maternal creatinine. *Gynecol. Obstet. Invest.* **1989**, *28*, 70–72. [CrossRef]
9. Gordjani, N.; Burghard, R.; Leititis, J.U.; Brandis, M. Serum creatinine and creatinine clearance in healthy neonates and prematures during the first 10 days of life. *Eur. J. Pediatr.* **1988**, *148*, 143–145. [CrossRef]

10. Walker, M.W.; Clark, R.H.; Spitzer, A.R. Elevation in plasma creatinine and renal failure in premature neonates without major anomalies: Terminology, occurrence and factors associated with increased risk. *J. Perinatol.* **2011**, *31*, 199–205. [CrossRef]
11. Lee, C.C.; Chan, O.W.; Lai, M.Y.; Hsu, K.H.; Wu, T.W.; Lim, W.H.; Wang, Y.C.; Lien, R. Incidence and outcomes of acute kidney injury in extremely-low-birth-weight infants. *PLoS ONE* **2017**, *12*, e0187764. [CrossRef] [PubMed]
12. Gilarska, M.; Raaijmakers, A.; Zhang, Z.Y.; Staessen, J.A.; Levtchenko, E.; Klimek, M.; Grudzien, A.; Starzec, K.; Allegaert, K.; Kwinta, P. Extremely Low Birth Weight Predisposes to Impaired Renal Health: A Pooled Analysis. *Kidney Blood Press. Res.* **2019**, *44*, 897–906. [CrossRef] [PubMed]
13. Thayyil, S.; Sheik, S.; Kempley, S.T.; Sinha, A. A gestation- and postnatal age-based reference chart for assessing renal function in extremely premature infants. *J. Perinatol.* **2008**, *28*, 226–229. [CrossRef] [PubMed]
14. Miall, L.S.; Henderson, M.J.; Turner, A.J.; Brownlee, K.G.; Brocklebank, J.T.; Newell, S.J.; Allgar, V.L. Plasma creatinine rises dramatically in the first 48 hours of life in preterm infants. *Pediatrics* **1999**, *104*, e76. [CrossRef]
15. Askenazi, D.; Abitbol, C.; Boohaker, L.; Griffin, R.; Raina, R.; Dower, J.; Davis, T.K.; Ray, P.E.; Perazzo, S.; DeFreitas, M.; et al. Optimizing the AKI definition during first postnatal week using Assessment of Worldwide Acute Kidney Injury Epidemiology in Neonates (AWAKEN) cohort. *Pediatr. Res.* **2019**, *85*, 329–338. [CrossRef]
16. Majed, B.; Bateman, D.A.; Uy, N.; Lin, F. Patent ductus arteriosus is associated with acute kidney injury in the preterm infant. *Pediatr. Nephrol.* **2019**, *34*, 1129–1139. [CrossRef]
17. Stojanovic, V.; Barisic, N.; Milanovic, B.; Doronjski, A. Acute kidney injury in preterm infants admitted to a neonatal intensive care unit. *Pediatr. Nephrol.* **2014**, *29*, 2213–2220. [CrossRef]
18. Jetton, J.G.; Boohaker, L.J.; Sethi, S.K.; Wazir, S.; Rohatgi, S.; Soranno, D.E.; Chishti, A.S.; Woroniecki, R.; Mammen, C.; Swanson, J.R.; et al. Incidence and outcomes of neonatal acute kidney injury (AWAKEN): A multicentre, multinational, observational cohort study. *Lancet Child Adolesc. Health* **2017**, *1*, 184–194. [CrossRef]
19. Shalaby, M.A.; Sawan, Z.A.; Nawawi, E.; Alsaedi, S.; Al-Wassia, H.; Kari, J.A. Incidence, risk factors, and outcome of neonatal acute kidney injury: A prospective cohort study. *Pediatr. Nephrol.* **2018**, *33*, 1617–1624. [CrossRef]
20. Viswanathan, S.; Manyam, B.; Azhibekov, T.; Mhanna, M.J. Risk factors associated with acute kidney injury in extremely low birth weight (ELBW) infants. *Pediatr. Nephrol.* **2012**, *27*, 303–311. [CrossRef]
21. Jetton, J.G.; Askenazi, D.J. Update on acute kidney injury in the neonate. *Curr. Opin. Pediatr.* **2012**, *24*, 191–196. [CrossRef] [PubMed]
22. Starr, M.C.; Boohaker, L.; Eldredge, L.C.; Menon, S.; Griffin, R.; Mayock, D.E.; Li, L.; Askenazi, D.; Hingorani, S.; Neonatal Kidney, C. Acute Kidney Injury and Bronchopulmonary Dysplasia in Premature Neonates Born Less than 32 Weeks' Gestation. *Am. J. Perinatol.* **2019**. [CrossRef] [PubMed]
23. Askenazi, D.; Patil, N.R.; Ambalavanan, N.; Balena-Borneman, J.; Lozano, D.J.; Ramani, M.; Collins, M.; Griffin, R.L. Acute kidney injury is associated with bronchopulmonary dysplasia/mortality in premature infants. *Pediatr. Nephrol.* **2015**, *30*, 1511–1518. [CrossRef]
24. Stoops, C.; Boohaker, L.; Sims, B.; Griffin, R.; Selewski, D.T.; Askenazi, D. The Association of Intraventricular Hemorrhage and Acute Kidney Injury in Premature Infants from the Assessment of the Worldwide Acute Kidney Injury Epidemiology in Neonates (AWAKEN) Study. *Neonatology* **2019**, *116*, 321–330. [CrossRef] [PubMed]
25. Rodriguez-Soriano, J.; Aguirre, M.; Oliveros, R.; Vallo, A. Long-term renal follow-up of extremely low birth weight infants. *Pediatr. Nephrol.* **2005**, *20*, 579–584. [CrossRef] [PubMed]
26. Hentschel, R.; Lodige, B.; Bulla, M. Renal insufficiency in the neonatal period. *Clin. Nephrol.* **1996**, *46*, 54–58. [PubMed]
27. Iacobelli, S.; Bonsante, F.; Ferdinus, C.; Labenne, M.; Gouyon, J.B. Factors affecting postnatal changes in serum creatinine in preterm infants with gestational age <32 weeks. *J. Perinatol.* **2009**, *29*, 232–236. [CrossRef]
28. Vanpee, M.; Ergander, U.; Herin, P.; Aperia, A. Renal function in sick, very low-birth-weight infants. *Acta Paediatr.* **1993**, *82*, 714–718. [CrossRef]
29. Weintraub, A.S.; Connors, J.; Carey, A.; Blanco, V.; Green, R.S. The spectrum of onset of acute kidney injury in premature infants less than 30 weeks gestation. *J. Perinatol.* **2016**, *36*, 474–480. [CrossRef]
30. Letshwiti, J.B.; Semberova, J.; Pichova, K.; Dempsey, E.M.; Franklin, O.M.; Miletin, J. A conservative treatment of patent ductus arteriosus in very low birth weight infants. *Early Hum. Dev.* **2017**, *104*, 45–49. [CrossRef]
31. Sung, S.I.; Chang, Y.S.; Chun, J.Y.; Yoon, S.A.; Yoo, H.S.; Ahn, S.Y.; Park, W.S. Mandatory closure versus nonintervention for patent ductus arteriosus in very preterm infants. *J. Pediatr.* **2016**, *177*, 66–71. [CrossRef] [PubMed]

32. Sung, S.I.; Chang, Y.S.; Kim, J.; Choi, J.H.; Ahn, S.Y.; Park, W.S. Natural evolution of ductus arteriosus with noninterventional conservative management in extremely preterm infants born at 23–28 weeks of gestation. *PLoS ONE* **2019**, *14*, e0212256. [CrossRef] [PubMed]
33. Kaempf, J.W.; Wu, Y.X.; Kaempf, A.J.; Kaempf, A.M.; Wang, L.; Grunkemeier, G. What happens when the patent ductus arteriosus is treated less aggressively in very low birth weight infants? *J. Perinatol.* **2012**, *32*, 344–348. [CrossRef] [PubMed]
34. Nemerofsky, S.L.; Parravicini, E.; Bateman, D.; Kleinman, C.; Polin, R.A.; Lorenz, J.M. The ductus arteriosus rarely requires treatment in infants >1000 grams. *Am. J. Perinatol.* **2008**, *25*, 661–666. [CrossRef]
35. Sung, S.I.; Ahn, S.Y.; Seo, H.J.; Yoo, H.S.; Han, Y.M.; Lee, M.S.; Chang, Y.S.; Park, W.S. Insensible water loss during the first week of life of extremely low birth weight infants less than 25 gestational weeks under high humidification. *Neonatal Med.* **2013**, *20*, 51–57. [CrossRef]
36. Park, J.H.; Chang, Y.S.; Sung, S.; Ahn, S.Y.; Park, W.S. Trends in overall mortality, and timing and cause of death among extremely preterm infants near the limit of viability. *PLoS ONE* **2017**, *12*, e0170220. [CrossRef]
37. Jobe, A.H.; Bancalari, E. Bronchopulmonary dysplasia. *Am. J. Respir. Crit. Care Med.* **2001**, *163*, 1723–1729. [CrossRef]
38. Papile, L.A.; Burstein, J.; Burstein, R.; Koffler, H. Incidence and evolution of subependymal and intraventricular hemorrhage: A study of infants with birth weights less than 1500 gm. *J. Pediatr.* **1978**, *92*, 529–534. [CrossRef]
39. Walsh, M.C.; Kliegman, R.M. Necrotizing enterocolitis: Treatment based on staging criteria. *Pediatr. Clin. N. Am.* **1986**, *33*, 179–201. [CrossRef]
40. International Committee for the Classification of Retinopathy of Prematurity. The International Classification of Retinopathy of Prematurity revisited. *Arch. Ophthalmol.* **2005**, *123*, 991–999. [CrossRef]
41. Bateman, D.A.; Thomas, W.; Parravicini, E.; Polesana, E.; Locatelli, C.; Lorenz, J.M. Serum creatinine concentration in very-low-birth-weight infants from birth to 34-36 wk postmenstrual age. *Pediatr. Res.* **2015**, *77*, 696–702. [CrossRef] [PubMed]
42. Velazquez, D.M.; Reidy, K.J.; Sharma, M.; Kim, M.; Vega, M.; Havranek, T. The effect of hemodynamically significant patent ductus arteriosus on acute kidney injury and systemic hypertension in extremely low gestational age newborns. *J. Matern. Fetal Neonatal Med.* **2019**, *32*, 3209–3214. [CrossRef] [PubMed]
43. Evans, N. Volume expansion during neonatal intensive care: Do we know what we are doing? *Semin. Neonatol.* **2003**, *8*, 315–323. [CrossRef]
44. Gawlowski, Z.; Aladangady, N.; Coen, P.G. Hypernatraemia in preterm infants born at less than 27 weeks gestation. *J. Paediatr. Child Health* **2006**, *42*, 771–774. [CrossRef]
45. Chow, J.M.; Douglas, D. Fluid and electrolyte management in the premature infant. *Neonatal Netw.* **2008**, *27*, 379–386. [CrossRef]
46. Awad, H.; el-Safty, I.; el-Barbary, M.; Imam, S. Evaluation of renal glomerular and tubular functional and structural integrity in neonates. *Am. J. Med. Sci.* **2002**, *324*, 261–266. [CrossRef]
47. Sutherland, M.R.; Gubhaju, L.; Moore, L.; Kent, A.L.; Dahlstrom, J.E.; Horne, R.S.; Hoy, W.E.; Bertram, J.F.; Black, M.J. Accelerated maturation and abnormal morphology in the preterm neonatal kidney. *J. Am. Soc. Nephrol.* **2011**, *22*, 1365–1374. [CrossRef]
48. Abbas, S.; Keir, A.K. In preterm infants, does fluid restriction, as opposed to liberal fluid prescription, reduce the risk of important morbidities and mortality? *J. Paediatr. Child Health* **2019**, *55*, 860–866. [CrossRef]
49. Cuzzolin, L.; Fanos, V.; Pinna, B.; di Marzio, M.; Perin, M.; Tramontozzi, P.; Tonetto, P.; Cataldi, L. Postnatal renal function in preterm newborns: A role of diseases, drugs and therapeutic interventions. *Pediatr. Nephrol.* **2006**, *21*, 931–938. [CrossRef]
50. Askenazi, D.J.; Koralkar, R.; Hundley, H.E.; Montesanti, A.; Patil, N.; Ambalavanan, N. Fluid overload and mortality are associated with acute kidney injury in sick near-term/term neonate. *Pediatr. Nephrol.* **2013**, *28*, 661–666. [CrossRef]
51. Foland, J.A.; Fortenberry, J.D.; Warshaw, B.L.; Pettignano, R.; Merritt, R.K.; Heard, M.L.; Rogers, K.; Reid, C.; Tanner, A.J.; Easley, K.A. Fluid overload before continuous hemofiltration and survival in critically ill children: A retrospective analysis. *Crit. Care Med.* **2004**, *32*, 1771–1776. [CrossRef] [PubMed]
52. Goldstein, S.L.; Currier, H.; Graf, C.; Cosio, C.C.; Brewer, E.D.; Sachdeva, R. Outcome in children receiving continuous venovenous hemofiltration. *Pediatrics* **2001**, *107*, 1309–1312. [CrossRef] [PubMed]

53. Goldstein, S.L.; Somers, M.J.; Baum, M.A.; Symons, J.M.; Brophy, P.D.; Blowey, D.; Bunchman, T.E.; Baker, C.; Mottes, T.; McAfee, N.; et al. Pediatric patients with multi-organ dysfunction syndrome receiving continuous renal replacement therapy. *Kidney Int.* **2005**, *67*, 653–658. [CrossRef] [PubMed]
54. Tammela, O.K.; Koivisto, M.E. Fluid restriction for preventing bronchopulmonary dysplasia? Reduced fluid intake during the first weeks of life improves the outcome of low-birth-weight infants. *Acta Paediatr.* **1992**, *81*, 207–212. [CrossRef] [PubMed]
55. Bell, E.F.; Acarregui, M.J. Restricted versus liberal water intake for preventing morbidity and mortality in preterm infants. *Cochrane Database Syst. Rev.* **2014**, *12*. [CrossRef] [PubMed]

5

Female Specific Association of Low Insulin-Like Growth Factor 1 (IGF1) Levels with Increased Risk of Premature Mortality in Renal Transplant Recipients

Frank Klont [1,*], Lyanne M. Kieneker [2], Antonio W. Gomes-Neto [2], Suzanne P. Stam [2], Nick H. T. ten Hacken [3], Ido P. Kema [4], André P. van Beek [5], Else van den Berg [2], Péter Horvatovich [1], Rainer Bischoff [1] and Stephan J. L. Bakker [2]

1 Department of Analytical Biochemistry, Groningen Research Institute of Pharmacy, University of Groningen, 9713 AV Groningen, The Netherlands; P.L.Horvatovich@rug.nl (P.H.); r.p.h.bischoff@rug.nl (R.B.)
2 Department of Internal Medicine, Division of Nephrology, University Medical Center Groningen, University of Groningen, 9700 RB Groningen, The Netherlands; l.m.kieneker@umcg.nl (L.M.K.); a.w.gomes.neto@umcg.nl (A.W.G.-N.); s.p.stam@umcg.nl (S.P.S.); elsevandenberg@hotmail.com (E.v.d.B.); s.j.l.bakker@umcg.nl (S.J.L.B.)
3 Department of Pulmonary Diseases, University Medical Center Groningen, University of Groningen, 9700 RB Groningen, The Netherlands; n.h.t.ten.hacken@umcg.nl
4 Department of Laboratory Medicine, University Medical Center Groningen, University of Groningen, 9700 RB Groningen, The Netherlands; i.p.kema@umcg.nl
5 Department of Endocrinology, University Medical Center Groningen, University of Groningen, 9700 RB Groningen, The Netherlands; a.p.van.beek@umcg.nl
* Correspondence: klont.frank@gmail.com

Abstract: Associations between insulin-like growth factor 1 (IGF1) and mortality have been reported to be female specific in mice and in human nonagenarians. Intervention in the growth hormone (GH)-IGF1 axis may particularly benefit patients with high risk of losing muscle mass, including renal transplant recipients (RTR). We investigated whether a potential association of circulating IGF1 with all-cause mortality in stable RTR could be female specific and mediated by variation in muscle mass. To this end, plasma IGF1 levels were measured in 277 female and 343 male RTR by mass spectrometry, and their association with mortality was assessed by Cox regression. During a median follow-up time of 5.4 years, 56 female and 77 male RTR died. In females, IGF1 was inversely associated with risk (hazard ratio (HR) per 1-unit increment in log2-transformed (doubling of) IGF1 levels, 95% confidence interval (CI)) of mortality (0.40, 0.24–0.65; $p < 0.001$), independent of age and the estimated Glomerular filtration rate (eGFR). In equivalent analyses, no significant association was observed for males (0.85, 0.56–1.29; $p = 0.44$), for which it should be noted that in males, age was negatively and strongly associated with IGF1 levels. The association for females remained materially unchanged upon adjustment for potential confounders and was furthermore found to be mediated for 39% by 24 h urinary creatinine excretion. In conclusion, low IGF1 levels associate with an increased risk of all-cause mortality in female RTR, which may link to conditions of low muscle mass that are known to be associated with poor outcomes in transplantation patients. For males, the strongly negative association of age with IGF1 levels may explain why low IGF1 levels were not found to be associated with an increased risk of all-cause mortality.

Keywords: insulin-like growth factor 1; growth hormone; muscle mass; patient survival; physical activity; renal transplant recipients

---

1. Introduction

The peptide hormone insulin-like growth factor 1 (IGF1) is a key mediator of the biochemical/endocrine effects of growth hormone (GH) [1]. Synthesis of IGF1 is regulated by GH and mainly takes place in the liver after which IGF1 is secreted and transported to other tissues, where it acts as an endocrine hormone [2,3]. IGF1 provides a stable, integrated measure of the activity of the somatotropic axis thereby contrasting with GH secretion which is highly variable [3].

Reduced GH and IGF1 signaling extends lifespan in many laboratory models, including worms, yeast, and drosophila [4]. A specific role for IGF1 receptor signaling in mammalian longevity was first established in IGF1 receptor-(haplo) insufficient mice. These mice lived 33% longer than their wildtype littermates, yet this effect was restricted to females [5], which was subsequently confirmed in two follow-up studies in mice [6,7]. A similar link between IGF1 receptor-insufficiency and longevity has been proposed for humans following observations in several studies [8–10]. Moreover, IGF1 levels predict better survival in nonagenarians (i.e., people between the age of 90 and 99), and, notably, the corresponding association between IGF1 levels and longevity was found to be female specific [11]. It remains, however, unclear whether circulating levels of IGF1 are also associated with longevity in middle-aged subjects and whether such association is female specific.

Studying the association between IGF1 levels and longevity (survival) in specific patient groups appears to be interesting as well, for example, following the growing interest in ghrelin receptor agonists targeting the GH-IGF1 axis to potentially reverse the anorexia–cachexia syndrome in a variety of conditions, including renal insufficiency [12–15]. An important mechanism by which stimulation of the GH-IGF1 axis may improve long-term outcome is through stimulation of muscle mass accretion [15,16]. To this regard, a large and growing group of patients that might be worthwhile studying is that of renal transplant recipients (RTR), in which protein–energy wasting is always lurking [17–19]. In fact, it has been found that the risk of premature mortality in this population is 6–7 times higher compared to the general population [20], and this risk was particularly high in RTR with low muscle mass, as reflected by low 24 h urinary creatinine excretion [21,22]. Recent studies furthermore suggested that 24 h urinary creatinine excretion may be a noninvasive, easily accessible, inexpensive, and direct measurement of total body muscle mass [19], while this measure is often not included in clinical studies to complement the imaging technique armamentarium which is applied for evaluation of muscle mass in observational and clinical intervention studies [23–25].

In this study, we aimed to investigate (1) the nature of the association between circulating levels of IGF1 and mortality in RTR, (2) whether such (potential) association is female specific, and (3) furthermore whether such (potential) association could, in part or as a whole, be mediated by variation in muscle mass, as reflected by 24 h urinary creatinine excretion.

2. Experimental Section

2.1. Study Population

All RTR (aged ≥ 18 years) that were transplanted at the University Medical Center Groningen (UMCG) and that were one year or longer post-transplantation were approached for participation in this study during outpatient clinic visits between 2008 and 2010, as described previously [26]. The RTR included in this study had no known or apparent systemic diseases (e.g., malignancies, active infections) at inclusion. Written informed consent was obtained from 707 (87%) of the 817 RTR that were initially invited, and plasma IGF1 levels were measured in 620 RTR (76%). For this study, ethical approval has been granted by the UMCG's review board (METc 2008/186), and the study adheres to the Declaration of Helsinki. The study is registered as 'TransplantLines Food and Nutrition Biobank and Cohort Study (TxL-FN)' at ClinicalTrials.gov (NCT identifier 'NCT02811835').

2.2. Data and Sample Collection

Measurement of clinical parameters has been described in detail previously [26]. Physical activity was assessed with the Short QUestionnaire to ASsess Health-enhancing physical activity (SQUASH) as developed and validated by the Dutch National Institute of Public Health and Environment to assess daily life physical activity in the Dutch adult population [27]. Information on medical history and medication use was obtained from patient records. Diabetes was defined as the use of antidiabetic medication or fasting plasma glucose of at least 7.0 mmol/L. Twenty-four h urine was collected (per strict protocol) a day before the outpatient clinic visits while blood was drawn in the morning on the day of the outpatient clinic visit, yet after completion of the 24 h urine collection.

2.3. Laboratory Procedures

Blood and urine markers were measured by routine laboratory procedures with the exception of serum creatinine which was assessed using a modified version of the Jaffé method (MEGA AU 510; Merck Diagnostica, Darmstadt, Germany), and the urine total protein concentration which was obtained using the Biuret reaction (MEGA AU 510; Merck Diagnostica). Renal function was estimated with the 2012 Chronic Kidney Disease Epidemiology (CKD-EPI) Collaboration equation using both serum creatinine and cystatin C [28]. IGF1 was assessed in plasma samples (which had not undergone any previous freeze–thaw cycle) using a semi-automated mass spectrometric IGF1 assay [29] which was validated according to FDA guidelines [30]. The samples were analyzed in 13 analytical runs containing up to 81 clinical samples per run, as well as nine calibration samples and duplicate quality control (QC) samples at three concentrations (i.e., low, midrange, and high IGF1 levels). All runs met the acceptance criteria stipulated in the FDA guidelines thereby featuring 75% (though at least six) of the calibration samples with back-calculated levels within 15% (or 20% for the lowest level calibration sample) of their expected value, and at least 67% of the QC samples (though at least one replicate per QC level) yielding IGF1 levels within 15% of their respective nominal value (see Figures S1 and S2 in the Supplementary Material).

2.4. Outcome Ascertainment

All-cause mortality was the primary outcome of this study and was recorded until the end of September 2015. Up-to-date information on patient status was obtained on the basis of a continuous surveillance system of the outpatient program. In case the status of a patient was unknown, general practitioners or referring nephrologists were contacted. There was no loss to follow-up for the outcome. Specific causes of mortality were secondary outcomes of this study. This information was obtained by linking patient numbers to the database of the Dutch Central Bureau of Statistics (CBS) to retrieve causes of mortality reported by physicians. Infectious mortality was defined as mortality from infectious causes [31]. Cardiovascular mortality was defined as mortality caused by cardiovascular pathology, coded by ICD-10 codes I10-I52 [32]. Mortality due to malignancies was defined as mortality caused by malignant diseases. Miscellaneous causes of mortality were defined as other causes of death, not included in mortality from infectious causes, cardiovascular mortality, or mortality due to malignancies.

2.5. Statistical Analyses

Data analyses were performed using IBM SPSS Statistics for Windows (version 23.0.0.0; IBM Corp., Armonk, NY, USA) and STATA/SE (version 15.1; StataCorp, College Station, TX, USA). All p-values are two-tailed, and a p-value lower than 0.050 was considered statistically significant. Baseline characteristics are presented according to tertiles of plasma IGF1 levels for female and male RTR. Continuous data are presented as mean with SD for normally distributed variables and as median with interquartile range (IQR) for variables with skewed distributions, whereas categorical variables are presented as percentages. Differences in baseline characteristics across the tertiles were tested by one-way ANOVA, Kruskal–Wallis test, and linear-by-linear association χ^2 test for normally distributed continuous, skewed continuous, and categorical variables, respectively. Multivariable linear regression was performed to assess associations between patients' characteristics and plasma IGF1 levels in female and male RTR. Models were included for analyses that were adjusted for age alone, for age and estimated glomerular filtration rate (eGFR), and for multiple variables selected following (automatic) stepwise backward elimination. The prospective associations of plasma IGF1 levels with all-cause mortality, as primary endpoint, and with cause-specific mortality, as secondary endpoint, were assessed by Cox proportional hazards regression. In order to verify the existence of effect modification by sex for the primary endpoint, we performed Cox regression analyses for the association of plasma IGF1 levels with all-cause mortality in which female and male RTR were grouped together, with additional inclusion of an interaction term of plasma IGF1 and sex in the Cox regression model. Hazard ratios (HR) and 95% confidence intervals (CIs) were calculated per 1 unit increment in log2-transformed IGF1 levels. Thereafter, we proceeded with sex-stratified prospective analyses for all-cause mortality as a primary endpoint. In addition to crude analyses, we performed analyses with adjustment for age and eGFR with and without additional physiological, lifestyle, routine clinical chemistry, transplantation, medication, and comorbidity related variables. Subsequently, we performed mediation analyses using the method as described by Preacher and Hayes, which allowed for testing the significance and magnitude of (potential) mediation [33]. In these analyses, mediation was assessed by computing bias-corrected confidence intervals upon running 2000 bootstrap samples. The proportion of mediation was obtained by dividing the indirect effect coefficient by the total effect coefficient, which were adjusted for age and eGFR. Mediation analyses were performed using IGF1 as a potential risk factor and 24 h urinary creatinine excretion, a marker of muscle mass, as potential mediator while also vice versa, because the observational nature of our study does not allow for drawing conclusions on cause–effect relationships. At last, we performed Cox-regression analyses for the association of plasma IGF1 levels with cause-specific mortality as secondary endpoints. Due to lower numbers of events, the exploratory nature of these analyses, and the generally accepted rule of thumb that allows for one variable to be included for each 7–10 events in Cox regression models [34], we performed sex-stratified crude analyses Cox regression analyses and sex-stratified age- and eGFR-adjusted analyses for the separate causes of mortality.

3. Results

3.1. RTR Characteristics

Baseline characteristics according to tertiles of plasma IGF1 levels for female and male RTR are shown in Table 1. At baseline, median IGF1 levels were 153 ng/mL (IQR: 118–196) in female and 168 ng/mL (IQR: 128–224) in male RTR (see Figure 1).

Female RTR who had higher IGF1 levels were more likely to have a larger waist circumference and a higher 24 h urinary creatinine excretion. In turn, the prevalence of diabetes mellitus as primary renal disease, the use of insulin therapy, the cumulative prednisolone dose, and the time between transplantation and baseline measurements were lower for these subjects.

For male RTR with higher levels of IGF1, subjects were more likely to be younger, to have a higher body weight and SQUASH score, and to have a lower waist circumference, prevalence of diabetes mellitus as primary renal disease, and cumulative prednisolone dose. Male RTR in the highest tertile of IGF1 levels were furthermore more likely to have received a graft from a living donor, to have undergone dialysis before transplantation, to have a shorter time between transplantation and baseline measurements, to use calcineurin inhibitors, whereas these subjects were less likely to use coumarin derivatives. Lastly, levels of serum creatinine, plasma albumin, plasma triglycerides, and 24 h urinary creatinine excretion were more likely to be higher whereas plasma aspartate transaminase (AST), gamma-glutamyltransferase (GGT), and high sensitivity C-reactive protein (hs-CRP) were more likely to be lower for these subjects.

Table 1. Baseline characteristics according to tertiles of plasma IGF1 levels in female and male RTR [1].

	Tertiles of Plasma IGF1 Levels for 277 Female RTR				Tertiles of Plasma IGF1 Levels for 343 Male RTR			
Variable	**<131 ng/mL**	**131–181 ng/mL**	**>181 ng/mL**	***p*-Value for Trend [2]**	**<141 ng/mL**	**141–202 ng/mL**	**>202 ng/mL**	***p*-Value for Trend [2]**
Age, y	56 (48–64)	54 (44–63)	54 (41–60)	0.42	59 (48–65)	55 (46–61)	49 (38–61)	<0.001
BMI, kg/m^2	25 (22–30)	26 (23–30)	27 (23–30)	0.31	25 (23–28)	26 (24–30)	26 (23–28)	0.07
Body weight, kg	67 (61–84)	73 (65–81)	74 (65–86)	0.20	80 (73–90)	86 (76–97)	84 (74–93)	0.03
Body length, cm	167 (161–171)	167 (162–173)	168 (163–171)	0.49	179 (174–183)	180 (174–184)	180 (174–185)	0.29
Waist circumference, cm	90 (78–104)	95 (87–106)	95 (88–105)	0.04	100 (91–108)	104 (94–112)	99 (89–107)	0.01
Blood pressure, systolic, mmHg	133 (121–147)	131 (120–142)	132 (124–145)	0.47	138 (127–151)	135 (124–145)	136 (125–145)	0.46
Blood pressure, diastolic, mmHg	80 ± 11	80 ± 12	82 ± 10	0.15	83 ± 10	84 ± 12	84 ± 10	0.27
Lifestyle:								
Smoking status, current, %	11.6	8.7	9.0	0.56	9.8	17.4	16.4	0.19
Alcohol consumption, yes, %	87.2	83.3	79.3	0.18	88.0	91.3	92.5	0.28
SQUASH score, ×1000	4.9 (2.6–7.6)	4.3 (1.7–7.1)	5.0 (2.0–6.7)	0.60	5.2 (1.8–7.3)	6.4 (3.0–10.7)	5.4 (2.5–9.6)	0.02
Primary renal disease:								
Primary glomerulosclerosis, %	23.9	20.4	27.2	0.60	28.9	39.5	32.2	0.61
Glomerulonephritis, %	10.9	8.6	4.3	0.10	9.6	4.4	8.7	0.79
Polycystic kidney disease, %	19.6	24.7	27.2	0.23	14.0	19.3	18.3	0.40
Renal hypoplasia/dysplasia, %	4.3	5.4	2.2	0.45	2.6	3.5	5.2	0.31
Diabetes mellitus, %	8.7	5.4	0.0	0.005	11.4	4.4	1.7	0.002
Other primary renal diseases, %	32.6	35.5	39.1	0.36	32.5	28.9	33.9	0.81
Kidney and transplantation related variables:								
eGFR, mL/min per 1.73 m^2	42 (27–57)	45 (32–57)	39 (25–51)	0.31	45 (32–61)	43 (29–55)	41 (31–55)	0.19
Serum creatinine, μmol/L	110 (87–148)	107 (87–140)	118 (96–162)	0.23	128 (102–167)	137 (115–171)	148 (116–175)	0.04
Living donor, %	28.3	40.2	39.1	0.13	26.3	31.9	42.6	0.009
Graft rejection, %	21.7	22.6	18.5	0.59	37.7	32.5	27.0	0.08
Dialysis before transplantation, %	87.0	75.3	78.3	0.14	91.2	89.5	79.1	0.007
Time between transplantation and baseline visit, y	7.5 (3.4–12.5)	5.0 (1.9–14.6)	3.7 (1.1–7.9)	0.003	7.5 (4.2–13.7)	7.0 (2.9–13.9)	2.6 (1.0–7.5)	<0.001

Table 1. *Cont.*

Variable	Tertiles of Plasma IGF1 Levels for 277 Female RTR				Tertiles of Plasma IGF1 Levels for 343 Male RTR			
	<131 ng/mL	131–181 ng/mL	>181 ng/mL	p-Value for Trend [2]	<141 ng/mL	141–202 ng/mL	>202 ng/mL	p-Value for Trend [2]
Blood markers:								
ALT, U/L	18 (13–25)	18 (13–22)	18 (13–23)	0.81	21 (16–29)	20 (16–27)	19 (14–27)	0.32
AST, U/L	23 (18–29)	22 (18–26)	20 (18–25)	0.08	24 (20–31)	22 (19–26)	21 (17–25)	<0.001
GGT, U/L	29 (19–49)	25 (16–37)	25 (18–34)	0.09	32 (21–48)	27 (19–43)	24 (18–33)	0.004
Albumin, g/L	42 (40–45)	42 (41–45)	43 (42–45)	0.10	42 (41–45)	43 (41–44)	44 (42–45)	0.003
Glucose, mmol/L	5.0 (4.6–6.2)	5.2 (4.7–5.9)	5.2 (4.7–5.6)	0.66	5.4 (4.9–6.2)	5.3 (4.9–6.2)	5.3 (5.0–5.9)	0.86
HbA1c, %	5.7 (5.4–6.0)	5.9 (5.5–6.3)	5.9 (5.5–6.3)	0.39	5.8 (5.5–6.2)	5.8 (5.5–6.3)	5.8 (5.5–6.2)	0.68
Triglycerides, mmol/L	1.7 (1.2–2.6)	1.7 (1.3–2.1)	1.7 (1.3–2.3)	0.97	1.6 (1.1–2.2)	1.7 (1.2–2.9)	1.8 (1.4–2.3)	0.03
Total cholesterol, mmol/L	5.5 (4.6–6.4)	5.1 (4.4–6.1)	5.2 (4.6–5.9)	0.32	5.1 (4.3–5.9)	4.8 (4.2–5.6)	4.8 (4.3–5.6)	0.29
HDL cholesterol, mmol/L	1.6 (1.1–1.9)	1.4 (1.2–1.8)	1.4 (1.2–1.8)	0.22	1.3 (1.1–1.6)	1.2 (0.9–1.4)	1.2 (1.0–1.4)	0.05
LDL cholesterol, mmol/L	3.0 (2.3–3.7)	3.0 (2.2–3.9)	3.0 (2.5–3.5)	0.94	2.9 (2.3–3.7)	2.8 (2.3–3.5)	2.8 (2.3–3.5)	0.43
hs-CRP, mg/L	1.8 (0.9–5.2)	2.0 (0.9–5.4)	1.7 (0.8–3.0)	0.23	1.8 (0.8–5.5)	1.9 (0.8–5.1)	1.3 (0.5–3.4)	0.03
Follicle-stimulating hormone, U/L	52 (7–90)	51 (5–81)	47 (5–78)	0.87	5.2 (3.0–11.0)	5.7 (3.8–10.7)	4.9 (2.9–8.3)	0.20
Follicle-stimulating hormone ≥ 34 U/L, yes, % [3]	64.0	65.2	63.6	0.95	3.8	5.8	1.8	0.43
Luteinizing hormone, U/L	32 (8–55)	28 (6–56)	32 (8–58)	0.95	5.0 (3.4–8.3)	5.1 (3.6–8.5)	5.1 (3.4–6.9)	0.52
Urine markers:								
Urinary creatinine excretion, mmol/24 h	8.6 (7.3–10.1)	9.6 (8.0–11.3)	10.1 (9.0–11.3)	<0.001	12.3 (10.3–14.5)	13.1 (11.0–15.4)	13.6 (11.4–15.7)	0.008
Urine total protein, g/24 h	0.14 (0.02–0.47)	0.15 (0.02–0.29)	0.15 (0.02–0.29)	0.67	0.24 (0.02–0.52)	0.25 (0.02–0.59)	0.21 (0.02–0.34)	0.29
Medication use:								
Proliferation inhibitors, yes, %	81.5	84.9	83.7	0.69	79.8	86.8	80.0	0.98
Coumarin derivatives, yes, %	14.1	9.7	7.6	0.15	16.7	11.4	7.8	0.04
Calcineurin inhibitors, yes, %	54.3	51.6	66.3	0.10	48.2	55.3	80.0	<0.001
Sirolimus, yes, %	1.2	4.5	0.0	0.55	4.6	0.9	1.0	0.07
Antihypertensive drugs, yes, %	87.0	81.7	89.1	0.67	88.6	92.1	91.3	0.48
Statins, yes, %	48.9	55.9	51.1	0.57	53.1	60.5	43.5	0.14
Diabetes, yes, %	28.3	23.7	26.1	0.74	27.2	22.8	20.0	0.20
Antidiabetics, yes, %	21.7	15.1	13.0	0.11	17.5	15.8	12.2	0.26
Metformin, yes, %	3.3	4.3	4.3	0.71	7.9	2.6	3.5	0.11
Insulin therapy, yes, %	17.4	10.8	7.6	0.04	10.5	7.9	6.1	0.22
Prednisolone, yes, %	97.8	98.9	98.9	0.54	100.0	97.4	100.0	1.00
Prednisolone, cumulative dose, g [4]	23 (10–37)	19 (6–40)	11 (4–25)	0.01	23 (14–42)	23 (10–46)	10 (4–28)	<0.001

[1] Continuous variables are reported as 'mean ± standard deviation' when normally distributed (Shapiro–Wilk test $p \geq 0.05$) or 'median (interquartile range)' when not normally distributed (Shapiro–Wilk test $p < 0.05$), and categorical variables are reported as percentage. [2] Determined by linear-by-linear association χ^2 test (categorical variables), Kruskal–Wallis test (continuous variables, not normally distributed), or one-way ANOVA (continuous variables, normally distributed). [3] A follicle-stimulating hormone cut-off level of ≥ 34 U/L was used to derive a surrogate marker of post-menopause [35]. Abbreviations: ALT: Alanine transaminase; AST: Aspartate transaminase; BMI: Body mass index; eGFR: Estimated glomerular filtration rate; GGT: Gamma-glutamyltransferase; HbA1c: Glycated hemoglobin; HDL: High-density lipoprotein; hs-CRP: High sensitivity C-reactive protein; LDL: Low-density lipoprotein; SQUASH: Short QUestionnaire to ASsess Health-enhancing physical activity [27]. [4] The cumulative dose of prednisolone was calculated as the sum of the maintenance dose of prednisolone until inclusion and the dose of prednisolone or methylprednisolone required for treatment of acute rejection (a conversion factor of 1.25 was used to convert methylprednisolone dose to its prednisolone dose equivalent).

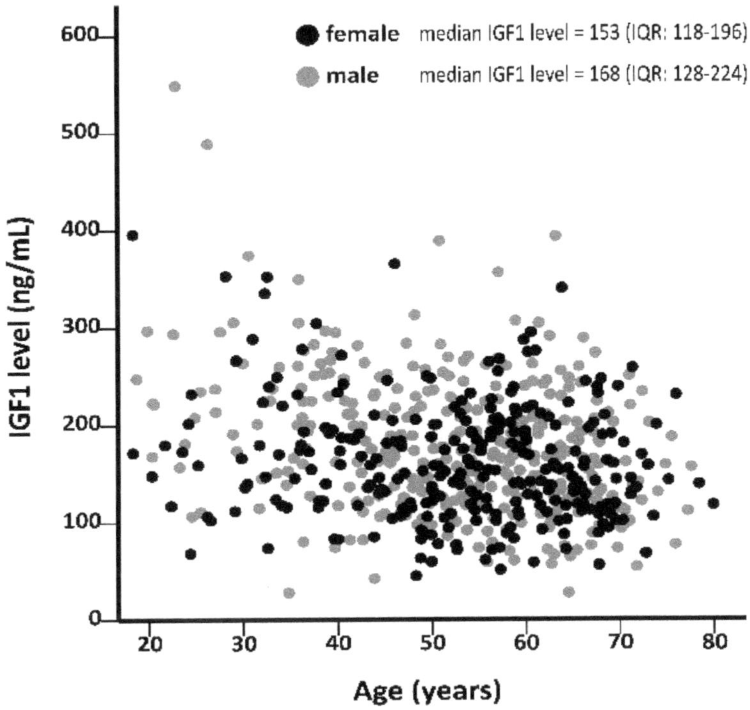

Figure 1. Association between insulin-like growth factor 1 (IGF1) levels and age for female and male renal transplant recipients (RTR).

3.2. Association of Plasma IGF1 with Selected Variables in RTR

Associations between plasma IGF1 levels and variables of interest adjusted for age alone, for age and eGFR, and for multiple variables which were selected following stepwise backward elimination are shown in Table 2.

For female RTR, the analyses adjusted for age featured positive and significant associations between plasma IGF1 and body weight, 24 h urinary creatinine excretion, and calcineurin inhibitor use. Significant inverse associations with plasma IGF1, independent of age, were observed for the prevalence of diabetes mellitus as primary renal disease, the time between transplantation and baseline measurements, the cumulative prednisolone dose, and GGT. After further adjustment for eGFR, the magnitude, direction, and significance of all associations generally remained the same. The final stepwise backward model featured an adjusted R^2 of 0.14 and revealed significant positive associations between plasma IGF1 and both 24 h urinary creatinine excretion and calcineurin inhibitor use, but also significant inverse associations with the prevalence of diabetes mellitus as primary renal disease, GGT, HDL cholesterol, and hs-CRP.

For male RTR, analyses adjusted for age showed significant positive associations between plasma IGF1 and both albumin and calcineurin inhibitor use. Significant inverse associations were observed between plasma IGF1 and eGFR, the prevalence of diabetes mellitus as primary renal disease, the cumulative prednisolone dose, AST, and GGT, and the time between transplantation and baseline measurements. Further adjustment for eGFR did not lead to major changes in the magnitude, direction, or significance of these associations. Lastly, an adjusted R^2 of 0.28 was obtained for the final stepwise backward model which featured significant positive associations between plasma IGF1 and both albumin and calcineurin inhibitor use. Significant inverse associations were furthermore revealed between plasma IGF1 and age, eGFR, the prevalence of diabetes mellitus as primary renal disease, and GGT.

Table 2. Multivariable linear regression analysis with plasma IGF1 as the dependent variable in female and male RTR [1].

	Female RTR (N = 277)						Male RTR (N = 343)					
	Age Adjusted		Age and eGFR Adjusted		Backward (adj. R^2 = 0.14)		Age Adjusted		Age and eGFR Adjusted		Backward (adj. R^2 = 0.28)	
Variable	Stand. β	*p*-Value	Stand. β	*p*-Value	Stand. β	*p*-Value	Stand. β	*p*-Value	Stand. β	*p*-Value	Stand. β	*p*-Value
Age, y	−0.16	0.007	−0.17	0.006			−0.32	<0.001	−0.35	<0.001	−0.27	<0.001
eGFR, mL/min per 1.73 m^2	−0.05	0.37	−0.05	0.37			−0.18	0.001	−0.18	0.001	−0.19	0.001
Body weight, kg	0.12	0.05	0.11	0.06			0.01	0.87	−0.01	0.88		
Body length, cm	0.09	0.14	0.09	0.14			0.00	0.97	−0.02	0.74		
SQUASH score	−0.05	0.43	−0.04	0.49	−0.11	0.09	0.02	0.64	0.05	0.38		
Diabetes mellitus, yes vs. no	−0.13	0.04	−0.13	0.03	−0.13	0.04	−0.12	0.02	−0.14	0.008	−0.13	0.009
Living donor, yes vs. no	0.02	0.71	0.03	0.63			0.02	0.66	0.04	0.44		
Graft rejection, yes vs. no	−0.05	0.37	−0.07	0.28			−0.10	0.06	−0.10	0.05	−0.09	0.06
Dialysis before transplantation, yes vs. no	0.07	0.28	0.07	0.23			0.05	0.39	0.06	0.26		
Time between transplantation and baseline visit, y	−0.14	0.02	−0.14	0.02			−0.15	0.003	−0.15	0.004		
AST, U/L	−0.09	0.16	−0.09	0.16			−0.21	<0.001	−0.15	0.005	−0.10	0.06
GGT, U/L	−0.12	0.04	−0.13	0.03	−0.14	0.02	−0.22	<0.001	−0.20	<0.001	−0.18	0.001
Albumin, g/L	0.09	0.15	0.10	0.11			0.12	0.03	0.17	0.003	0.15	0.01
Triglycerides, mmol/L	−0.06	0.36	−0.07	0.23	−0.11	0.10	0.09	0.08	0.06	0.26		
HDL cholesterol, mmol/L	−0.08	0.20	−0.07	0.27	−0.14	0.03	−0.09	0.08	−0.05	0.32		
hs-CRP, mg/L	−0.10	0.09	−0.10	0.09	−0.15	0.01	−0.04	0.49	−0.06	0.22		
Urinary creatinine excretion, mmol/24 h	0.24	<0.001	0.25	<0.001	0.25	<0.001	0.07	0.19	0.06	0.22		
Coumarin derivatives, yes vs. no	−0.09	0.13	−0.10	0.11			−0.02	0.67	−0.05	0.34		
Calcineurin inhibitors, yes vs. no	0.15	0.01	0.15	0.02	0.16	0.01	0.20	<0.001	0.16	0.003	0.18	0.001
Sirolimus, yes vs. no	−0.07	0.23	−0.07	0.23			−0.06	0.24	−0.05	0.30		
Insulin therapy, yes vs. no	−0.10	0.10	−0.11	0.08			−0.06	0.26	−0.07	0.19		
Prednisolone, cumulative dose, g [2]	−0.12	0.05	−0.12	0.05			−0.13	0.01	−0.13	0.01		

[1] Variables showing *p*-values below 0.10 for the trend of tertiles of IGF1 in at least one of the sexes (see Table 1), with the exception of highly correlated variables (e.g., BMI, waist circumference, serum creatinine), as well as body weight and body height were included for multivariable linear regression analysis. Abbreviations: AST: Aspartate transaminase; eGFR: Estimated glomerular filtration rate; GGT: Gamma-glutamyltransferase; HDL: High-density lipoprotein; hs-CRP: High sensitivity C-reactive protein; SQUASH: Short QUestionnaire to ASsess Health-enhancing physical activity [27]. [2] The cumulative dose of prednisolone was calculated as the sum of the maintenance dose of prednisolone until inclusion and the dose of prednisolone or methylprednisolone required for treatment of acute rejection (a conversion factor of 1.25 was used to convert the methylprednisolone dose to its prednisolone dose equivalent).

3.3. *Association of Plasma IGF1 with All-Cause Mortality in RTR*

Median follow-up was 5.4 years (IQR: 4.8–6.0 years) for female and 5.4 years (IQR: 4.8–6.3 years) for male RTR. During this prospective follow-up, 56 female and 77 male RTR died. We first investigated whether the association of plasma IGF1 levels with all-cause mortality was modified by sex. In these analyses, with data of female and male RTR combined, we found that higher plasma IGF1 levels were associated with a significantly decreased risk (HR per log2 increment of plasma IGF1, 95% CI) of all-cause mortality (0.61, 0.47–0.80; $p < 0.001$). Furthermore, inclusion of a product-term of (log2-transformed plasma) IGF1 levels and sex in the basic multivariable model (i.e., with adjustment for age and eGFR) revealed the existence of significant effect modification by sex (p for interaction = 0.02). After finding this significant interaction by sex, we proceeded with sex-stratified analyses of the association of (log2-transformed) plasma IGF1 levels with all-cause mortality. For female RTR, the crude analyses showed that higher plasma IGF1 levels were associated with a significantly decreased risk of all-cause mortality (0.42, 0.26–0.66; $p < 0.001$; see Figure 2 and Table 3), while a nonsignificant trend towards a decreased risk was observed for male RTR (0.74, 0.52–1.04; $p = 0.09$; see Table 3 and Figure 2).

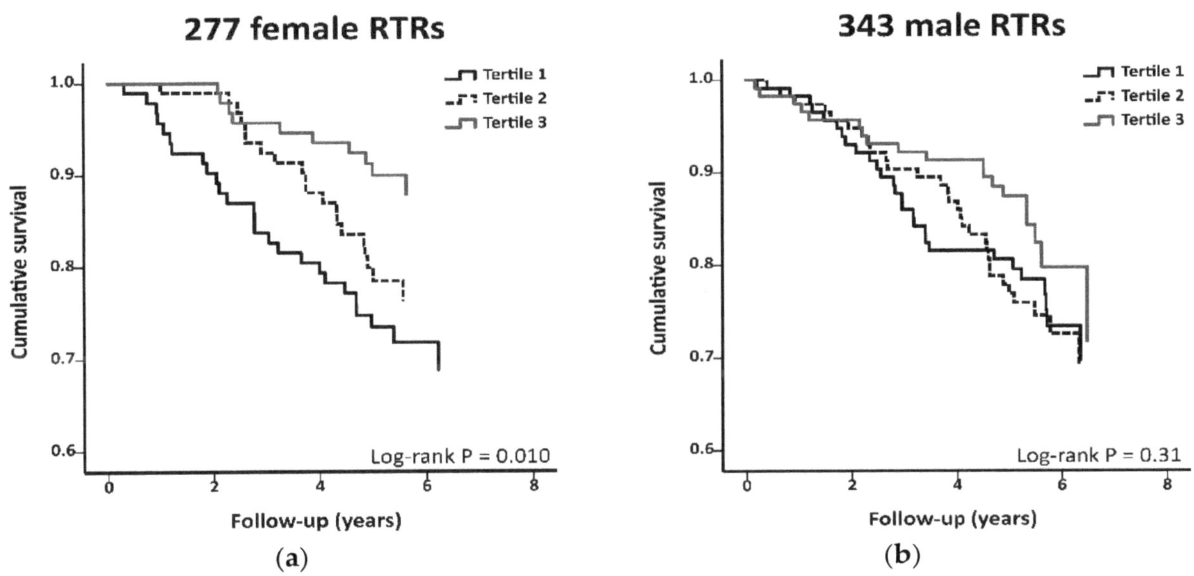

Figure 2. Kaplan–Meier curves for all-cause mortality according to tertiles of plasma insulin-like growth factor 1 (IGF1) in (**a**) female and (**b**) male renal transplant recipients (RTR). For female RTR, IGF1 levels of the tertiles 1, 2, and 3 are below 131 ng/mL, range between 131 and 181 ng/mL, and are above 181 ng/mL, respectively. For male RTR, IGF1 levels of the tertiles 1, 2, and 3 are below 141 ng/mL, range between 141 and 202 ng/mL, and are above 202 ng/mL, respectively.

In the model with adjustment for age and eGFR, the significant inverse association of IGF1 with all-cause mortality remained in female RTR (0.40, 0.24–0.65; $p < 0.001$) and the association in male RTR remained insignificant (0.85, 0.56–1.29; $p = 0.44$). Further adjustment for potential confounders, which was assessed based on seven different multivariable models, did not substantially affect the associations between plasma IGF1 and mortality for both female and male subjects (see Table 3). Lastly, mediation analysis (according to the procedures of Preacher and Hayes [33]) was carried out for the female subjects and revealed 24 h urinary creatinine excretion as significant mediator (p-value for indirect effect < 0.05) accounting for 39% on the association between plasma IGF1 and all-cause mortality (see Table 4). Since the observational nature of our study does not allow for drawing conclusions regarding cause–effect relationships, we also performed alternative mediation analyses with 24 h urinary creatinine excretion as potential risk factors and plasma IGF1 levels as potential mediators. In these analyses, we found that plasma IGF1 levels as significant mediators (p-value for indirect effect

< 0.05) accounted for 9% on the association between 24 h urinary creatinine excretion and all-cause mortality (see Supplemental Table S5).

Table 3. Association between log2-transformed plasma IGF1 levels and the risk of all-cause mortality in female and male RTR [1].

	277 Female RTR (56 Events)			343 Male RTR (77 Events)		
Variable	**HR (log2)**	**95% CI**	***p*-Value**	**HR (log2)**	**95% CI**	***p*-Value**
Crude model	0.42	0.26–0.66	<0.001	0.74	0.52–1.04	0.09
Model 1 [2]	0.40	0.24–0.65	<0.001	0.85	0.56–1.29	0.44
Model 2 [3]	0.47	0.27–0.81	0.006	0.88	0.58–1.34	0.55
Model 3 [4]	0.33	0.16–0.64	0.001	0.88	0.54–1.42	0.60
Model 4 [5]	0.38	0.23–0.63	<0.001	0.81	0.51–1.27	0.35
Model 5 [6]	0.39	0.24–0.65	<0.001	0.87	0.57–1.32	0.50
Model 6 [7]	0.34	0.20–0.57	<0.001	0.94	0.61–1.45	0.78
Model 7 [8]	0.36	0.21–0.61	<0.001	1.06	0.66–1.69	0.82
Model 8 [9]	0.41	0.24–0.69	0.001	0.85	0.55–1.29	0.44

[1] Hazard ratios (HR) per 1 unit increment in log2-transformed plasma IGF1 levels and corresponding 95% confidence intervals (CI) were derived from Cox proportional hazards models. [2] Multivariable model adjusted for age and estimated glomerular filtration rate (eGFR). [3] Multivariable model adjusted for age, eGFR, body length, body weight, waist circumference, systolic blood pressure, and diastolic blood pressure. [4] Multivariable model adjusted for age, eGFR, smoking status, alcohol consumption, and Short QUestionnaire to ASsess Health-enhancing physical activity (SQUASH) score [27]. [5] Multivariable model adjusted for age, eGFR, glucose, glycated hemoglobin (HbA1c), triglycerides, serum total cholesterol, high-density lipoprotein (HDL) cholesterol, and low-density lipoprotein (LDL) cholesterol. [6] Multivariable model adjusted for age, eGFR, serum creatinine, and urine total protein. [7] Multivariable model adjusted for age, eGFR, primary renal disease, graft rejection, dialysis before transplantation, time between transplantation and baseline visit, and donor status. [8] Multivariable model adjusted for age, eGFR, aspartate transaminase (AST), gamma-glutamyltransferase (GGT), serum albumin, high sensitivity C-reactive protein (hs-CRP), follicle-stimulating hormone, and luteinizing hormone. [9] Multivariable model adjusted for age, eGFR, antidiabetics, antihypertensive drugs, coumarin derivatives, proliferation inhibitors, calcineurin inhibitors, insulin, and prednisolone.

Table 4. Mediation analysis of the relationship between plasma IGF1, 24 h urinary creatinine excretion, and all-cause mortality in female RTR.

		Multivariable Model [1]	
Potential Mediator	**Effect [2]**	**Coefficient (95% CI, *bc*) [3]**	**Proportion Mediated [4]**
24 h urinary creatinine excretion	indirect effect (*ab* path)	−0.11 (−0.18–−0.06)	39.3%
	direct effect (*c′* path)	−0.17 (−0.33–−0.02)	
	total effect (*ab* + *c′* path)	−0.28 (−0.44–−0.12)	

[1] Coefficients and corresponding 95% confidence intervals (CI) of the indirect and total effects are standardized for the standard deviations of the potential mediator, plasma IGF1, and all-cause mortality. [2] Coefficients are adjusted for age and estimated glomerular filtration rate (eGFR). [3] 95% CIs for the indirect and total effects are bias-corrected confidence intervals after running 2000 bootstrap samples. [4] The size of (statistically significant) mediated effects is calculated by dividing the standardized indirect effect by the standardized total effect followed by multiplication by 100.

3.4. *Association of Plasma IGF1 with Cause-Specific Mortality in RTR*

Next, we performed sex-stratified analyses of the association of log2-transformed plasma IGF1 levels with mortality from specific causes of death, namely death from infectious diseases, cardiovascular mortality, death from malignancies, and other, miscellaneous causes of death. In females, we found that higher plasma IGF1 levels were strongly associated with a significantly decreased risk of infectious disease-related mortality (0.17, 0.07–0.38; $p < 0.001$; see Supplemental Table S1, Model 1). In females, we also found a borderline significant association of higher plasma IGF1 levels with cardiovascular mortality (0.43, 0.18–1.00; $p = 0.05$; see Supplemental Table S2, Model 1), but neither a significant association with cancer-related mortality (1.50, 0.45–4.93; $p = 0.51$; see Supplemental Table S3, Model 1), nor with mortality from miscellaneous causes (0.43, 0.10–1.78; $p = 0.24$; see Supplemental Table

S4, Model 1). In males, no significant associations with cause-specific mortality were encountered (see respective Supplemental Tables S1–S4).

4. Discussion

This study showed that low plasma IGF1 levels were independently associated with an increased risk of all-cause mortality in female RTR. Such association was less pronounced and insignificant in male RTR, which should be seen in the context of IGF1 levels being negatively and strongly associated with age in males, which may explain why low plasma IGF1 levels were not associated with mortality in males. Adjustment for potential confounders did not alter the association observed in women, and 39% of this association was found to be mediated by 24 h urinary creatinine excretion, a marker of muscle mass. In alternative analyses, we found that 9% of the association of urinary creatinine excretion with mortality in women was mediated by plasma IGF1 levels. In secondary analyses, in which the association of plasma IGF1 with cause-specific mortality was assessed, we found a particularly strong association of low plasma IGF1 levels with increased risk of mortality due to infectious causes in females.

To our knowledge, this is the first study that investigated the association between IGF1 and long-term outcomes in RTR, hence we were limited in comparing our study with existing literature. Studies addressing associations between IGF1 and outcomes in other clinical settings are available, yet such studies are scarce and generally do not assess female and male subjects separately. When attempting to compare our results to studies on IGF1 in which both sexes were analyzed separately, we found inconsistent evidence. For example, in a cross-sectional study of 5388 US adults, the magnitude of the (positive) association between high IGF1 levels and the risk of chronic kidney disease was found to be stronger for males than for females [36]. In addition, a study of 183 healthy nonagenarians (i.e., people between the age of 90 and 99) reported a significant association between low IGF1 levels and longer survival in female subjects which was not observed for males [11]. Recently, a prospective population-based study on 1618 elderly adults reported that men featured greater decreases in IGF1 and its most important binding protein (i.e., IGF binding protein 3) with age as compared to females [37]. A recently described cross-sectional study on 200 elderly subjects furthermore reported a (negative) association between IGF1 levels and co-existent frailty and low muscle mass in female subjects whereas such association was not found for male subjects [38]. The difference between females and males as we observed in our study therefore links to previous data but also connects to why gender-specific reference ranges for IGF1 are being employed in routine clinical practice [39–41]. It should, however, be noted that all these results were obtained using different analytical methods, and it is known that different methods may yield different analyte levels, particularly in the case of IGF1 [42,43]. Moreover, IGF1 predominantly circulates being bound to IGF binding proteins [44], and the efficiency of dissociating such complexes may vary between (immuno)assays from different vendors and thereby lead to biased, or at least to incomparable results [45].

With respect to the observed association between IGF1 and mortality in female RTR, several other findings which were put forward in our study should be taken into consideration. Firstly, the identification of 24 h urinary creatinine excretion as a strong mediator in this association represents an interesting finding of our study. The fact that 24 h urinary creatinine is a widely available and accepted marker reflecting muscle mass [46–48] and the recognition of IGF1 as a growth hormone involved in muscle growth [49,50] support the biological plausibility of a link between IGF1 and physical fitness. Low physical activity is, in fact, known to be a risk factor for morbidity and mortality in RTR [51–53], hence further studies on IGF1 in this context are warranted. Secondly, the significant association between IGF1 and the use of calcineurin inhibitors should be viewed in this context as well. The target of these drugs, calcineurin, has been described as a regulator of muscle mass, although it should be noted that much is still unknown about the underlying mechanisms [54–56]. Thirdly, the observed strongly significant association of higher plasma IGF1 levels with lower risk for infectious disease-related mortality may be interesting as well in this regard. At last, it should be noted that evidence for a potential link between IGF1 and physical fitness is currently still circumstantial and that further research is needed to verify and explore our findings.

Important limitations of this study include the facts that it represents a single-center study and that it addresses a population consisting mainly of Caucasian participants. It is unknown whether our findings can be extrapolated to other populations, and repeating this study in other populations is therefore desirable. Moreover, there may be untested or residual confounding relevant for the observed association, as is often true for observational studies. Moreover, laboratory markers were analyzed only once at baseline, hence corresponding changes over time could not be addressed in the present study. With respect to the IGF1 measurements, it should be noted that measurements were carried out using biobanked samples which had been stored for several years at −80 °C. Sample stability parameters (e.g., freeze-thaw stability, benchtop stability) were addressed during validation of our IGF1 method thereby following the US Food and Drug Administration (FDA) guidelines on bioanalytical method validation [30]. Nonetheless, storage conditions comparable to those applying to the long-term stored plasma samples could not possibly be addressed during validation, as is often the case when targeting biobanked samples. We could, however, monitor the extent of IGF1 oxidation which represents a prominent feature of our mass spectrometric IGF1 assay [29] considering that protein oxidation is a (unwanted) chemical modification occurring during storage of proteins [57]; yet, no abnormalities in IGF1 oxidation were observed. In order to reduce the (potential) impact of corresponding pre-analytical variability on the quality of our data, we only included samples which had not undergone any previous freeze–thaw cycle and we verified that the samples had not been exposed to deviating storage conditions, for example caused by power outages or freezer malfunctions.

Strengths of this study are its prospective design, the relatively large cohort of well-characterized, stable RTR, the complete follow-up for all-cause mortality, the availability of detailed data on potential confounders, and the use of a mass spectrometric IGF1 assay which allowed for highly selective IGF1 quantification.

In conclusion, low plasma IGF1 levels were found to be associated with an increased risk of all-cause mortality in female RTR, and this association was not found (to be significant) for male RTR. The association in females was mediated for a substantial proportion by 24 h urinary creatinine excretion which hints at a possible link with conditions of low muscle mass (e.g., poor physical fitness, poor nutritional state). Secondary analyses pointed towards a particularly strong association of low plasma IGF1 levels with mortality from infectious causes. Further research is, however, needed to explore the existence and/or relevance of such a link, and also to investigate whether IGF1 can be useful as a (predictive) marker of mortality in female RTR possibly by reflecting physical fitness in this population.

Supplementary Materials:
Figure S1: Overview of calibration data for the thirteen runs carried out for quantification of insulin-like growth factor 1 (IGF1) in the clinical samples. Figure S2: Overview of the quality control data obtained during the thirteen runs carried out for quantification of insulin-like growth factor 1 (IGF1) in the clinical samples. Table S1: Association between log2-transformed plasma IGF1 levels and the risk of infectious disease-related mortality in female and male RTR. Table S2: Association between log2-transformed plasma IGF1 levels and the risk of cardiovascular mortality in female and male RTR. Table S3: Association between log2-transformed plasma IGF1 levels and the risk of cancer-related mortality in female and male RTR. Table S4: Association between log2-transformed plasma IGF1 levels and the risk of miscellaneous-cause mortality in female and male RTR. Table S5: Mediation analysis of the relationship between 24 h urinary creatinine excretion, plasma IGF1 levels, and all-cause mortality in female RTR.

Author Contributions: F.K., N.H.T.t.H., P.H., R.B., and S.J.L.B.; Methodology, F.K., L.M.K., A.W.G.-N., S.P.S., N.H.T.t.H., I.P.K., A.P.v.B., E.v.d.B., P.H., R.B., and S.J.L.B.; Formal analysis, F.K., L.M.K., P.H., and S.J.L.B.; Data curation, F.K., L.M.K., A.W.G.-N., S.P.S., E.v.d.B., and S.J.L.B.; Writing—original draft preparation, F.K., L.M.K.,

R.B., and S.J.L.B.; Writing—review and editing, F.K., L.M.K., A.W.G.-N., S.P.S., N.H.T.t.H., I.P.K., A.P.v.B., E.v.d.B., P.H., R.B., and S.J.L.B.; Supervision, R.B. and S.J.L.B.; Funding acquisition, N.H.T.t.H., R.B., and S.J.L.B. All authors have read and agreed to the published version of the manuscript.

Acknowledgments: The authors gratefully acknowledge the Dutch Biomarker Development Center (BDC; http://www.biomarkerdevelopmentcenter.nl/) for support of this work.

References

1. Sowers, M.R.; Zheng, H.; McConnell, D.; Nan, B.; Harlow, S.; Randolph, J.F., Jr. Follicle stimulating hormone and its rate of change in defining menopause transition stages. *J. Clin. Endocrinol. Metab.* **2008**, *93*, 3958–3964. [CrossRef] [PubMed]
2. Ketha, H.; Singh, R.J. Clinical assays for quantitation of insulin-like-growth-factor-1 (IGF1). *Methods* **2015**, *81*, 93–98. [CrossRef] [PubMed]
3. Laron, Z. Insulin-like growth factor 1 (IGF-1): A growth hormone. *Mol. Pathol.* **2001**, *54*, 311–316. [CrossRef]
4. Bidlingmaier, M. Pitfalls of insulin-like growth factor I assays. *Horm. Res.* **2009**, *71* (Suppl. S1), 30–33. [CrossRef]
5. Mao, K.; Quipildor, G.F.; Tabrizian, T.; Novaj, A.; Guan, F.; Walters, R.O.; Delahaye, F.; Hubbard, G.B.; Ikeno, Y.; Ejima, K.; et al. Late-Life targeting of the IGF-1 receptor improves healthspan and lifespan in female mice. *Nat. Commun.* **2018**, *9*, 2394. [CrossRef]
6. Holzenberger, M.; Dupont, J.; Ducos, B.; Leneuve, P.; Geloen, A.; Even, P.C.; Cervera, P.; Le Bouc, Y. IGF-1 receptor regulates lifespan and resistance to oxidative stress in mice. *Nature* **2003**, *421*, 182–187. [CrossRef]
7. Bokov, A.F.; Garg, N.; Ikeno, Y.; Thakur, S.; Musi, N.; DeFronzo, R.A.; Zhang, N.; Erickson, R.C.; Gelfond, J.; Hubbard, G.B.; et al. Does reduced IGF-1R signaling in Igf1r+/− mice alter aging? *PLoS ONE* **2011**, *6*, e26891. [CrossRef]
8. Xu, J.; Gontier, G.; Chaker, Z.; Lacube, P.; Dupont, J.; Holzenberger, M. Longevity effect of IGF-1R(+/−) mutation depends on genetic background-specific receptor activation. *Aging Cell* **2014**, *13*, 19–28. [CrossRef]
9. Suh, Y.; Atzmon, G.; Cho, M.O.; Hwang, D.; Liu, B.; Leahy, D.J.; Barzilai, N.; Cohen, P. Functionally significant insulin-like growth factor I receptor mutations in centenarians. *Proc. Natl. Acad. Sci. USA* **2008**, *105*, 3438–3442. [CrossRef]
10. Tazearslan, C.; Huang, J.; Barzilai, N.; Suh, Y. Impaired IGF1R signaling in cells expressing longevity-associated human IGF1R alleles. *Aging Cell* **2011**, *10*, 551–554. [CrossRef]
11. Milman, S.; Huffman, D.M.; Barzilai, N. The somatotropic axis in human aging: Framework for the current state of knowledge and future research. *Cell. Metab.* **2016**, *23*, 980–989. [CrossRef] [PubMed]
12. Milman, S.; Atzmon, G.; Huffman, D.M.; Wan, J.; Crandall, J.P.; Cohen, P.; Barzilai, N. Low insulin-like growth factor-1 level predicts survival in humans with exceptional longevity. *Aging Cell* **2014**, *13*, 769–771. [CrossRef]
13. Pietra, C.; Takeda, Y.; Tazawa-Ogata, N.; Minami, M.; Yuanfeng, X.; Duus, E.M.; Northrup, R. Anamorelin HCl (ONO-7643), a novel ghrelin receptor agonist, for the treatment of cancer anorexia-cachexia syndrome: Preclinical profile. *J. Cachexia Sarcopenia Muscle* **2014**, *5*, 329–337. [CrossRef] [PubMed]
14. Esposito, A.; Criscitiello, C.; Gelao, L.; Pravettoni, G.; Locatelli, M.; Minchella, I.; Di Leo, M.; Liuzzi, R.; Milani, A.; Massaro, M.; et al. Mechanisms of anorexia-cachexia syndrome and rational for treatment with selective ghrelin receptor agonist. *Cancer Treat. Rev.* **2015**, *41*, 793–797. [CrossRef] [PubMed]
15. Borner, T.; Loi, L.; Pietra, C.; Giuliano, C.; Lutz, T.A.; Riediger, T. The ghrelin receptor agonist HM01 mimics the neuronal effects of ghrelin in the arcuate nucleus and attenuates anorexia-cachexia syndrome in tumor-bearing rats. *Am. J. Physiol. Regul. Integr. Comp. Physiol.* **2016**, *311*, R89–R96. [CrossRef] [PubMed]
16. Campbell, G.A.; Patrie, J.T.; Gaylinn, B.D.; Thorner, M.O.; Bolton, W.K. Oral ghrelin receptor agonist MK-0677 increases serum insulin-like growth factor 1 in hemodialysis patients: A randomized blinded study. *Nephrol. Dial. Transplant.* **2018**, *33*, 523–530. [CrossRef]
17. Florini, J.R.; Ewton, D.Z.; Magri, K.A. Hormones, growth factors, and myogenic differentiation. *Annu. Rev. Physiol.* **1991**, *53*, 201–216. [CrossRef]

18. Molnar, M.Z.; Czira, M.E.; Rudas, A.; Ujszaszi, A.; Haromszeki, B.; Kosa, J.P.; Lakatos, P.; Beko, G.; Sarvary, E.; Varga, M.; et al. Association between the malnutrition-inflammation score and post-transplant anaemia. *Nephrol. Dial. Transplant.* **2011**, *26*, 2000–2006. [CrossRef]
19. Molnar, M.Z.; Czira, M.E.; Rudas, A.; Ujszaszi, A.; Lindner, A.; Fornadi, K.; Kiss, I.; Remport, A.; Novak, M.; Kennedy, S.H.; et al. Association of the malnutrition-inflammation score with clinical outcomes in kidney transplant recipients. *Am. J. Kidney Dis.* **2011**, *58*, 101–108. [CrossRef]
20. Stam, S.P.; Eisenga, M.F.; Gomes Neto, A.W.; Van Londen, M.; De Meijer, V.E.; Van Beek, A.P.; Gansevoort, R.T.; Bakker, S.J.L. Muscle mass determined from urinary creatinine excretion rate, and muscle performance in renal transplant recipients. *J. Cachexia Sarcopenia Muscle* **2019**, *10*, 621–629. [CrossRef]
21. Oterdoom, L.H.; de Vries, A.P.; van Ree, R.M.; Gansevoort, R.T.; van Son, W.J.; van der Heide, J.J.; Navis, G.; de Jong, P.E.; Gans, R.O.; Bakker, S.J. N-terminal pro-B-type natriuretic peptide and mortality in renal transplant recipients versus the general population. *Transplantation* **2009**, *87*, 1562–1570. [CrossRef] [PubMed]
22. Oterdoom, L.H.; van Ree, R.M.; de Vries, A.P.; Gansevoort, R.T.; Schouten, J.P.; van Son, W.J.; Homan van der Heide, J.J.; Navis, G.; de Jong, P.E.; Gans, R.O.; et al. Urinary creatinine excretion reflecting muscle mass is a predictor of mortality and graft loss in renal transplant recipients. *Transplantation* **2008**, *86*, 391–398. [CrossRef] [PubMed]
23. Said, M.Y.; Deetman, P.E.; de Vries, A.P.; Zelle, D.M.; Gans, R.O.; Navis, G.; Joosten, M.M.; Bakker, S.J. Causal path analyses of the association of protein intake with risk of mortality and graft failure in renal transplant recipients. *Clin. Transplant.* **2015**, *29*, 447–457. [CrossRef] [PubMed]
24. Tyrovolas, S.; Koyanagi, A.; Olaya, B.; Ayuso-Mateos, J.L.; Miret, M.; Chatterji, S.; Tobiasz-Adamczyk, B.; Koskinen, S.; Leonardi, M.; Haro, J.M. Factors associated with skeletal muscle mass, sarcopenia, and sarcopenic obesity in older adults: A multi-continent study. *J. Cachexia Sarcopenia Muscle* **2016**, *7*, 312–321. [CrossRef]
25. Chu, M.P.; Lieffers, J.; Ghosh, S.; Belch, A.; Chua, N.S.; Fontaine, A.; Sangha, R.; Turner, R.A.; Baracos, V.E.; Sawyer, M.B. Skeletal muscle density is an independent predictor of diffuse large B-cell lymphoma outcomes treated with rituximab-based chemoimmunotherapy. *J. Cachexia Sarcopenia Muscle* **2017**, *8*, 298–304. [CrossRef] [PubMed]
26. Makizako, H.; Shimada, H.; Doi, T.; Tsutsumimoto, K.; Lee, S.; Lee, S.C.; Harada, K.; Hotta, R.; Nakakubo, S.; Bae, S.; et al. Age-dependent changes in physical performance and body composition in community-dwelling Japanese older adults. *J. Cachexia Sarcopenia Muscle* **2017**, *8*, 607–614. [CrossRef]
27. Van den Berg, E.; Pasch, A.; Westendorp, W.H.; Navis, G.; Brink, E.J.; Gans, R.O.; van Goor, H.; Bakker, S.J. Urinary sulfur metabolites associate with a favorable cardiovascular risk profile and survival benefit in renal transplant recipients. *J. Am. Soc. Nephrol.* **2014**, *25*, 1303–1312. [CrossRef]
28. Wendel-Vos, G.C.; Schuit, A.J.; Saris, W.H.; Kromhout, D. Reproducibility and relative validity of the short questionnaire to assess health-enhancing physical activity. *J. Clin. Epidemiol.* **2003**, *56*, 1163–1169. [CrossRef]
29. Inker, L.A.; Schmid, C.H.; Tighiouart, H.; Eckfeldt, J.H.; Feldman, H.I.; Greene, T.; Kusek, J.W.; Manzi, J.; Van Lente, F.; Zhang, Y.L.; et al. Estimating glomerular filtration rate from serum creatinine and cystatin C. *N. Engl. J. Med.* **2012**, *367*, 20–29. [CrossRef]
30. Klont, F.; Ten Hacken, N.H.T.; Horvatovich, P.; Bakker, S.J.L.; Bischoff, R. Assuring consistent performance of an insulin-like growth factor 1 MALDImmunoassay by monitoring measurement quality indicators. *Anal. Chem.* **2017**, *89*, 6188–6195. [CrossRef]
31. Food and Drug Administration (FDA). *Guidance for Industry: Bioanalytical Method Validation*; The United States Department of Health and Human Services: Washington, DC, USA, 2001.
32. Tubben, A.; Sotomayor, C.G.; Post, A.; Minovic, I.; Frelink, T.; de Borst, M.H.; Said, M.Y.; Douwes, R.M.; van den Berg, E.; Rodrigo, R.; et al. Urinary oxalate excretion and long-term outcomes in kidney transplant recipients. *J. Clin. Med.* **2019**, *8*, 2104. [CrossRef] [PubMed]
33. Minović, I.; van der Veen, A.; van Faassen, M.; Riphagen, I.J.; van den Berg, E.; van der Ley, C.; Gomes-Neto, A.W.; Geleijnse, J.M.; Eggersdorfer, M.; Navis, G.J.; et al. Functional vitamin B-6 status and long-term mortality in renal transplant recipients. *Am. J. Clin. Nutr.* **2017**, *106*, 1366–1374. [CrossRef] [PubMed]
34. Preacher, K.J.; Hayes, A.F. SPSS and SAS procedures for estimating indirect effects in simple mediation models. *Behav. Res. Methods Instrum. Comput.* **2004**, *36*, 717–731. [CrossRef] [PubMed]

35. Burkitt, W.; Domann, P.; O'Connor, G. Conformational changes in oxidatively stressed monoclonal antibodies studied by hydrogen exchange mass spectrometry. *Protein Sci.* **2010**, *19*, 826–835. [CrossRef]
36. Harrell, F.E., Jr.; Lee, K.L.; Califf, R.M.; Pryor, D.B.; Rosati, R.A. Regression modelling strategies for improved prognostic prediction. *Stat. Med.* **1984**, *3*, 143–152. [CrossRef]
37. Teppala, S.; Shankar, A.; Sabanayagam, C. Association between IGF-1 and chronic kidney disease among US adults. *Clin. Exp. Nephrol.* **2010**, *14*, 440–444. [CrossRef]
38. Wennberg, A.M.V.; Hagen, C.E.; Petersen, R.C.; Mielke, M.M. Trajectories of plasma IGF-1, IGFBP-3, and their ratio in the Mayo Clinic study of aging. *Exp. Gerontol.* **2018**, *106*, 67–73. [CrossRef]
39. Chew, J.; Tay, L.; Lim, J.P.; Leung, B.P.; Yeo, A.; Yew, S.; Ding, Y.Y.; Lim, W.S. Serum myostatin and IGF-1 as gender-specific biomarkers of frailty and low muscle mass in community-dwelling older adults. *J. Nutr. Health Aging* **2019**, *23*, 979–986. [CrossRef]
40. Kong, A.P.; Wong, G.W.; Choi, K.C.; Ho, C.S.; Chan, M.H.; Lam, C.W.; Tong, P.C.; Ozaki, R.; So, W.Y.; Ma, R.C.; et al. Reference values for serum levels of insulin-like growth factor (IGF-1) and IGF-binding protein 3 (IGFBP-3) and their ratio in Chinese adolescents. *Clin. Biochem.* **2007**, *40*, 1093–1099. [CrossRef]
41. Friedrich, N.; Alte, D.; Volzke, H.; Spilcke-Liss, E.; Ludemann, J.; Lerch, M.M.; Kohlmann, T.; Nauck, M.; Wallaschofski, H. Reference ranges of serum IGF-1 and IGFBP-3 levels in a general adult population: Results of the study of health in Pomerania (SHIP). *Growth Horm. IGF Res.* **2008**, *18*, 228–237. [CrossRef]
42. Alberti, C.; Chevenne, D.; Mercat, I.; Josserand, E.; Armoogum-Boizeau, P.; Tichet, J.; Leger, J. Serum concentrations of insulin-like growth factor (IGF)-1 and IGF binding protein-3 (IGFBP-3), IGF-1/IGFBP-3 ratio, and markers of bone turnover: Reference values for French children and adolescents and z-score comparability with other references. *Clin. Chem.* **2011**, *57*, 1424–1435. [CrossRef] [PubMed]
43. Chanson, P.; Arnoux, A.; Mavromati, M.; Brailly-Tabard, S.; Massart, C.; Young, J.; Piketty, M.L.; Souberbielle, J.C.; VARIETE Investigators. Reference values for IGF-I serum concentrations: Comparison of six immunoassays. *J. Clin. Endocrinol. Metab.* **2016**, *101*, 3450–3458. [CrossRef] [PubMed]
44. Bonert, V.; Carmichael, J.; Wu, Z.; Mirocha, J.; Perez, D.A.; Clarke, N.J.; Reitz, R.E.; McPhaul, M.J.; Mamelak, A. Discordance between mass spectrometry and immunometric IGF-1 assay in pituitary disease: A prospective study. *Pituitary* **2018**, *21*, 65–75. [CrossRef] [PubMed]
45. Endogenous Hormones and Breast Cancer Collaborative Group; Key, T.J.; Appleby, P.N.; Reeves, G.K.; Roddam, A.W. Insulin-like growth factor 1 (IGF1), IGF binding protein 3 (IGFBP3), and breast cancer risk: Pooled individual data analysis of 17 prospective studies. *Lancet Oncol.* **2010**, *11*, 530–542. [CrossRef]
46. Heijboer, A.C.; Blankenstein, M.A.; Kema, I.P.; Buijs, M.M. Accuracy of 6 routine 25-hydroxyvitamin D assays: Influence of vitamin D binding protein concentration. *Clin. Chem.* **2012**, *58*, 543–548. [CrossRef]
47. Di Micco, L.; Quinn, R.R.; Ronksley, P.E.; Bellizzi, V.; Lewin, A.M.; Cianciaruso, B.; Ravani, P.; Alberta Kidney Disease Network (AKDN). Urine creatinine excretion and clinical outcomes in CKD. *Clin. J. Am. Soc. Nephrol.* **2013**, *8*, 1877–1883. [CrossRef]
48. Kalantari, K.; Bolton, W.K. A good reason to measure 24-h urine creatinine excretion, but not to assess kidney function. *Clin. J. Am. Soc. Nephrol.* **2013**, *8*, 1847–1849. [CrossRef]
49. Oterdoom, L.H.; Gansevoort, R.T.; Schouten, J.P.; de Jong, P.E.; Gans, R.O.; Bakker, S.J. Urinary creatinine excretion, an indirect measure of muscle mass, is an independent predictor of cardiovascular disease and mortality in the general population. *Atherosclerosis* **2009**, *207*, 534–540. [CrossRef]
50. Yakar, S.; Isaksson, O. Regulation of skeletal growth and mineral acquisition by the GH/IGF-1 axis: Lessons from mouse models. *Growth Horm. IGF Res.* **2016**, *28*, 26–42. [CrossRef]
51. Clemmons, D.R. Role of IGF-I in skeletal muscle mass maintenance. *Trends Endocrinol. Metab.* **2009**, *20*, 349–356. [CrossRef]
52. Zelle, D.M.; Corpeleijn, E.; Stolk, R.P.; de Greef, M.H.; Gans, R.O.; van der Heide, J.J.; Navis, G.; Bakker, S.J. Low physical activity and risk of cardiovascular and all-cause mortality in renal transplant recipients. *Clin. J. Am. Soc. Nephrol.* **2011**, *6*, 898–905. [CrossRef] [PubMed]
53. Rosas, S.E.; Reese, P.P.; Huan, Y.; Doria, C.; Cochetti, P.T.; Doyle, A. Pretransplant physical activity predicts all-cause mortality in kidney transplant recipients. *Am. J. Nephrol.* **2012**, *35*, 17–23. [CrossRef] [PubMed]
54. Bellizzi, V.; Cupisti, A.; Capitanini, A.; Calella, P.; D'Alessandro, C. Physical activity and renal transplantation. *Kidney Blood Press. Res.* **2014**, *39*, 212–219. [CrossRef] [PubMed]

55. Dunn, S.E.; Burns, J.L.; Michel, R.N. Calcineurin is required for skeletal muscle hypertrophy. *J. Biol. Chem.* **1999**, *274*, 21908–21912. [CrossRef]
56. Michel, R.N.; Dunn, S.E.; Chin, E.R. Calcineurin and skeletal muscle growth. *Proc. Nutr. Soc.* **2004**, *63*, 341–349. [CrossRef]
57. Hudson, M.B.; Price, S.R. Calcineurin: A poorly understood regulator of muscle mass. *Int. J. Biochem. Cell Biol.* **2013**, *45*, 2173–2178. [CrossRef]

6

Prognostic Value of Neutrophil-To-Lymphocyte Ratio and Platelet-To-Lymphocyte Ratio for Renal Outcomes in Patients with Rapidly Progressive Glomerulonephritis

Yukari Mae, Tomoaki Takata *, Ayami Ida, Masaya Ogawa, Sosuke Taniguchi, Marie Yamamoto, Takuji Iyama, Satoko Fukuda and Hajime Isomoto

Division of Medicine and Clinical Science, Faculty of Medicine, Tottori University, Yonago, Tottori 683-8504, Japan

* Correspondence: t-takata@tottori-u.ac.jp

Abstract: Background: Rapidly progressive glomerulonephritis (RPGN) is a syndrome characterized by a rapid decline in renal function that often causes end-stage renal disease. Although it is important to predict renal outcome in RPGN before initiating immunosuppressive therapies, no simple prognostic indicator has been reported. The aim of this study was to investigate the associations of neutrophil-to-lymphocyte ratio (NLR) and platelet-to-lymphocyte ratio (PLR) to renal outcomes in patients with RPGN. Methods: Forty-four patients with a clinical diagnosis of RPGN who underwent renal biopsy were enrolled. The relationships between NLR and PLR and renal outcome after 1 year were investigated. Results: NLR and PLR were significantly higher in patients with preserved renal function in comparison to patients who required maintenance hemodialysis ($p < 0.05$ and $p < 0.01$, respectively). An NLR of 4.0 and a PLR of 137.7 were the cutoff values for renal outcome (area under the curve, 0.782 and 0.819; sensitivity, 78.4% and 89.2%; specificity, 71.4% and 71.4%, respectively). Furthermore, an NLR of 5.0 could predict recovery from renal injury in patients requiring hemodialysis (area under the curve, 0.929; sensitivity, 83.3%; specificity, 85.7%). Conclusion: NLR and PLR could be candidates for predicting renal outcomes in patients with RPGN.

Keywords: NLR; PLR; RPGN; predictive value; hemodialysis; withdrawal; cellular crescent; global sclerosis

---

1. Introduction

Rapidly progressive glomerulonephritis (RPGN) is a syndrome characterized by hematuria, proteinuria, anemia, and a rapid decline in renal function [1]. The diagnosis of RPGN is made when renal dysfunction occurs within a short period of time and is complicated with proteinuria or hematuria [2]. The etiology of RPGN is divided into three classifications: immune complex crescentic glomerulonephritis, pauci-immune crescentic glomerulonephritis, and anti-glomerular basement membrane (GBM) crescentic glomerulonephritis. In Japan, the number of end-stage renal disease (ESRD) cases caused by RPGN has increased approximately 3.1 times between 1994 and 2018, which represents the fifth most common etiology of ESRD [2,3]. Since RPGN causes a progressive decline in renal function, patients with RPGN require aggressive treatment with steroids and immunosuppressive agents [4]. However, these treatments are not always effective and, in such cases, RPGN is refractory and requires maintenance hemodialysis (HD). Considering that steroids and immunosuppressive agents can cause life-threatening infections, conservative treatment is also considered for patients with RPGN. Although it is critically important to predict renal outcomes in the early stages of RPGN [5], a simple prognostic marker for RPGN is yet to be established.

In recent years, neutrophil-to-lymphocyte ratio (NLR) and platelet-to-lymphocyte ratio (PLR) have received attention as potential new markers of systemic inflammation. In previous studies, NLR and PLR have been reported to be useful in systemic inflammatory diseases such as aortitis syndrome [6], Behçet's disease [7], Kawasaki disease [8], Henoch–Schönlein purpura [9], systemic lupus erythematosus [10], and anti-neutrophil cytoplasmic antibody (ANCA)-associated vasculitis (AAV) [11,12]. Furthermore, NLR and PLR have been proposed as markers of inflammation in patients with ESRD [13,14]. Therefore, we speculated that NLR and PLR could be simple predictors of renal decline in RPGN. The purpose of this study was to investigate the associations of NLR and PLR to renal outcome in patients with RPGN.

2. Materials and Methods

2.1. Study Population

In this study, we enrolled 501 patients who underwent renal biopsy at the Tottori University Hospital between 2009 and 2019. Renal biopsies were performed according to the indications of the guidelines from the Japanese Society of Nephrology [15]; persistent hematuria and/or proteinuria, proteinuria more than 0.5 g/day, a rapid decline in renal function, or gross hematuria. Among the 501 patients enrolled, 47 patients were clinically diagnosed with RPGN based on the guidelines from the Japanese Society of Nephrology [16]. Excluding 2 cases with an active bacterial infection and 1 case with a relapse of the glomerulonephritis, 44 patients were included in the analyses (Figure 1). None of the patients included had a history of cancer or prescribed corticosteroids. Immunosuppressive therapies were determined according to the guidelines [16]. This study was conducted in accordance with the Declaration of Helsinki and approved by the Ethics Committee of Tottori University Hospital (approval number: 19A138).

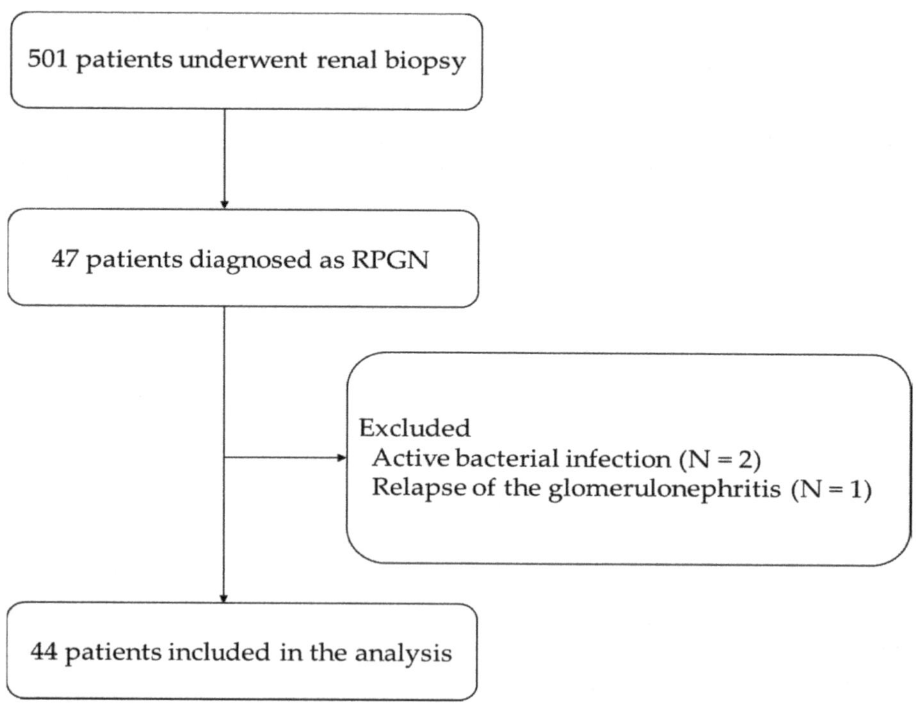

Figure 1. Study design. Of the 501 patients who underwent renal biopsy, 44 patients were included in the analysis.

2.2. Clinical and Laboratory Findings

The patient's characteristics and laboratory findings on admission, including white blood cell count (WBC), neutrophil count (Neu), lymphocyte count (Lym), platelet count (Plt), creatinine (Cr), estimated glomerular filtration rate (eGFR) [17], C-reactive protein (CRP), erythrocyte sedimentation rate (ESR), myeloperoxidase (MPO)-ANCA, proteinase 3 (PR3)-ANCA, and the anti-GBM antibody, were acquired retrospectively. NLR was calculated as the ratio of neutrophil count to lymphocyte count (NLR = Neu/Lym), and PLR was calculated as the ratio of platelet count to lymphocyte count (PLR = Plt/Lym). Renal outcomes 1 year from diagnosis were also recorded.

2.3. *Histological Findings*

Ultrasound-guided renal biopsy was performed as previously described [18]. In brief, renal tissue was obtained using a 16-gauge biopsy gun (Acecut; TSK Laboratory, Tochigi, Japan). The specimen was fixed in 10% formalin and embedded in paraffin. Sections (4 μm thickness) were stained with periodic acid-Schiff (PAS). Pathological changes in glomeruli were defined as global sclerosis, cellular crescent, fibrocellular crescent, fibrous crescent, and others. Pathological analyses were performed by an experienced nephrologist (S.F.), who was independent of the acquisition and analysis of the clinical information.

2.4. *Statistical Analyses*

Continuous variables were expressed as the mean ± standard deviation or the median (range) according to the distribution. The Kolmogorov–Smirnov test was used to assess normal distribution. Differences between groups were analyzed using the Student's t test for normally distributed variables, the Mann–Whitney U test for non-normally distributed variables, or the chi-square test for categorical variables. In addition, receiver operating characteristic (ROC) curve analysis was performed to determine the optimal cutoff values for NLR and PLR. The optimal cutoff point was determined by minimizing the square of the distance between the point (sensitivity of 1, 1-specificity of 0) and any point on the ROC curve. Multivariate regression analysis was carried out, in which age, eGFR, CRP, and NLR or PLR were selected, with the stepwise forward selection method, to investigate independent predictors of renal outcomes in the 44 patients. StatFlex Ver7 for Windows (Artec, Osaka, Japan) was used for the statistical analyses. A two-tailed p-value of < 0.05 was considered statistically significant.

3. Results

3.1. *Differences between Patients with Preserved Renal Function and Renal Failure*

All patients enrolled in this study were ethnically homogenous. The etiology of the 44 patients was as follows: ANCA-associated vasculitis ($n = 34$), ANCA-negative vasculitis ($n = 6$), and anti-GBM disease ($n = 4$). We first divided the patients into two groups according to their renal outcomes at 1 year post diagnosis. The characteristics of the 37 cases with preserved renal function (pre-dialysis group) and 7 cases with renal failure (maintenance HD group) are shown in Table 1 and Figure 2. WBC, Neu, Plt, Cr, eGFR and the anti-GBM antibody all showed significant differences between the groups. We also observed significant differences in NLR (8.2 (2.0–32.0) vs. 3.9 (2.8–8.4), $p = 0.019$) and PLR (265.7 (82.9–2255.0) vs. 126.0 (107.1–269.0), $p = 0.008$) between the pre-dialysis and maintenance HD groups, respectively. Multivariate regression analysis revealed that renal function was the strongest influencing factor for renal outcome (stdβ = 0.363, $p = 0.012$). There was also a trend suggesting the significance of NLR as a predictive value (stdβ = 0.276, $p = 0.052$); PLR, however, did not display this significance (stdβ = 0.207, $p = 0.148$).

Table 1. Patient's characteristics between the pre-dialysis and maintenance hemodialysis (HD) groups.

	Pre-dialysis (n = 37)	Maintenance HD (n = 7)	p Value
Sex (Male/Female)	22/15	5/2	0.132
Age (years)	71.4 ± 11.6	65.7 ± 7.8	0.222
Classifications of RPGN			
Immune complex CGN	33 (89.2%)	1 (14.3%)	
Pauci-immune CGN	4 (10.8%)	2 (28.6%)	
Anti-GBM CGN	0 (0%)	4 (57.1%)	
Immunosuppressive therapy			
Pulse corticosteroids	29/8	6/1	0.557
Cyclophosphamide	13/24	0/7	0.069
Plasma exchange	0/37	3/4	0.003
White blood cell count (10^3/μL)	10.2 (4.9–23.5)	6.2 (4.7–12.4)	0.037
Neutrophil count (10^3/μL)	8.5 (3.6–22.1)	4.6 (3.3–8.4)	0.012
Lymphocyte count (10^3/μL)	1.17 ± 0.59	1.31 ± 0.43	0.550
Platelet count (10^3/μL)	327 (98–808)	189 (117–269)	0.015
Creatinine (mg/dL)	2.80 ± 2.01	8.74± 1.80	<0.001
eGFR (mL/min/1.73 m^2)	27.3 ± 21.2	5.4 ± 2.0	<0.001
CRP (mg/dL)	5.0 (0–24.8)	4.0 (0.4–26.9)	0.987
ESR (mm/h)	99 (10–140)	111 (62–134)	0.771
MPO-ANCA (U/mL)	166 (0–860)	0 (0–2440)	0.109
PR3-ANCA (U/mL)	0 (0–35.8)	0 (0–0)	0.308
anti-GBM antibody (U/mL)	0 (0–0)	42.3 (0–858.0)	<0.001
NLR	8.2 (2.0–32.0)	3.9 (2.8–8.4)	0.019
PLR	265.7 (82.9–2255.0)	126.0 (107.1–269.0)	0.008

Data are presented as the mean ± standard deviation, median (range), or number (%). HD—hemodialysis; RPGN—rapidly progressing glomerulonephritis; CGN—crescentic glomerulonephritis; eGFR—estimated glomerular filtration rate; CRP—C-reactive protein; ESR—erythrocyte sedimentation rate; MPO—myeloperoxidase; ANCA—anti-neutrophil cytoplasmic antibody; PR3—proteinase 3; GBM—glomerular basement membrane; NLR—neutrophil-to-lymphocyte ratio; PLR—platelet-to-lymphocyte ratio.

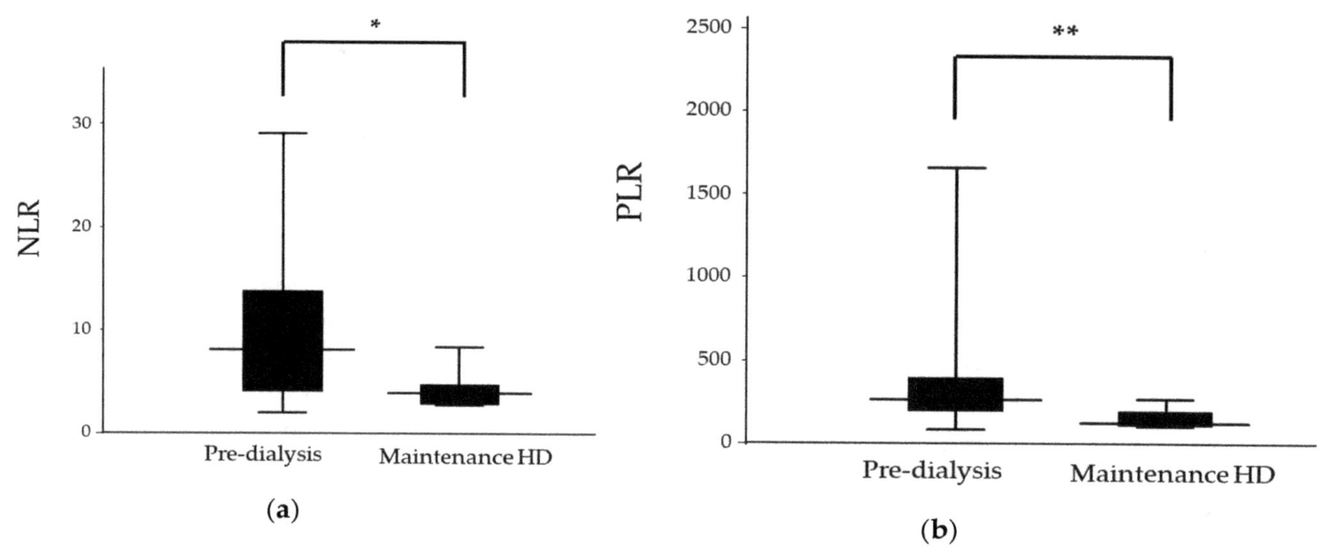

Figure 2. Neutrophil-to-lymphocyte ratios (NLR) and platelet-to-lymphocyte ratios (PLR) in the pre-dialysis and maintenance hemodialysis (HD) groups. (**a**) NLR in the pre-dialysis and maintenance HD groups. (**b**) PLR in the pre-dialysis and maintenance HD groups. The top and the bottom of the boxes are the first and third quartile, respectively. The length of the box represents the interquartile range. The line through the middle of each box represents the median. The error bars show the minimum and maximum values (range). *, $p < 0.05$; ** $p < 0.01$. NLR—neutrophil-to-lymphocyte ratio; PLR—platelet-to-lymphocyte ratio; HD—hemodialysis.

The ROC curves analyses were performed to define the cutoff value of PLR and NLR for predicting renal outcomes after 1 year (Figure 3). Both NLR and PLR were accurate predictors of renal outcomes, with an area under the curve (AUC) of 0.782 in NLR and 0.819 in PLR. The cutoff values defined were 4.0 in NLR, with a sensitivity of 78.4% and specificity of 71.4%, and 137.7 in PLR, with a sensitivity of 89.2% and specificity of 71.4%.

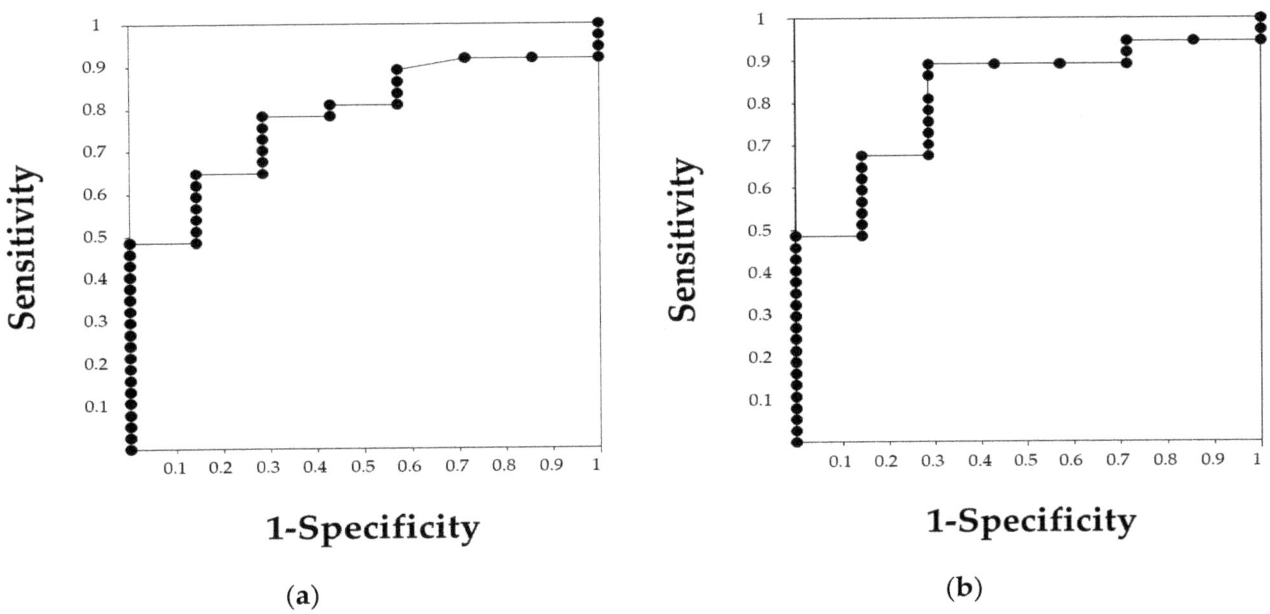

Figure 3. The receiver operating characteristic (ROC) curve of neutrophil-to-lymphocyte ratio (NLR) and platelet-to-lymphocyte ratio (PLR) for predicting renal outcome. (**a**) The ROC curve of NLR showing an area under the curve (AUC) of 0.782. An NLR of 4.0 was the cutoff value with a sensitivity of 78.4% and a specificity of 71.4%. (**b**) The ROC curve of PLR showing an AUC of 0.819. The cutoff value of 137.7 was determined with a sensitivity of 89.2% and a specificity of 71.4%.

3.2. Differences between Patients with Temporary Hemodialysis and Maintenance Hemodialysis

Since renal function on admission was a strong predicting factor for renal outcome, we divided the 13 patients who required HD into two groups as follows: 6 patients with recovery of renal function (temporary HD group) and 7 patients with persistent renal failure (maintenance HD group). Sex, WBC and Neu showed significant differences between the groups (Table 2). NLR was significantly higher in the temporary HD group compared to the maintenance HD group (12.4 (4.1–21.4) vs. 3.9 (2.8–8.4), $p = 0.008$, respectively, Figure 4). However, no significant difference was observed in PLR between the temporary HD group and the maintenance HD group (341.7 ± 217.7 vs. 156.1 ± 62.6, $p = 0.053$, respectively). The ROC curve analysis showed that an NLR of 5.0 could predict withdrawal from HD with a sensitivity of 83.3% and a specificity of 85.7%, with an AUC of 0.929 (Figure 5).

Table 2. Patient's characteristics between temporary the HD and maintenance HD groups.

	Temporary HD ($n = 6$)	Maintenance HD ($n = 7$)	p Value
Sex (Male/Female)	1/5	5/2	0.048
Age (years)	72.7 ± 18.4	65.7 ± 7.8	0.381
Classifications of RPGN			
Immune complex CGN	0 (0%)	1 (14.3%)	
Pauci-immune CGN	6 (100%)	2 (28.6%)	
Anti-GBM CGN	0 (0%)	4 (57.1%)	
Immunosuppressive therapy			
Pulse corticosteroids	6/0	6/1	0.538
Cyclophosphamide	1/5	0/7	0.462
Plasma exchange	6/0	3/4	0.049
White blood cell count ($10^3/\mu L$)	12.6 ± 5.1	7.6 ± 2.9	0.048
Neutrophil count ($10^3/\mu L$)	11.0 ± 5.0	5.3 ± 2.1	0.018
Lymphocyte count ($10^3/\mu L$)	1.10 ± 0.58	1.31 ± 0.43	0.470
Platelet count ($10^3/\mu L$)	289.7 ± 112.7	191.4 ± 55.6	0.066
CRP (mg/dL)	11.2 ± 7.0	8.1 ± 10.3	0.554
ESR (mm/h)	104 ± 32	103 ± 27	0.985
MPO-ANCA (U/mL)	160 (17.0–469.0)	0 (0–2440)	0.138
anti-GBM antibody (U/mL)	0 (0–0)	42.3 (0–858.0)	0.065
NLR	12.4 (4.1–21.4)	3.9 (2.8–8.4)	0.008
PLR	341.7 ± 217.7	156.1 ± 62.6	0.053

Data are presented as the mean ± standard deviation, median (range), or number (%). HD—hemodialysis; RPGN—rapidly progressing glomerulonephritis; CGN—crescentic glomerulonephritis; eGFR—estimated glomerular filtration rate; CRP—C-reactive protein; ESR—erythrocyte sedimentation rate; MPO—myeloperoxidase; ANCA—anti-neutrophil cytoplasmic antibody; PR3—proteinase 3; GBM—glomerular basement membrane; NLR—neutrophil-to-lymphocyte ratio; PLR—platelet-to-lymphocyte ratio.

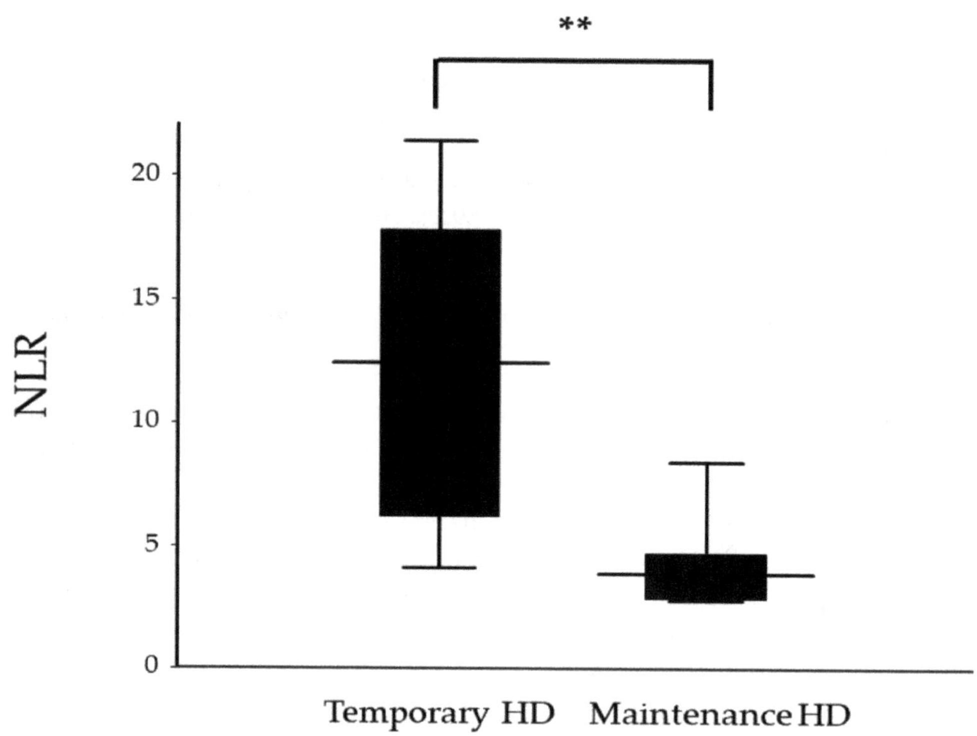

Figure 4. Neutrophil-to-lymphocyte ratios (NLR) of the temporary and maintenance hemodialysis (HD) groups. The top and the bottom of the boxes are the first and third quartile, respectively. The length of the box represents the interquartile range. The line through the middle of each box represents the median. The error bars show the minimum and maximum values (range). ** $p < 0.01$. NLR—neutrophil-to-lymphocyte ratio; HD—hemodialysis.

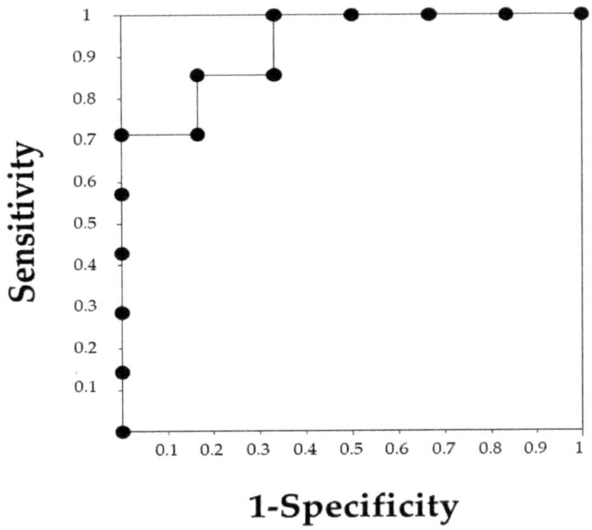

Figure 5. The receiver operating characteristic (ROC) curve for neutrophil-to-lymphocyte ratio (NLR) for recovery from renal failure. The NLR of 5.0 was determined to be a cutoff value with a sensitivity of 83.3% and a specificity of 85.7%, and the area under the curve was 0.929.

We further investigated histological changes in the temporary HD group and maintenance HD group (Table 3, Figures 6 and 7). The number of globally sclerotic glomeruli was significantly lower in the temporary HD group (9.0% ± 10.1% vs. 53.0% ± 9.7%, $p < 0.001$), whereas the number of glomeruli with cellular crescent was significantly higher in the temporary HD group (27.9 (0–73.3) vs. 0 (0–13.3), $p = 0.022$).

Table 3. Histological changes in the temporary hemodialysis (HD) and maintenance HD groups.

	Temporary HD ($n = 6$)	Maintenance HD ($n = 7$)	p Value
Cellular crescent (%)	30.4 ± 24.1	4.4 ± 5.7	0.022
Fibrocellular crescent (%)	11.9 ± 14.1	10.2 ± 9.4	0.945
Fibrous crescent (%)	19.0 ± 22.9	20.1 ± 16.3	0.921
Global sclerosis (%)	9.0 ± 10.1	53.0 ± 9.7	<0.001

Data are presented as the mean ± standard deviation. HD—hemodialysis.

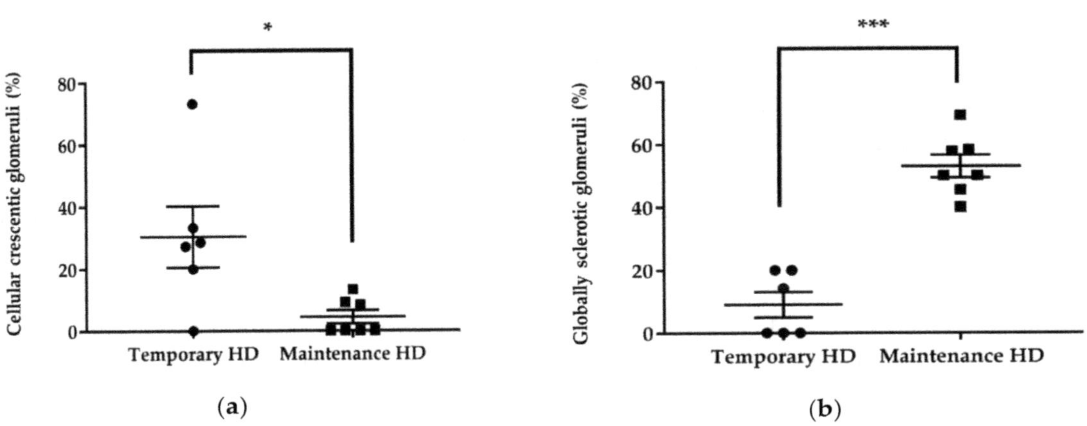

Figure 6. Quantification of histological findings in the temporary and maintenance hemodialysis (HD) groups. (**a**) Comparison of the percentage of glomeruli with cellular crescent between the temporary and maintenance HD groups. (**b**) Comparison of the percentage of globally sclerotic glomeruli between the temporary and maintenance HD groups. Bars indicate mean ± SEM. *, $p < 0.05$; *** $p < 0.001$. HD—hemodialysis.

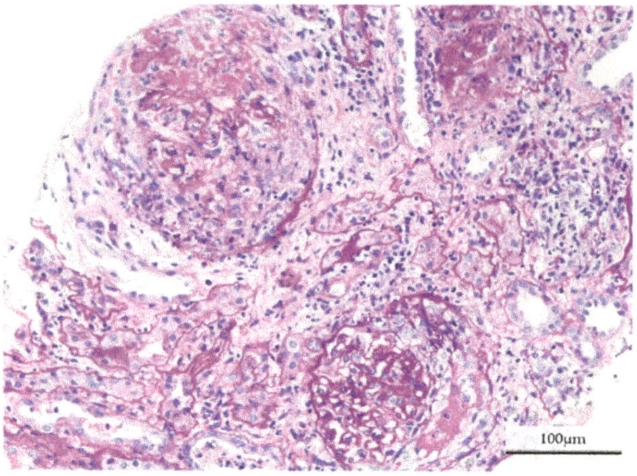

(a)

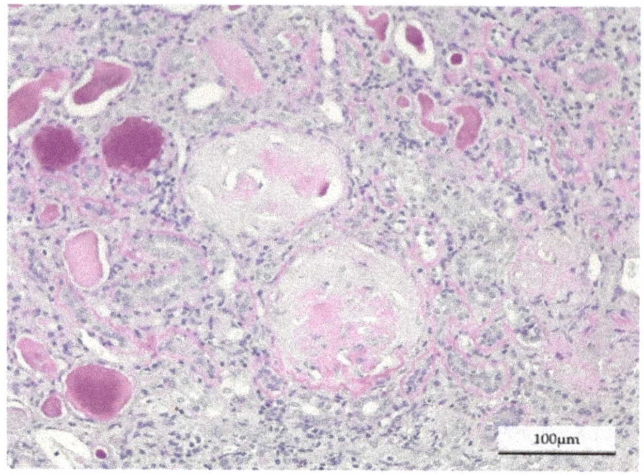

(b)

Figure 7. Histological findings in each group. Representative images of Periodic acid-Schiff staining on paraffin-embedded kidney sections, from patients in (**a**) the temporary hemodialysis (HD) group, and (**b**) the maintenance HD group. Cellular crescentic glomeruli were dominant in the temporary HD group, whereas most of the glomeruli were globally sclerotic in the maintenance HD group.

4. Discussion

In this study, we found that NLR and PLR at the point of diagnosis of RPGN are associated with renal outcome. In particular, NLR was considered to be a useful prognostic indicator for the recovery from HD in patients with RPGN.

RPGN often causes a progressive decline in renal function that leads to ESRD at a high rate. In this study, we observed that around 16% of the cases resulted in ESRD. Several renal prognostic indicators of RPGN, such as the degree of decline in renal function on admission, histological classification, and the level of the anti-GBM antibody, have been suggested in previous reports [4,19]. However, it is difficult to accurately predict renal outcome without a renal biopsy or in patients who require HD. Therefore, it is important to establish a simple renal prognostic indicator other than renal function or histological assessment.

NLR and PLR are simple and cost-effective markers, that represent the ratio of the number of cells with two different hemocytes. Neu and Plt increase with inflammation [11,20], while Lym may decrease with inflammation in autoimmune diseases [21]. Since the majority of the patients included in this study had an etiology of autoimmune vasculitis, it was expected that the increase in Neu and Plt, and the decrease in Lym, would be proportionate to the degree of inflammation. Therefore, we considered that NLR and PLR could be more reliable than a single hemocyte number. Infection, cancers, ischemic heart disease and peripheral vascular disease affect NLR and PLR [22]. In addition, steroids increase Neu, while immunosuppressive agents may reduce Neu by myelosuppression. Thus, in this study, we excluded patients who had infectious diseases and who were already administered steroids or immunosuppressive drugs at diagnosis, and confirmed no patient had a history of malignancy, ischemic heart disease or peripheral vascular disease.

NLR and PLR have been reported to be associated with AAV disease activity; high NLR and PLR indicate a higher disease activity [11,12,20,22]. On the other hand, several studies have mentioned that the application of NLR and PLR is limited. It has been demonstrated that NLR is a good predictor of the relapse rate, but not of death in patients with AAV [22]. PLR is also able to predict the disease activity but cannot predict relapse in AAV patients [20]. In this study, both NLR and PLR at diagnosis were significantly higher in patients with preserved renal function than in patients with maintenance HD. We speculate that a higher NLR and PLR indicate acute disease and an active phase, sustaining the possibility of a positive response to immunosuppressive therapy, whereas a lower NLR and PLR may suggest a chronic phase with irreversible renal injury. This was confirmed by the histological analysis, which revealed significant differences in glomerular changes. The majority of the glomeruli in the maintenance HD group were globally sclerosing, indicating irreversible renal injury. Cellular crescent presence, suggesting a possibility of improvement, was highly observed in the temporary HD group. We demonstrated that an NLR < 4.0 or PLR < 137.7 at diagnosis were associated with negative renal outcomes, especially in patients requiring HD. An NLR < 5.0 at diagnosis could predict irreversible renal failure.

Since the patients in the pre-dialysis group showed variable renal function, and the multivariate analysis revealed that renal function was the strongest influencing factor, we investigated the predictive abilities of NLR and PLR in patients requiring HD. Among the 13 patients, NLR at diagnosis was significantly higher in the temporary HD group than in the maintenance HD group. Although PLR showed an increased presence in the temporary HD group, the difference was not significant. The half-life of Neu and Plt could affect this result. Neu can survive for less than 24 h, while Plt survives for 10 days, and their lifespans are controlled by endogenous apoptosis [23,24]. Plt, which is increased by inflammation, circulates for a longer period than Neu. In predicting the course of patients requiring HD, it would be desirable to evaluate the acute phase of inflammation and disease activity. Therefore, NLR would be a better predictor than PLR for withdrawal of HD.

There are some limitations to our study. First, all the patients were treated based on the clinical guidelines for the ANCA-associated RPGN [25]; thus, the treatment strategy differed in each patient. Since all four patients with an anti-GBM disease required maintenance HD, this may affect the result of our study. However, we observed a significant difference in NLR between the temporary and maintenance HD groups when these patients were eliminated. In addition to the variations in NLR and PLR, this study was a retrospective study, with a small number of subjects. Therefore, the results of the present study should be carefully interpreted, and a prospective study with a larger number of patients is required to confirm the suitability of NLR and PLR as predicative factors in renal outcomes.

5. Conclusions

In conclusion, we revealed that the NLR and PLR at diagnosis could predict renal outcomes in patients with RPGN, and that NLR could predict withdrawal from HD in patients requiring HD. Treatment strategies could be modified according to the NLR and PLR, especially in patients whose renal function is unlikely to recover, which may reduce the risk of treatment-related complications.

Author Contributions: Conceptualization, Y.M. and T.T.; Methodology, Y.M. and T.T.; Formal analysis, Y.M.; Investigation, Y.M.; Data Curation, Y.M., A.I., M.O., S.T., M.Y., T.I., and S.F.; Writing—Original Draft Preparation, Y.M.; Writing—Review & Editing, T.T.; Supervision, T.T. and H.I. All authors have read and agreed to the published version of the manuscript.

References

1. Nachman, P.H.; Jennette, J.C.; Falk, R.J. Primary glomerular disease. In *Brenner and Rector's The Kidney*, 9th ed.; Taal, M.W., Chertow, G.M., Marsden, P.A., Skorecki, K., Yu, A.S.L., Brenner, B.M., Eds.; Elsevier Inc.: Philadelphia, PA, USA, 2012; Volume 1, pp. 1153–1154.
2. Usui, J.; Yamagata, K. Progressive renal diseases: Recent advances in diagnosis and treatments. Topics: II. Pathophysiology and treatments; 4. Crescentic glomerulonephritis. *J. Jpn. Soc. Int. Med.* **2013**, *102*, 1128–1135. (In Japanese) [CrossRef] [PubMed]
3. Nitta, K.; Masakane, I.; Hanafusa, N.; Goto, S.; Abe, M.; Nakai, S.; Taniguchi, M.; Hasegawa, T.; Wada, A.; Hamano, T.; et al. 2018 annual dialysis data report, JSDT renal data registry. *J. Jpn. Soc. Dial. Ther.* **2018**, *52*, 679–754. (In Japanese) [CrossRef]
4. Toraman, A.; Neşe, N.; Özyurt, B.C.; Kürşat, S. Association between neutrophil-lymphocyte & platelet lymphocyte ratios with prognosis & mortality in rapidly progressive glomerulonephritis. *Indian J. Med. Res.* **2019**, *150*, 399–406. [PubMed]

5. Xu, P.C.; Chen, T.; Wu, S.J.; Yang, X.; Gao, S.; Hu, S.Y.; Wei, L.; Yan, T.K. Pathological severity determines the renal recovery for anti-myeloperoxidase antibody-associated vasculitis requiring dialysis at disease onset: A retrospective study. *BMC Nephrol.* **2019**, *20*, 287. [CrossRef] [PubMed]
6. Pan, L.; Du, J.; Li, T.; Liao, H. Platelet-to-lymphocyte ratio and neutrophil-to-lymphocyte ratio associated with disease activity in patients with Takayasu's arteritis: A case-control study. *BMJ Open* **2017**, *7*, e014451. [CrossRef]
7. Yuksel, M.; Yildiz, A.; Oylumlu, M.; Turkcu, F.M.; Bilik, M.Z.; Ekinci, A.; Elbey, B.; Tekbas, E.; Alan, S. Novel markers of endothelial dysfunction and inflammation in Behçet's disease patients with ocular involvement: Epicardial fat thickness, carotid intima media thickness, serum ADMA level, and neutrophil-to-lymphocyte ratio. *Clin. Rheumatol.* **2016**, *35*, 701–708. [CrossRef]
8. Chantasiriwan, N.; Silvilairat, S.; Makonkawkeyoon, K.; Pongprot, Y.; Sittiwangkul, R. Predictors of intravenous immunoglobulin resistance and coronary artery aneurysm in patients with Kawasaki Disease. *Paediatr. Int. Child. Health* **2018**, *38*, 209–212. [CrossRef]
9. Park, C.H.; Han, D.S.; Jeong, J.Y.; Eun, C.S.; Yoo, K.S.; Jeon, Y.C.; Sohn, J.H. The optimal cut-off value of neutrophil-to-lymphocyte ratio for predicting prognosis in adult patients with Henoch-Schönlein purpura. *PLoS ONE* **2016**, *11*, e0153238. [CrossRef]
10. Wu, Y.; Chen, Y.; Yang, X.; Chen, L.; Yang, Y. Neutrophil-to-lymphocyte ratio (NLR) and platelet-to-lymphocyte ratio (PLR) were associated with disease activity in patients with systemic lupus erythematosus. *Int. Immunopharmacol.* **2016**, *36*, 94–99. [CrossRef]
11. Küçük, H.; Göker, B.; Varan, Ö.; Dumludag, B.; Haznedaroğlu, Ş.; Öztürk, M.A.; Tufan, A.; Emiroglu, T.; Erten, Y. Predictive value of neutrophil/lymphocyte ratio in renal prognosis of patients with granulomatosis with polyangiitis. *Ren. Fail.* **2017**, *39*, 273–276. [CrossRef]
12. Abaza, N.M.; El-Latif, E.M.; Gheita, T.A. Clinical significance of neutrophil/lymphocyte ratio in patients with granulomatosis with polyangiitis. *Reumatol. Clin.* **2019**, *15*, 363–367. [CrossRef] [PubMed]
13. Turkmen, K.; Guney, I.; Yerlikaya, F.H.; Tonbul, H.Z. The relationship between neutrophil-to- lymphocyte ratio and inflammation in end-stage renal disease patients. *Ren. Fail.* **2012**, *34*, 155–159. [CrossRef] [PubMed]
14. Turkmen, K.; Erdur, F.M.; Ozcicek, F.; Ozcicek, A.; Akbas, E.M.; Ozbicer, A.; Demirtas, L.; Turk, S.; Tonbul, H.Z. Platelet-to-lymphocyte ratio better predicts inflammation than neutrophil-to-lymphocyte ratio in end-stage renal disease patients. *Hemodial. Int.* **2013**, *17*, 391–396. [CrossRef] [PubMed]
15. Sakai, H.; Kurokawa, K.; Koyama, A.; Arimura, Y.; Kida, H.; Shigematsu, H.; Suzuki, S.; Nihei, H.; Makino, H.; Ueda, N.; et al. Guidelines for the management of rapidly progressive glomerulonephritis. *Nihon Jinzo Gakkai Shi* **2002**, *44*, 55–82. (In Japanese) [PubMed]
16. Japanese Society of Nephrology. Clinical practice guidebook for diagnosis and treatment of chronic kidney disease 2012. *Nihon Jinzo Gakkai Shi* **2012**, *54*, 1034–1191.
17. Matsuo, S.; Imai, E.; Horio, M.; Yasuda, Y.; Tomita, K.; Nitta, K.; Yamagata, K.; Tomino, Y.; Yokoyama, H.; Hishida, A. Revised equations for estimated GFR from serum creatinine in Japan. *Am. J. kidney. Dis.* **2009**, *53*, 982–992. [CrossRef]
18. Iyama, T.; Takata, T.; Koda, M.; Fukuda, S.; Hoi, S.; Mae, Y.; Fukui, T.; Munemura, C.; Isomoto, H. Renal shear wave elastography for the assessment of nephron hypertrophy: A cross-sectional study in chronic kidney disease. *J. Med. Ultrason.* **2018**, *45*, 571–576. [CrossRef]
19. Jennette, J.C. Rapidly progressive crescentic glomerulonephritis. *Kidney Int.* **2003**, *63*, 1164–1177. [CrossRef]
20. Park, H.J.; Jung, S.M.; Song, J.J.; Park, Y.B.; Lee, S.W. Platelet to lymphocyte ratio is associated with the current activity of ANCA-associated vasculitis at diagnosis: A retrospective monocentric study. *Rheumatol. Int.* **2018**, *38*, 1865–1871. [CrossRef]
21. Schulze-Koops, H. Lymphopenia and autoimmune diseases. *Arthritis Res. Ther.* **2004**, *6*, 178–180. [CrossRef]
22. Ahn, S.S.; Jung, S.M.; Song, J.J.; Park, Y.B.; Lee, S.W. Neutrophil to lymphocyte ratio at diagnosis can estimate vasculitis activity and poor prognosis in patients with ANCA-associated vasculitis: A retrospective study. *BMC Nephrol.* **2018**, *19*, 187. [CrossRef] [PubMed]
23. McCracken, J.M.; Allen, L.A. Regulation of human neutrophil apoptosis and lifespan in health and disease. *J. Cell Death* **2014**, *7*, 15–23. [CrossRef] [PubMed]
24. Lebois, M.; Josefsson, E.C. Regulation of platelet lifespan by apoptosis. *Platelets* **2016**, *27*, 497–504. [CrossRef] [PubMed]

7

C3d-Positive Preformed DSAs Tend to Persist and Result in a Higher Risk of AMR after Kidney Transplants

Sooin Choi [1,†], Kyo Won Lee [2,†], Jae Berm Park [2], Kyunga Kim [3], Hye-Ryeon Jang [4], Wooseong Huh [4] and Eun Suk Kang [5,*]

1 Department of Laboratory Medicine, Soonchunhyang University Hospital Cheonan, Soonchunhyang University College of Medicine, Cheonan 31151, Korea; sooin2@schmc.ac.kr

2 Department of Surgery, Samsung Medical Center, Sungkyunkwan University School of Medicine, Seoul 06351, Korea; kw1980.lee@gmail.com (K.W.L.); jbparkmd@gmail.com (J.B.P.)

3 Statistics and Data Center, Research Institute for Future Medicine, Samsung Medical Center, Seoul 06351, Korea; kyunga.j.kim@samsung.com

4 Division of Nephrology, Department of Medicine, Samsung Medical Center, Sungkyunkwan University School of Medicine, Seoul 06351, Korea; shinehr@skku.edu (H.-R.J.); whuh03@skku.edu (W.H.)

5 Department of Laboratory Medicine and Genetics, Samsung Medical Center, Sungkyunkwan University School of Medicine, Seoul 06351, Korea

* Correspondence: eskang@skku.edu

† Contributed equally to this study.

Abstract: C3d-binding assays have been introduced as methods for the prediction of the presence of complement-binding functional antibodies; however, the prognostic value of C3d-positive preformed donor-specific antibodies (pDSAs) has not been fully evaluated. In this study, we performed a retrospective investigation of the association of pDSAs and their C3d-binding capacity with one-year clinical outcomes. pDSAs were defined as donor-specific antibodies (DSAs) that were produced before kidney transplants (KTs) (pre-pDSAs) or within the first four weeks after KTs, owing to rebound immune response (post-pDSAs). Of 455 adult KT recipients, pre-pDSAs and post-pDSAs were found in 56 (12.3%) and 56 (12.3%) recipients, respectively, and C3d-positive post-pDSAs were found in 13 recipients (2.9%) in total. Approximately half of the C3d-negative pre-pDSAs (37/73, 50.7%) disappeared after transplantation; however, all C3d-positive pre-pDSAs (8/8, 100%) persisted after transplantation despite desensitization (p = 0.008). C3d-positive pDSAs were significantly associated with a higher incidence and risk of AMR (p < 0.001, OR 94.467–188.934). Identification of the C3d-binding activity of pDSAs before and early after KT is important for predicting the persistence of pDSAs and the risk of AMR induced by the presence of pDSAs.

Keywords: kidney transplant (KT); donor-specific antibodies (DSA); C3d-binding assay; antibody-mediated rejection (AMR)

---

1. Introduction

Donor-specific human leukocyte antigen antibodies (DSAs) are a critical factor in kidney transplantation (KT), as antibody-mediated rejection (AMR) induced by the binding of DSAs to the allograft represents a major post-transplant complication. If DSAs are detected before transplantation, desensitization procedures, such as the administration of rituximab or intravenous immunoglobulin (IVIG), or plasmapheresis, may be performed to reduce the DSA titer and lower the risk of AMR [1].

Single antigen bead-based antibody identification (SAB) assays are generally used as the standard for DSA monitoring. However, the clinical relevance of all the detected DSAs remains unclear because the presence of DSAs does not always correlate with complement-mediated cytotoxicity crossmatching and may not induce AMR. Recently, C1q- and C3d-binding assays were introduced as methods for predicting the presence of complement-binding functional antibodies; however, the prognostic value of these tests remains controversial [2–8]. In particular, the clinical significance of preformed DSAs (pDSAs) with complement-binding activities has been not fully evaluated.

Human leukocyte antigen (HLA) antibodies at a titer below the SAB assay cut-off level or diluted across multiple beads that share target epitopes may not be appropriately detected in SAB assays. The titer of those cryptic antibodies can be elevated by immunological memory response shortly after KT [9]. Wiebe et al. suggested that false-negative pDSAs and their increased titer after transplantation, due to memory B cell activation, may create the false impression of de novo DSA (dnDSA) early post-transplantation. They suggested that no dnDSA was detected prior to 6 months when using two strict definitions: (1) all historic and current samples were DSA-negative, with an MFI cut-off of 300 and special attention to grouped epitopes; (2) no AMR in protocol biopsies at 6 months after transplantation [10]. Therefore, we thought that DSAs that were found only before KT should not be defined as pDSAs. In this study, we considered all of the DSAs produced within one month following KT as pDSAs and then investigated the production of pDSAs in pre- and post-transplantation and evaluated their effect on the occurrence of acute rejection and clinical outcome associated with their C3d-binding activity.

2. Materials and Methods

2.1. Study Population

Of the 560 adult recipients who underwent KT between January 2013 and July 2017 at the Samsung Medical Centre, Seoul, Korea, 455 patients (279 men and 176 women) were included in this study. Multi-organ, ABO-incompatible, or combined kidney and bone marrow transplantation cases were excluded (Figure 1). Recipients who underwent desensitization owing to a high level of panel reactive antibodies (PRA) (over 50%) without DSAs were excluded. All cases were negative for complement-dependent cytotoxicity (CDC), crossmatched on the day of transplantation. DSA status was monitored pre-transplantation (within 1 month before KT) and post-transplantation (at 1 and 4 weeks after KT). The recipients were divided into four groups according to the presence of DSAs before (pre-pDSA) and after transplantation (post-pDSA): Group 1, the pDSA-negative group (recipients without pre- and post-pDSAs); Group 2, the cryptic pDSA rebound group (comprising recipients with post-pDSA only); Group 3, the pDSA reversed group (recipients with pre-pDSA only); and Group 4, the pDSA persistent group (recipients with both pre- and post-pDSAs). To determine the effect of C3d-binding capacity on clinical outcomes, the post-pDSA positive groups (Groups 2 and 4) were subdivided according to their C3d-binding capacity. A schematic of the study is shown in Figure 2. This study was approved by the Institutional Review Board of Samsung Medical Centre, Seoul, Korea (SMC-2016-07-140-003), and the requirement for the subjects' informed consent was waived.

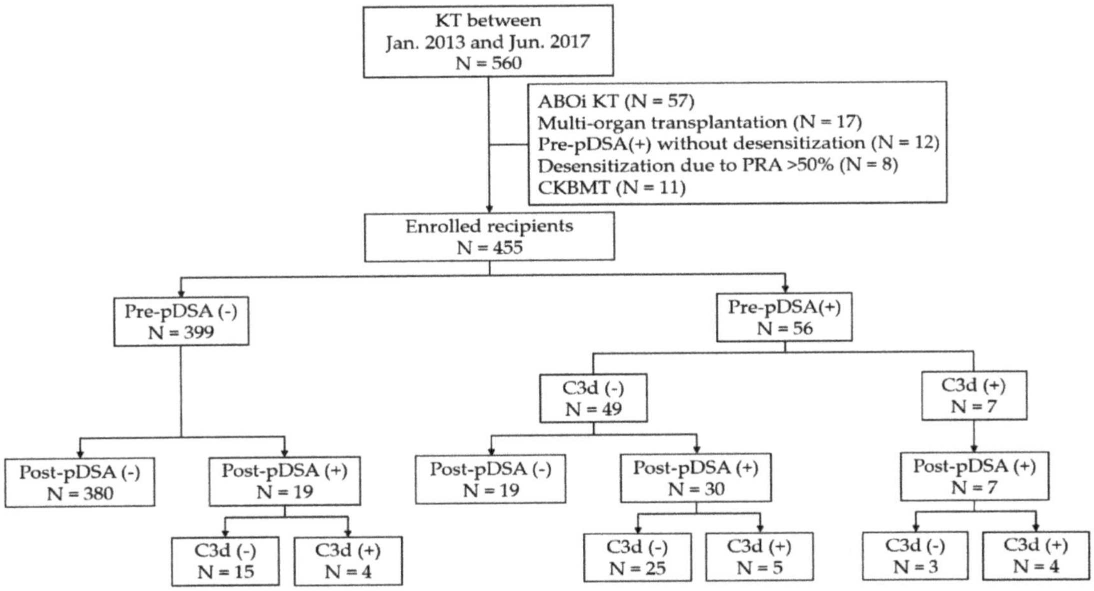

Figure 1. Study population and recipient groups according to donor-specific antibody (DSA) presence and C3d-binding capacity. Pre-pDSA, DSA confirmed before transplantation; Post-pDSA, DSA confirmed within 1 month of KT; KT, kidney transplantation; ABOi, ABO-incompatible; pDSA, preformed donor-specific HLA antibody; PRA, panel-reactive antibody; CKBMT, combined kidney and bone marrow transplantation.

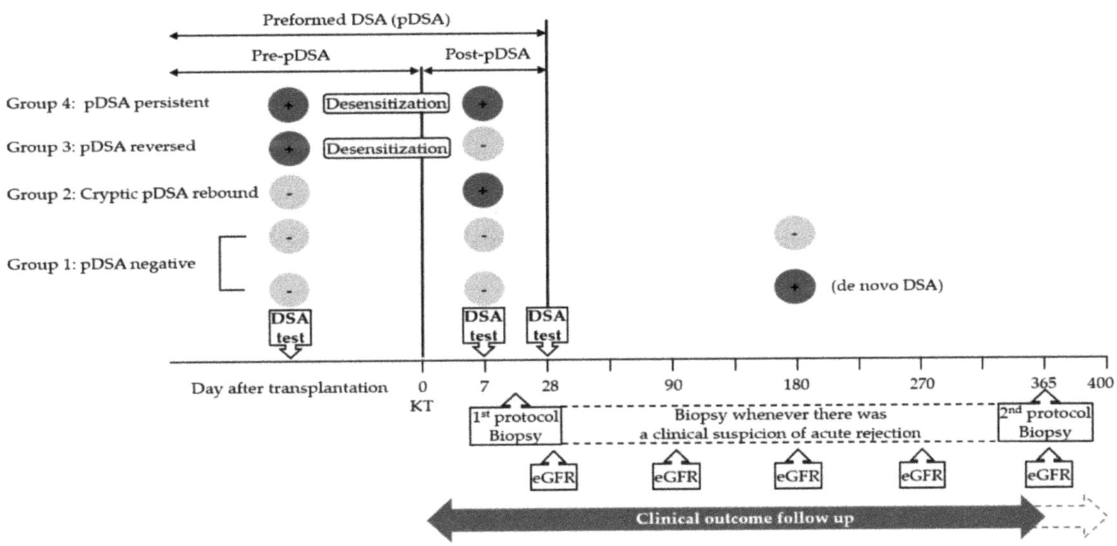

Figure 2. The study scheme showing definitions of recipient groups and a summary of clinical outcome follow up. All DSAs presented within 1 month before KT and produced within 1 month after KT were considered as preformed DSAs (pDSAs). Pre-pDSA, DSAs confirmed before transplantation; Post-pDSA, DSAs confirmed at 1 week and/or 4 weeks after KT; KT, kidney transplantation; pDSA, preformed donor-specific HLA antibody; SAB, single antigen bead-based antibody identification assay; eGFR, estimated glomerular filtration rate.

2.2. Desensitization and Immunosuppression

The desensitization protocol consisted of the administration of rituximab (Genentech Inc., San Francisco, CA, USA), treatment with intravenous immunoglobulin (IVIG) (Green Cross, Seoul, Korea), and plasmapheresis by using a COBE Spectra (Gambro BCR, Lakewood, CO, USA) before transplantation. In recipients with a pre-pDSA mean fluorescence intensity (MFI) of ≥2,500 by SAB assay, all three desensitization protocols were performed; in recipients with a low pre-pDSA MFI of

<2,500 by SAB assay, only rituximab was administered. For the induction of immunosuppression, recombinant anti-thymocyte globulin (rATG) (Genzyme, Cambridge, MA, USA) was administered on Day 0; it was administered post-transplantation on Days 1 and 2. Basiliximab (Simulect, Novartis, Basel, Switzerland) was used to induce immunosuppression in recipients without pre-pDSA. Desensitization and immunosuppression protocol details have been described elsewhere [11].

2.3. *Immunologic Assays*

HLA-A, -B, -C, -DRB1, and -DQB1 loci HLA typing for donors and recipients was performed by using polymerase chain reaction with sequence-specific primer (PCR-SSP) (One Lambda, Canoga Park, CA, USA) or reverse sequence-specific oligonucleotide probes (rSSOP) (Immucor, Peachtree Corners, GA, USA).

Anti-HLA antibody measurements were performed at 1 and 4 weeks after KT. Anti-HLA class I and II IgG antibodies were tested by using a Luminex bead-based detection assay. The LABScreen Mixed kit (One Lambda, Waltham, MA, USA) was used to screen for class I and II antibodies in conjunction with the HLA Fusion software v3.0 (One Lambda, Canoga Park, CA, USA). Sera that were positive in the screening test were subsequently tested for HLA antibody specificities and the presence of DSA using the LIFECODES LSA Class I and Class II SAB kit (Immucor, Stamford, CT, USA) in accordance with the manufacturer's recommendations; the results were analyzed by using Match-It software v1.2 (Immucor, Norcross, GA, USA). All sera were subjected to SAB treatment with 50 mM dithiothreitol (DTT) for 30 min. Antibody-positive results were assigned when more than two criteria were calculated from background MFI, control MFI was calculated, and the normalization factors recommended by the manufacturer were met.

The complement-binding capacity of DSAs in sera stored at −70 °C was measured using the LIFECODES C3d assay kit (Immucor, Stamford, CT, USA) in accordance with the manufacturer's instructions.

2.4. *Data Collection and Statistical Methods*

Data describing patient characteristics and their clinical outcomes were obtained from medical records. Categorical variables were summarized by number and percentage (%) and compared among groups by using Fisher's exact test or the chi-square test as appropriate. For continuous variables, the Shapiro–Wilks test was performed beforehand to examine the normality of distributions, and then summarized with mean (SD, standard deviation) or median (IQR, interquartile range) and compared among groups using one-way ANOVA or the Kruskal–Wallis test according to the normality of their distribution.

2.4.1. Recipient Characteristics

Data on demography, underlying diseases, transplantation conditions, conditioning, and immunosuppression regimens were included in the analysis.

2.4.2. HLA Antibody Characterization

Preformed DSAs (pDSAs) were defined as DSAs that were produced before KT (pre-pDSAs), including Groups 3 and 4, or within the first 4 weeks after KT due to rebound immune response (post-pDSAs), such as Group 2. One of our hypotheses was that the cryptic pDSA rebound group (Group 2) would be useful for the assessment of the effects of pDSAs that were undetectable before transplantation using current antibody tests, and patients were therefore not subjected to the pre-transplant desensitization, in contrast to the sensitization in the pre-pDSA positive groups (Groups 3 and 4). Receiver operating curves (ROC) were plotted to assess SAB MFI performance in an effort to predict the C3d-binding activities of HLA antibodies. Optimal cut-offs exhibiting maximal sensitivity and specificity (Youden index) were obtained for risk assessment of the presence of DSAs.

2.4.3. Clinical Outcome

To assess clinical outcomes, graft rejection rate, rejection-free survival, and graft function were evaluated. Graft biopsy was performed on Day 14 and 1 year post-KT, or whenever there was clinical suspicion of acute rejection. Biopsy results up to 400 days after KT were included in the analysis because the protocol-mandated biopsy schedule was delayed for some patients due to hospital or patient circumstances. Acute cellular rejection (ACR) and AMR were diagnosed in accordance with the Banff Criteria 2013 [12]. The rates of ACR and AMR occurrence were compared among recipient groups using Fisher's exact test or the chi-square test, as appropriate. The univariable logistic regression was repeatedly used for the four-group comparison (Groups 1, 2, 3, and 4) and also for two- or four-subgroup comparisons: Group 1, Group 4 C3d (-) subgroup, and Group 4 C3d (+) subgroup. Wald's chi-square test was used for pairwise comparison with Bonferroni's correction. Rejection-free survival rates were estimated by using the Kaplan–Meier method, and the four groups were compared via the stratified log-rank test. Graft function was evaluated using the estimated glomerular filtration rate (eGFR) at 1, 3, 6, 9, and 12 months post-KT. eGFR was calculated using the modification of diet in renal disease (MDRD) study equation. Generalized estimating equation (GEE) analyses were applied to repeated measurements of eGFR. $p < 0.05$ was considered statistically significant.

2.4.4. Statistical Software

Statistical analyses were computed by using SAS v9.4 (SAS Institute, Cary, NC, USA) and SPSS v22.0 (IBM, Armonk, NY, USA). Analyse-it v5.10 (Analyse-it Software, Leeds, UK) was used for graphical analyses.

3. Results

3.1. Recipient Characteristics

Fifty-six recipients (12.3%) had detectable DSAs prior to KT (re-pDSA; Figure 1). The patients were divided into four groups according to their pre- and post-KT DSA status: the pDSA negative group (Group 1; $n = 380$, 83.5%), the cryptic pDSA rebound group (Group 2; $n = 19$, 4.2%), a pDSA reversed group (Group 3; $n = 19$, 4.2%), and a pDSA persistent group (Group 4; $n = 37$, 8.1%). All recipients with pre-pDSA (Groups 3 and 4) underwent desensitization. The recipient characteristics for each group are summarized in Table 1.

In pre-transplantation, seven recipients (12.5%) had C3d-positive pDSAs; however, the number of recipients having C3d-positive pDSAs increased to 13 recipients (23.2%) within the first month after KT. Five recipients exhibited persistently C3d-positive pDSAs before and after transplantation. HLA classes of total and C3d (+) DSAs in Groups 2, 3, and 4 are summarized in Table 2. Class II DSAs were assessed with limited loci, as –DR and -DQB1. In contrast with the higher frequencies of class I HLAs in pre-transplantation, class II HLAs were more frequent in post-transplantation, not only among total DSAs but also among C3d (+) DSAs. However, there were no significant differences in the distribution of post-pDSA class and SAB MFI between Groups 2 and 4 ($p = 1.000$; $p = 0.327$ in class I and $p = 0.882$ in class II, respectively; Supplementary Table S1).

Table 1. Patient characteristics.

Characteristics	Total	Group 1: pDSA negative	Group 2: Cryptic pDSA rebound	Group 3: pDSA reversed	Group 4: pDSA persistent	*p*-Value *
Number	455	380	19	19	37	
Age, median (IQR)	52.0 (43.0–59.0)	52.0 (42.0–59.0)	49.0 (40.0–56.3)	51.0 (44.2–57.7)	52.0 (48.0–60.0)	0.635
Sex (male) (%)	279 (61.3)	259 (68.2)	7 (36.8)	1 (5.3)	12 (32.4)	<0.001
Dialysis duration, median (IQR)	810.0 (50.2–2173.7)	843.5 (51.4–2164.1)	260.0 (47.3–2107.2)	172.0 (1.2–1652.7)	1305.0 (82.7–2428.3)	0.333
Underlying diseases (%)						
DM	125 (27.5)	114 (37.1)	3 (15.8)	3 (15.8)	5 (13.5)	0.034
GN (1 – 3)	71 (15.6)	61 (16.1)	1 (5.3)	1 (5.3)	8 (21.6)	
IgA	62 (13.6)	49 (12.9)	4 (21.1)	6 (31.6)	3 (8.1)	
Other	176 (38.7)	141 (37.1)	10 (52.6)	5 (26.3)	20 (54.1)	
Re-transplantation (%)	46 (10.1)	28 (7.4)	4 (21.1)	0 (0.0)	14 (37.8)	<0.001
DDKT (%)	230 (50.5)	192 (50.5)	10 (52.6)	9 (47.4)	19 (51.4)	0.989
Desensitization						
RTX	46 (10.1)	0 (0.0)	0 (0.0)	13 (68.4)	33 (89.2)	NA
RTX + PP	10 (2.2)	0 (0.0)	0 (0.0)	6 (31.6)	4 (10.8)	
Induction therapy						
rATG	291 (64.0)	226 (59.5)	10 (52.6)	19 (100.0)	36 (97.3)	NA
Basiliximab	164 (36.0)	154 (40.5)	9 (47.4)	0 (0.0)	1 (2.7)	
Maintenance regimen						
CsA + MMF (PD)	6 (1.3)	6 (1.6)	0 (0.0)	0 (0.0)	0 (0.0)	NA
FK + MMF (PD)	446 (98.0)	372 (97.9)	18 (94.7)	19 (100)	37 (100)	
Sirolimus/Everolimus combination	3 (0.7)	2 (0.5)	1 (5.3)	0 (0.0)	0 (0.0)	
Pre-sensitization (PRA %)						
Class I	0.0 (0.0–0.0)	0.0 (0.0–0.0)	0.0 (0.0–11.7)	37.0 (5.4–77.0)	54.0 (0.0–87.7)	<0.001
Class II	0.0 (0.0–0.0)	0.0 (0.0–0.0)	0.0 (0.0–14.0)	0.0 (0.0–63.8)	36.0 (0.0–74.3)	<0.001
HLA mismatches, median (IQR)	3.0 (2.0–4.0)	3.0 (2.0–4.0)	4.0 (2.0–4.0)	3.0 (2.2–4.8)	3.0 (2.0–4.0)	0.642

* $p < 0.05$ was considered statistically significant. IQR, interquartile range; DM, diabetes mellitus; GN, glomerulonephritis; IgA, IgA nephropathy; DDKT, deceased donor kidney transplantation; pDSA, preformed donor-specific HLA antibody; NA, not applicable; MFI, mean fluorescence intensity; RTX, rituximab; PP, plasmapheresis; rATG, recombinant anti-thymocyte globulin; CsA, cyclosporine A; MMF, Mycophenolate mofetil; PD, prednisolone; FK, FK506; PRA, panel reactive antibody.

Table 2. HLA classes and complement binding activities of pre- and post-transplantation donor-specific HLA antibodies in recipient groups.

HLA Classes of pDSA	Group 2: Cryptic pDSA Rebound		Group 3: pDSA Reversed		Group 4: pDSA Persistent	
	Total pDSA	**C3d (+) pDSA**	**Total pDSA**	**C3d (+) pDSA**	**Total pDSA**	**C3d (+) pDSA**
Pre-transplantation			19	**0 (0.0)**	37	7 (18.9)
Class I only	NA	NA	13 (68.4)	0 (0.0)	13 (35.1)	0 (0.0)
Class II* only	NA	NA	5 (26.3)	0 (0.0)	14 (37.8)	7 (18.9)
Class I + II*	NA	NA	1 (0.53)	0 (0.0)	10 (27.0)	0 (0.0)
Post-transplantation	19	4 (21.1)			37	9 (24.3)
Class I only	6 (31.6)	1 (5.3)	NA	NA	11 (29.7)	0 (0.0)
Class II* only	11 (57.9)	3 (15.8)	NA	NA	21 (56.8)	9 (24.3)
Class I + II*	2 (10.5)	0 (0.0)	NA	NA	5 (13.5)	0 (0.0)

* Class II pDSAs were assessed limited loci; as –DR, and -DQB1. Bold letters indicate significant results. pDSA, preformed donor-specific HLA antibody; MFI, mean fluorescent intensity; NA, not applicable.

3.2. *HLA Antibody Characteristics, Including Complement Binding Capacities*

In total, 105 pDSAs derived from 75 recipients (Groups 2, 3, and 4) were identified; the median number per recipient was 1.4 (range: 1–6) (Supplementary Table S2). Of these pDSAs, 81 (77.1%) were persistent pre-pDSA, and 24 (22.9%) were rebound cryptic pDSAs that were newly produced within 4 weeks post-KT. C3d-binding capacities were observed in 9.9% (8/81) of pre-pDSA and 20.6% (14/68) of post-pDSA. Among the 73 C3d-negative pre-pDSAs derived from 49 recipients, 50.7% (37/73) became negative (pDSA reversed), 43.8% (32/73) persisted as C3d-negative, and 5.5% (4/73) became C3d-positive after transplantation. Pre-pDSA SAB MFIs were significantly higher in Group 4 than in Group 3 ($p < 0.001$). Importantly, all 8 C3d-positive pre-pDSAs identified in 7 recipients persisted after transplantation, although 25% (2/8) became C3d-negative, which was significant when compared with the C3d-negative pre-pDSAs ($p = 0.008$; Figure 3, red lines).

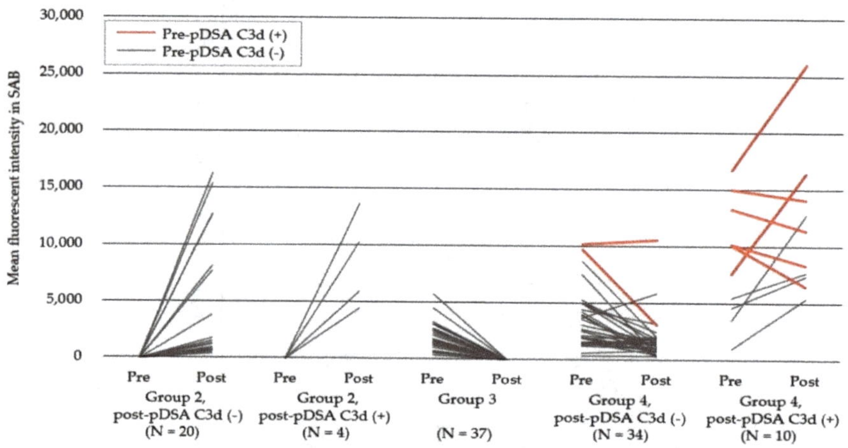

Figure 3. Production and MFI changes of pDSAs within 4 weeks of kidney transplantation in different patient groups. The red lines indicate cases of C3d-positive pDSAs and the grey lines highlight cases of C3d-negative pDSAs. pDSA, preformed donor-specific HLA antibody; MFI, mean fluorescence intensity.

To determine the SAB MFI cut-offs for HLA antibodies predicting C3d-binding activities, all 1515 HLA antibodies from 112 recipients were analyzed (Figure 4). The numbers of observed HLA antibodies to A, B, C, DR, DQB1, and DPB1 were 322, 526, 71, 370, 159, and 67, respectively. SAB MFIs of C3d-positive antibodies were significantly higher than those of C3d-negative antibodies in all loci. For class I antibodies, 15.1% (139/919) of the HLA antibodies were C3d-positive, and their median SAB MFI was 9429 (IQR: 5457–16,016), whereas that of the C3d-negative antibodies was 1988 (IQR: 1271–3190). The optimal cut-off value of the total class I loci for predicting C3d-binding activities was 7797, and the area under the curve (AUC) was 0.908. For class II antibodies, 42.6% (254/596) of the HLA antibodies were C3d-positive, and their median SAB MFI was 10,341 (IQR: 6693–14,207), whereas that of the C3d-negative antibodies was 1,711 (IQR: 1002–3401). The optimal cut-off value of total class II loci was 4460, and the AUC was 0.914 (Supplementary Table S3, Supplementary Figure S1).

3.3. *Rejection Episodes and Graft Function*

Overall, 177 recipients (38.9%) were diagnosed with rejection episodes, including ACR and AMR, with an incidence of 168 (36.9%) and 13 (2.9%), respectively; in addition, 4 (1.7%) recipients were diagnosed with both ACR and AMR (Table 3). The incidence of ACR among the four groups was not significantly different. In contrast, the incidence of AMR among the four groups was significantly different. In both Groups 2 and 4, recipients with C3d-positive post-pDSA exhibited a significantly higher incidence of AMR (2/4, 50.0% and 3/9, 33.3%, respectively) than recipients with C3d-negative post-pDSA (1/15, 6.7% and 4/28, 14.3%, respectively). The odds ratio (OR) of AMR risk was significantly increased in the Group 2 C3d (+) subgroup and both C3d (-) and (+) subgroups in Group 4 compared with Group 1 (Table 4). Although it had marginal statistical significance (adjusted $p = 0.0876$), the C3d-positive subgroup, but not the C3d-negative subgroup in Group 2, exhibited quite different OR (OR = 0.056 and OR = 0.778, respectively) compared with Group 3.

The 1-year AMR-free survival was also significantly different among all groups (Figure 5a), and it was the lowest in the C3d-positive subgroup of Group 2, the cryptic pDSA rebound cases (Figure 5b).

During the maximum 400 day follow-up period (median 17.5, IQR 12.0–330.0), graft failure was not observed in any recipients, and the eGFR differences observed among the groups were not significantly different at any time point ($p = 0.575$; Supplementary Figure S2).

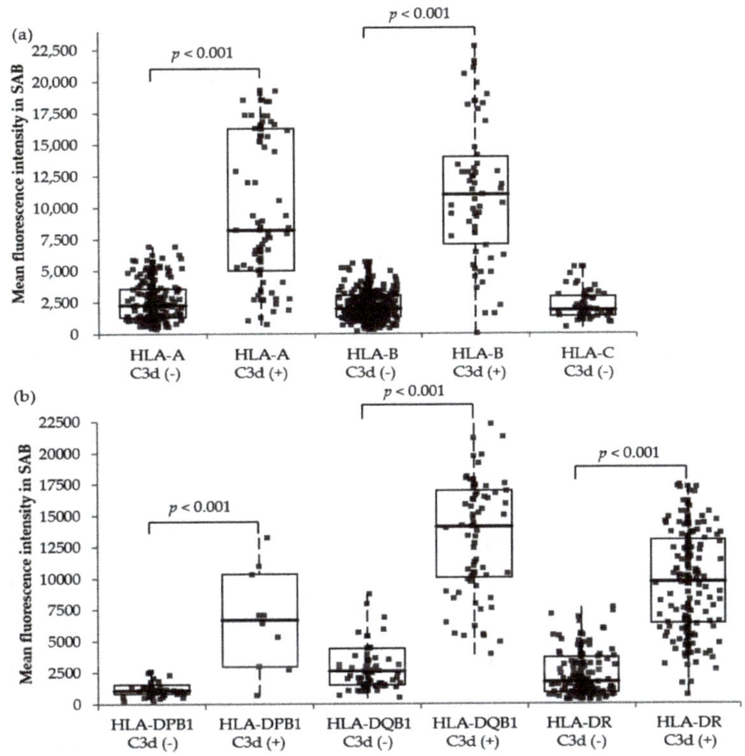

Figure 4. Mean fluorescence intensity distribution of 1522 Class I and II HLA antibodies according to their loci and C3d-binding capacities (**a**,**b**). Box plot, 1st to 3rd quartile range and whiskers extend to the furthest observation within 1.5× interquartile range from the quartiles. SAB, single antigen bead-based antibody identification assay.

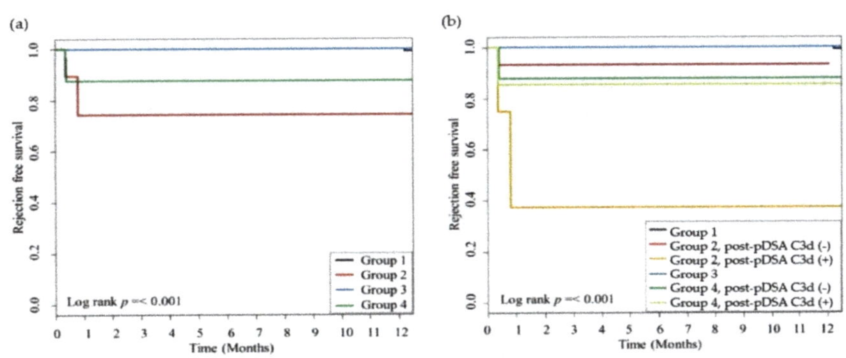

Figure 5. AMR-free survival according to the presence of pre-and post-pDSAs and C3d-binding capacities. The incidences of AMR were significantly different among the groups (**a**) and when considering the presence of post-pDSA C3d-binding capacities (**b**) ($p < 0.001$, respectively). The statistical difference between the Kaplan–Meier survival curves was evaluated by using the log-rank test, and p-values of <0.05 were considered statistically significant. AMR, antibody-mediated rejection; pDSA, preformed donor-specific HLA antibody.

4. Discussion

Both preformed DSAs present before (pre-pDSAs) and early after KT (post-pDSAs) were associated with the risk of AMR when they had C3d-binding activities. In particular, C3d-positive pre-pDSAs tended to persist after transplantation, despite the pretransplant desensitization.

4.1. Cryptic DSAs

pDSAs that were produced within 1 month of transplantation were considered as cryptic pDSAs with anamnestic reactions [10]. Using this study design, we compared the clinical effect of pDSAs with or without pre-transplantation desensitization. Our results indicated that the presence of rebound pDSA was primarily associated with AMR, followed by that of persistent pDSA, reversed pDSA, and negative pDSA.

The incidence of newly produced DSAs after transplantation, which usually occurs within 1 year of KT, with a variable median time between 6 months and 4.6 years, has been reported in 13% to 30% of pDSA-negative recipients before KT [10,13,14]. Several studies have analyzed the effect of early produced DSAs, which were defined as those produced within 1 year of transplantation [15,16], but it remained unclear whether this was dnDSA or pDSA [16]. King et al. reported that DSAs that were produced sooner than 1 month after transplantation exerted more pronounced effects on recipients and allografts than the effects of those produced later [16]. Cryptic DSAs may exist below the detection limit of the current antibody tests and can be induced rapidly by anamnestic reactions after re-stimulation by the donor graft. This is in contrast with dnDSAs, which develop gradually through the primary immune reaction associated with an indirect pathway after encountering new alloantigens [9,10]. Anamnestic reactions lead to the production of C3d-positive pDSAs, and this was related to the highest incidence of AMR in this study. Therefore, further studies regarding the management of cryptic pDSAs are necessary.

4.2. Persistent pDSAs

pDSA persistence is known to be associated with AMR. Kimball et al. reported a higher AMR incidence in persistent pDSA groups than in negatively converted groups (43% and 3%, respectively) [17]. In addition, Marfo et al. demonstrated that recipients with persistent pDSAs experienced more acute and chronic rejection ($p = 0.006$) than recipients with reversed pDSA [18]. The independent risk factor associated with persistence of pDSA was pre-transplant MFI, as shown by Redondo-Pachon et al., and class II DSAs persisted more frequently [19]. Similarly, we found that persistent pDSAs possessed higher MFIs. Although the risk of AMR was not statistically different between the persistent pDSA group and reversed pDSA group, it tended to be higher in the persistent pDSA group. The C3d-positivity (33.3%, 3/9) of persistent pDSA resulted in an increased risk of AMR (OR = 9.000, $p = 0.0781$) compared with C3d-negative group (OR = 3.000, $p = 0.3439$).

Table 3. Comparison of the occurrence of rejection in recipient groups.

	Total	Group 1: pDSA Negative	Group 2: Cryptic pDSA Rebound			Group 3: pDSA Reversed	Group 4: pDSA Persistent			*p*-Value*
			Post-pDSA C3d (-)	Post-pDSA C3d (+)	*p*-Value		Post-pDSA C3d (-)	Post-pDSA C3d (+)	*p*-Value	
Number	455	380	15	4		19	28	9		
ACR (%)	168 (36.9)	142 (37.4)	7 (46.7)	2 (50.0)	0.906	7 (36.8)	7 (25.0)	3 (33.3)	0.624	0.479
AMR (%)	13 (2.9)	2 (0.5)	1 (6.7)	2 (50.0)	**0.035**	1 (5.3)	4 (14.3)	3 (33.3)	0.204	< **0.001**

* p-values among the four groups without consideration of post-DSA C3d-binding activity. $p < 0.05$ was considered statistically significant. Bold letters indicate significant results. pDSA, preformed donor-specific HLA antibody; ACR, acute cellular rejection; AMR, antibody-mediated rejection.

Table 4. Estimated risk of antibody-mediated rejection between recipient groups according to C3d-binding activities of post-transplant pDSAs.

Comparison groups	Odds ratio (95% CI)	95% Confidence limits		*p*-Value*	Adjusted *p*-value*
Group 1 vs. Group 2	**35.425**	5.528	227.022	**< 0.001**	**0.001**
Group 1 vs. Group 2 C3d (-)	**13.495**	1.154	157.782	**0.038**	0.076
Group 1 vs. Group 2 C3d (+)	**188.934**	17.098	>999.999	**<0.001**	**<0.001**
Group 1 vs. Group 3	10.496	0.909	121.203	0.060	0.358
Group 1 vs. Group 4	**44.084**	8.771	221.57	**<0.001**	**<0.001**
Group 1 vs. Group 4 C3d (-)	**31.489**	5.491	180.593	**<0.001**	**<0.001**
Group 1 vs. Group 4 C3d (+)	**94.467**	13.275	672.252	**<0.001**	**<0.001**
Group 2 vs. Group 3	0.296	0.028	3.142	0.313	0.999
Group 2 C3d (-) vs. Group 3	0.778	0.045	13.559	0.863	0.999
Group 2 C3d (+) vs. Group 3	**0.056**	0.003	0.923	**0.044**	0.088
Group 2 vs. Group 4	1.244	0.283	5.48	0.773	0.999
Group 2 C3d (-) vs. Group 4 C3d (-)	2.333	0.237	22.999	0.468	0.999
Group 2 C3d (-) vs. Group 4 C3d (+)	7.000	0.6	81.674	0.121	0.965
Group 2 C3d (+) vs. Group 4 C3d (-)	0.167	0.018	1.546	0.115	0.919
Group 2 C3d (+) vs. Group 4 C3d (+)	0.500	0.045	5.514	0.571	0.999
Group 3 vs. Group 4	4.200	0.477	36.978	0.196	0.999
Group 3 vs. Group 4 C3d (-)	3.000	0.308	29.182	0.344	0.688
Group 3 vs. Group 4 C3d (+)	9.000	0.781	103.723	0.078	0.156

* p-values of < 0.05 were considered statistically significant; bold letters indicate significant results; adjusted p-values were computed with Bonferroni's correction for multiple comparisons. pDSA, preformed donor-specific HLA antibody; CI, confidence interval.

4.3. Complement-Binding Capacities and Clinical Outcome

SAB was designed to detect all IgG antibody isotypes, irrespective of their complement-binding capacity. IgG3 was the most potent complement binder among the subclasses of IgG and significantly affected the occurrence of rejection and graft loss after transplantation via IgG3-induced C1q-binding [20]. Honger et al. reported that IgG pre-pDSA was composed of 39% IgG1 and/or IgG3, 7% IgG2 and/or IgG4, and a 54% mixture of both complement-binding and weak/non-complement-binding subclasses [21]. These findings suggested that not all SAB-positive antibodies promoted complement activation, rejection, and graft loss. Therefore, two modified SAB assays targeting different complement derivatives were recently introduced (the C1q- and C3d-binding assays). dnDSAs harboring C1q-binding capacity were known to affect clinical outcomes such as graft survival, acute AMR, and transplant glomerulopathy [8,22–27], but the role of pDSA in AMR or poor graft survival prediction is controversial [28–31]. C3d-positive dnDSA increased the risk of graft loss, AMR, proteinuria, C4d histological staining, and rapid progression to graft dysfunction [3,6,32,33]; however, C3d-positive pre-pDSA was reported not to increase the risk of graft failure significantly [34]. In the present study, we performed a C3d-binding assay, rather than a C1q-binding assay, for two reasons. First, targeting C3d is more relevant because C3d is derived after the initiation of the complement activation cascade, so it may reflect more of the functional aspects of antibodies [7]. Second, less data are available on the significance of C3d-positive pDSAs than that of C1q-positive pDSAs. We also found that C3d-positive pDSAs tended to persist after KT, and were associated with higher AMR incidence, regardless of desensitization.

The threshold of SAB MFI, which was correlated with C1q- and C3d-binding capacities, has been reported [3,7], with the purpose of estimating the risk of identified antibodies in a timely manner before carrying out the subsequent complement binding assay. The suggested cut-off MFIs for predicting C3d-binding capacities in previous reports ranged from 4225–17,057 and 8356–15,027 for HLA class I and class II antibodies, respectively [6,32,35]. Class II HLA antibodies were reported to possess higher MFIs than those of class I in regard to C3d-binding capacity. In this study, the median MFI of C3d-positive antibodies also tended to be higher in class II than those of class I, but the optimal cut-off value of class I (MFI, 7797; sensitivity, 61.9%; specificity, 97.9%) was higher than that of class II (MFI, 4460; sensitivity, 88.9%; specificity, 83.9%). Such a discrepancy may be due to different sensitivities and specificities, as determined by different studies or the limited number of HLA antibodies analyzed in our study. Kamburova et al. reported that 95% of C3d-positive antibodies exhibit SAB MFI values of 4000 or more, but only 56% of antibodies exhibiting an MFI of 4000 or more possessed C3d-binding capacity. Based on this, they suggested that the C3d-binding capacity was correlated with the SAB MFI; however, positivity cannot be completely predicted based on SAB MFI [34].

This study has a few limitations. First, the definition of pDSAs, which included cryptic pDSAs, was not verified by using donor-specific mBCs, and the possibility of rapidly produced dnDSAs cannot be excluded. Second, the number of recipients who progressed to AMR was small, although the study was able to determine statistical significance from these data. Finally, the contribution of HLA-DP DSAs could not be estimated, as donor and recipient DP typing was not performed.

5. Conclusions

The monitoring of pDSA persistence, particularly that with C3d-binding capacities that occurred despite desensitization, and of DSA production immediately following KT likely reflects that elevated cryptic pDSAs, due to the anamnestic response, are critical for the prediction of AMR. This approach would aid the initiation of timely therapeutic intervention to reduce the risk of DSAs.

identification assay performance in an effort to predict complement binding capability in class I (a) and class II (b); Figure S2: eGFR differences observed among the groups were not significantly different. eGFR was calculated by the modification of diet in renal disease (MDRD) study equation.

Author Contributions: E.S.K. conceived the study; S.C., K.W.L., J.B.P., H.-R.J., W.H., and E.S.K. conducted the research described; C.S. and K.K. performed the statistical analysis; all authors contributed to writing the final manuscript. All authors have read and agreed to the published version of the manuscript.

Acknowledgments: The authors wish to acknowledge the contributions of Bok Ryo Kim, R.N., and the technical support of Jun Woo Park, M.T.

References

1. Montgomery, R.A.; Lonze, B.E.; King, K.E.; Kraus, E.S.; Kucirka, L.M.; Locke, J.E.; Warren, D.S.; Simpkins, C.E.; Dagher, N.N.; Singer, A.L. Desensitization in hla-incompatible kidney recipients and survival. *N. Engl. J. Med.* **2011**, *365*, 318–326. [CrossRef] [PubMed]
2. Sicard, A.; Ducreux, S.; Rabeyrin, M.; Couzi, L.; McGregor, B.; Badet, L.; Scoazec, J.Y.; Bachelet, T.; Lepreux, S.; Visentin, J.; et al. Detection of c3d-binding donor-specific anti-hla antibodies at diagnosis of humoral rejection predicts renal graft loss. *J. Am. Soc. Nephrol.* **2015**, *26*, 457–467. [CrossRef] [PubMed]
3. Comoli, P.; Cioni, M.; Tagliamacco, A.; Quartuccio, G.; Innocente, A.; Fontana, I.; Trivelli, A.; Magnasco, A.; Nocco, A.; Klersy, C. Acquisition of c3d-binding activity by de novo donor-specific hla antibodies correlates with graft loss in nonsensitized pediatric kidney recipients. *Am. J. Transp.* **2016**, *16*, 2106–2116. [CrossRef] [PubMed]
4. Kovandova, B.; Slavcev, A.; Sekerkova, Z.; Honsova, E.; Trunecka, P. Antibody-mediated rejection after liver transplantation-relevance of c1q and c3d-binding antibodies. *HLA* **2018**, *92*, 34–37. [CrossRef]
5. Lee, D.R.; Kim, B.C.; Kim, J.P.; Kim, I.G.; Jeon, M.Y. C3d-binding donor-specific hla antibody is associated with a high risk of antibody-mediated rejection and graft loss in stable kidney transplant recipients: A single-center cohort study. *Transp. Proc.* **2018**, *50*, 3452–3459. [CrossRef]
6. Pelletier, R.P.; Balazs, I.; Adams, P.; Rajab, A.; DiPaola, N.R.; Henry, M.L. Clinical utility of c3d binding donor-specific anti-human leukocyte antigen antibody detection by single antigen beads after kidney transplantation-a retrospective study. *Transp. Int.* **2018**, *31*, 424–435. [CrossRef]
7. Claisse, G.; Absi, L.; Cognasse, F.; Alamartine, E.; Mariat, C.; Maillard, N. Relationship between mean fluorescence intensity and c1q/c3d-fixing capacities of anti-hla antibodies. *Hum. Immunol.* **2017**, *78*, 336–341. [CrossRef]
8. Calp-Inal, S.; Ajaimy, M.; Melamed, M.L.; Savchik, C.; Masiakos, P.; Colovai, A.; Akalin, E. The prevalence and clinical significance of c1q-binding donor-specific anti-hla antibodies early and late after kidney transplantation. *Kidney Int.* **2016**, *89*, 209–216. [CrossRef]
9. Wiebe, C.; Nickerson, P. Posttransplant monitoring of de novo human leukocyte antigen donor-specific antibodies in kidney transplantation. *Curr. Opin. Organ Transp.* **2013**, *18*, 470–477. [CrossRef]
10. Wiebe, C.; Gibson, I.; Blydt-Hansen, T.; Karpinski, M.; Ho, J.; Storsley, L.; Goldberg, A.; Birk, P.; Rush, D.; Nickerson, P. Evolution and clinical pathologic correlations of de novo donor-specific hla antibody post kidney transplant. *Am. J. Transp.* **2012**, *12*, 1157–1167. [CrossRef]
11. Lee, K.W.; Park, J.B.; Cho, C.W.; Lee, N.; Yoo, H.; Kim, K.; Park, H.; Kang, E.S.; Huh, W.; Kim, S. The impact of donor-specific anti-human leukocyte antigen (hla) antibody rebound on the risk of antibody mediated rejection in sensitized kidney transplant recipients. *Ann. Transp.* **2017**, *22*, 166–176. [CrossRef] [PubMed]
12. Solez, K.; Racusen, L.C. The banff classification revisited. *Kidney Int.* **2013**, *83*, 201–206. [CrossRef] [PubMed]
13. Zhang, R. Donor-specific antibodies in kidney transplant recipients. *Clin. J. Am. Soc. Nephrol.* **2018**, *13*, 182–192. [CrossRef] [PubMed]
14. Hirai, T.; Furusawa, M.; Omoto, K.; Ishida, H.; Tanabe, K. Analysis of predictive and preventive factors for de novo dsa in kidney transplant recipients. *Transplantation* **2014**, *98*, 443–450. [CrossRef] [PubMed]
15. Heilman, R.L.; Nijim, A.; Desmarteau, Y.M.; Khamash, H.; Pando, M.J.; Smith, M.L.; Chakkera, H.A.; Huskey, J.; Valdez, R.; Reddy, K.S. De novo donor-specific human leukocyte antigen antibodies early after kidney transplantation. *Transplantation* **2014**, *98*, 1310–1315. [CrossRef] [PubMed]

16. King, C.S.; Cochrane, A.B. The impact of early de novo donor-specific antibodies on lung transplant outcomes: Is timing everything? *J. Heart Lung Transp.* **2016**, *35*, 1057–1058. [CrossRef] [PubMed]
17. Kimball, P.M.; Baker, M.A.; Wagner, M.B.; King, A. Surveillance of alloantibodies after transplantation identifies the risk of chronic rejection. *Kidney Int.* **2011**, *79*, 1131–1137. [CrossRef]
18. Marfo, K.; Ajaimy, M.; Colovai, A.; Kayler, L.; Greenstein, S.; Lubetzky, M.; Gupta, A.; Kamal, L.; de Boccardo, G.; Masiakos, P.; et al. Pretransplant immunologic risk assessment of kidney transplant recipients with donor-specific anti-human leukocyte antigen antibodies. *Transplantation* **2014**, *98*, 1082–1088. [CrossRef]
19. Redondo-Pachon, D.; Perez-Saez, M.J.; Mir, M.; Gimeno, J.; Llinas, L.; Garcia, C.; Hernandez, J.J.; Yelamos, J.; Pascual, J.; Crespo, M. Impact of persistent and cleared preformed hla dsa on kidney transplant outcomes. *Hum. Immunol.* **2018**, *79*, 424–431. [CrossRef]
20. Lefaucheur, C.; Viglietti, D.; Bentlejewski, C.; van Huyen, J.-P.D.; Vernerey, D.; Aubert, O.; Verine, J.; Jouven, X.; Legendre, C.; Glotz, D. Igg donor-specific anti-human hla antibody subclasses and kidney allograft antibody-mediated injury. *J. Am. Soc. Nephrol.* **2016**, *27*, 293–304. [CrossRef]
21. Honger, G.; Hopfer, H.; Arnold, M.L.; Spriewald, B.M.; Schaub, S.; Amico, P. Pretransplant igg subclasses of donor-specific human leukocyte antigen antibodies and development of antibody-mediated rejection. *Transplantation* **2011**, *92*, 41–47. [CrossRef] [PubMed]
22. Loupy, A.; Lefaucheur, C.; Vernerey, D.; Prugger, C.; van Huyen, J.-P.D.; Mooney, N.; Suberbielle, C.; Frémeaux-Bacchi, V.; Méjean, A.; Desgrandchamps, F. Complement-binding anti-hla antibodies and kidney-allograft survival. *N. Engl. J. Med.* **2013**, *369*, 1215–1226. [CrossRef] [PubMed]
23. Bamoulid, J.; Roodenburg, A.; Staeck, O.; Wu, K.; Rudolph, B.; Brakemeier, S.; Halleck, F.; Lehner, L.; Schönemann, C.; Lachmann, N. Clinical outcome of patients with de novo c1q-binding donor-specific hla antibodies after renal transplantation. *Transplantation* **2017**, *101*, 2165–2174. [CrossRef] [PubMed]
24. Malheiro, J.; Santos, S.; Tafulo, S.; Dias, L.; Martins, L.S.; Fonseca, I.; Almeida, M.; Pedroso, S.; Beirão, I.; Castro-Henriques, A. Detection of complement-binding donor-specific antibodies, not igg-antibody strength nor c4d status, at antibody-mediated rejection diagnosis is an independent predictor of kidney graft failure. *Transplantation* **2018**, *102*, 1943–1954. [CrossRef] [PubMed]
25. Yabu, J.M.; Higgins, J.P.; Chen, G.; Sequeira, F.; Busque, S.; Tyan, D.B. C1q-fixing human leukocyte antigen antibodies are specific for predicting transplant glomerulopathy and late graft failure after kidney transplantation. *Transplantation* **2011**, *91*, 342–347. [CrossRef]
26. Fichtner, A.; Süsal, C.; Höcker, B.; Rieger, S.; Waldherr, R.; Westhoff, J.H.; Sander, A.; Opelz, G.; Tönshoff, B. Association of c1q-fixing dsa with late graft failure in pediatric renal transplant recipients. *Pediatr. Nephrol.* **2016**, *31*, 1157–1166. [CrossRef]
27. Bailly, E.; Anglicheau, D.; Blancho, G.; Gatault, P.; Vuiblet, V.; Chatelet, V.; Morelon, E.; Malvezzi, P.; Parissiadis, A.; Tourret, J. Prognostic value of the persistence of c1q-binding anti-hla antibodies in acute antibody-mediated rejection in kidney transplantation. *Transplantation* **2018**, *102*, 688–698. [CrossRef]
28. Malheiro, J.; Tafulo, S.; Dias, L.; Martins, L.S.; Fonseca, I.; Beirão, I.; Castro-Henriques, A.; Cabrita, A. Determining donor-specific antibody c1q-binding ability improves the prediction of antibody-mediated rejection in human leucocyte antigen-incompatible kidney transplantation. *Transp. Int.* **2017**, *30*, 347–359. [CrossRef]
29. Molina, J.; Navas, A.; Agüera, M.-L.; Rodelo-Haad, C.; Alonso, C.; Rodríguez-Benot, A.; Aljama, P.; Solana, R. Impact of preformed donor-specific anti-human leukocyte antigen antibody c1q-binding ability on kidney allograft outcome. *Front. Immunol.* **2017**, *8*, 1310. [CrossRef]
30. Otten, H.G.; Verhaar, M.C.; Borst, H.P.; Hene, R.J.; van Zuilen, A.D. Pretransplant donor-specific hla class-i and -ii antibodies are associated with an increased risk for kidney graft failure. *Am. J. Transp.* **2012**, *12*, 1618–1623. [CrossRef]
31. Crespo, M.; Torio, A.; Mas, V.; Redondo, D.; Pérez-Sáez, M.J.; Mir, M.; Faura, A.; Guerra, R.; Montes-Ares, O.; Checa, M.D. Clinical relevance of pretransplant anti-hla donor-specific antibodies: Does c1q-fixation matter? *Transpl. Immunol.* **2013**, *29*, 28–33. [CrossRef] [PubMed]
32. Lee, H.; Han, E.; Choi, A.-R.; Ban, T.H.; Chung, B.H.; Yang, C.W.; Choi, Y.J.; Oh, E.-J. Clinical impact of complement (c1q, c3d) binding de novo donor-specific hla antibody in kidney transplant recipients. *PLoS ONE* **2018**, *13*, e0207434. [CrossRef] [PubMed]

33. Kim, J.J.; Shaw, O.; Martin, C.; Michaelides, G.; Balasubramaniam, R.; Sebire, N.J.; Mamode, N.; Dorling, A.; Vaughan, R.; Marks, S.D. Clinical risk stratification of paediatric renal transplant recipients using c1q and c3d fixing of de novo donor-specific antibodies. *Pediatr. Nephrol.* **2018**, *33*, 167–174. [CrossRef] [PubMed]
34. Kamburova, E.G.; Wisse, B.W.; Joosten, I.; Allebes, W.A.; Van Der Meer, A.; Hilbrands, L.B.; Baas, M.C.; Spierings, E.; Hack, C.E.; Van Reekum, F.E. Pretransplant c3d-fixing donor-specific anti-hla antibodies are not associated with increased risk for kidney graft failure. *J. Am. Soc. Nephrol.* **2018**, *29*, 2279–2285. [CrossRef] [PubMed]
35. Ko, S.Y.; Lee, W.; Jung, C.W.; Cho, Y. C3d assay in correlation with single antigen bead assay for human leukocyte antigen antibodies. *Transp. Proc.* **2018**, *50*, 2354–2358. [CrossRef] [PubMed]

8

Acute Kidney Injury Patterns Following Transplantation of Steatotic Liver Allografts

Caroline Jadlowiec [1,*], Maxwell Smith [2], Matthew Neville [3], Shennen Mao [4], Dina Abdelwahab [5], Kunam Reddy [1], Adyr Moss [1], Bashar Aqel [6] and Timucin Taner [7]

1 Division of Transplant Surgery, Mayo Clinic, Phoenix, AZ 85054, USA; Reddy.Kunam@mayo.edu (K.R.); Moss.Adyr@mayo.edu (A.M.)
2 Division of Anatomic Pathology, Mayo Clinic, Phoenix, AZ 85054, USA; Smith.Maxwell@mayo.edu
3 Instructor in Biostatistics, Mayo Clinic College of Medicine, Phoenix, AZ 85054, USA; Neville.Matthew@mayo.edu
4 Division of Transplant Surgery, Mayo Clinic, Jacksonville, FL 32224, USA; Mao.Shennen@mayo.edu
5 Division of Nephrology, Mayo Clinic, Phoenix, AZ 85054, USA; elhamahmi.dina@mayo.edu
6 Division of Transplant Hepatology, Mayo Clinic, Phoenix, AZ 85054, USA; Aqel.Bashar@mayo.edu
7 Division of Transplant Surgery, William J von Liebig Transplant Center, Rochester, MN 55902, USA; Taner.timucin@mayo.edu
* Correspondence: Jadlowiec.Caroline@mayo.edu

Abstract: Background: Steatotic grafts are increasingly being used for liver transplant (LT); however, the impact of graft steatosis on renal function has not been well described. Methods: A total of 511 allografts from Mayo Clinic Arizona and Minnesota were assessed. We evaluated post-LT acute kidney injury (AKI) patterns, perioperative variables and one-year outcomes for patients receiving moderately steatotic allografts (>30% macrovesicular steatosis, $n = 40$) and compared them to non-steatotic graft recipients. Results: Post-LT AKI occurred in 52.5% of steatotic graft recipients versus 16.7% in non-steatotic recipients ($p < 0.001$). Ten percent of steatotic graft recipients required new dialysis post-LT ($p = 0.003$). At five years, there were no differences for AKI vs. no AKI patient survival (HR 0.95, 95% CI 0.08–10.6, $p = 0.95$) or allograft survival (HR 1.73, 95% CI 0.23–13.23, $p = 0.59$) for those using steatotic grafts. Lipopeliosis on biopsy was common in those who developed AKI (61.0% vs. 31.6%, $p = 0.04$), particularly when the Model for End-Stage Liver Disease (MELD) was ≥20 (88.9%; $p = 0.04$). Lipopeliosis was a predictor of post-LT AKI (OR 6.0, 95% CI 1.1–34.6, $p = 0.04$). Conclusion: One-year outcomes for moderately steatotic grafts are satisfactory; however, a higher percentage of post-LT AKI and initiation of dialysis can be expected. Presence of lipopeliosis on biopsy appears to be predictive of post-LT AKI.

Keywords: acute kidney injury; allograft steatosis; lipopeliosis

---

1. Introduction

Due to the ongoing organ shortage, there has been an increased interest in utilizing moderately steatotic donor liver allografts to maximize opportunities for transplantation. Historically, the use of liver allografts with significant steatosis has been associated with increased risk of primary nonfunction, poor early graft function, and decreased patient and allograft survival [1–5]. The degree of steatosis, as well as its histological pattern, appears to impact patient and allograft survival [2,6]. While allografts with severe macrovesicular steatosis (>60%) carry a very high risk of primary non-function, those with mild macrovesicular steatosis (<30%) yield results similar to those of non-steatotic liver allografts [2]. The outcomes of liver allografts with moderate steatosis (30% to 60%) remain variable and the impact of graft steatosis on renal function has not been well described [7,8]. As such, the objectives of this study were to: (1) evaluate postoperative acute kidney injury (AKI) patterns in recipients of steatotic grafts; (2) assess biopsy-findings predictive of AKI in the use of steatotic livers; (3) examine one-year patient and allograft outcomes.

2. Materials and Methods

2.1. Study Population

This was an eight-year, two-center retrospective study of patients who underwent a liver transplant at Mayo Clinic Arizona and Mayo Clinic Minnesota between January 2009 and December 2016 ($n = 810$). This study was approved by the Mayo Clinic Institutional Review Board. Outcomes were compared between moderately steatotic (>30% macrovesicular steatosis) and non-steatotic (<30% macrovesicular steatosis) grafts. In order to assess post-liver transplant (LT) acute kidney injury (AKI) patterns, patients with pre-LT acute kidney injury (AKI) ($n = 143$) were excluded. The majority of LT were performed via piggyback technique; 2.7% ($n = 14$) were performed via caval interposition. The data that supports the findings of this study is available from the corresponding author upon reasonable request.

Pre-LT AKI was defined using the Kidney Disease Improving Global Outcomes (KDIGO) guidelines by an increase in serum creatinine > 0.3 mg/dL or 1.5–1.9 times baseline. Post-LT AKI was defined by those patients satisfying the KDIGO guidelines within 48 h post-LT and maintaining the criteria for > 48 h. Patients with pre-existing chronic kidney disease were not excluded unless they had pre-LT AKI. Mean follow-up was 4.2 years.

All liver allografts were biopsied at the time of transplant and the biopsies were reviewed by a group of designated liver pathologists. Biopsy reports were retrospectively reviewed and macrovesicular steatosis percentage was recorded (less than 30% vs. greater than 30%). Early allograft dysfunction was defined as an aspartate aminotransferase (AST) greater than 2000 U/L within the first 7 days post-LT.

Liver biopsies reported as having moderate (>30% macrovesicular) steatosis were prospectively re-reviewed by a single liver pathologist (M.S.) to specifically assess for macro- and microvesicular steatosis, the percentage of small- and large droplet macrovesicular steatosis, zonation, features of steatohepatitis, fibrosis, preservation reperfusion injury (PRI), and lipopeliosis. Percentages of steatosis were based on the percentage of hepatic parenchyma involved by fat and were estimated using previously published reference figures [9].

Operative hemodynamics were quantified using a modified operative inotrope score (inotrope score = dopamine (×1) + dobutamine (×1) + amrinone (×1) + milrinone (×15) + epinephrine (×100) + norepinephrine (×100) + phenylephrine (×1) + vasopressin (×1), with each drug dosed in μg/kg/min). The inotrope score was calculated during the pre-anhepatic, anhepatic, and post-reperfusion phases for the moderately macrovesicular steatosis cohort [10]. An average of systolic blood pressure (SBP) and mean arterial pressure (MAP) was also recorded for these operative periods.

Immunosuppression was maintained per our center's protocol. All recipients were started on mycophenolate mofetil (MMF), tacrolimus, and prednisone post-LT. MMF was withdrawn at 2–4 months; prednisone was discontinued at 4 months. Tacrolimus trough levels were set at 7–10 ng/mL for the first 2 months post-LT; at one-year post-LT, trough levels were reduced to 4–6 ng/mL. By protocol at our centers, tacrolimus is typically started immediately following transplant unless there are concerns for renal insufficiency. In the setting of post-LT renal insufficiency (defined as creatinine >2.0 mg/dL, estimated glomerular filtration rate (eGFR) <40 mL/minute or dialysis), Basiliximab 20 mg is given on post-operative days 0 and 4 to allow for a delay in tacrolimus initiation. In this setting, tacrolimus initiation is delayed until postoperative day 5.

2.2. Statistical Methods

Descriptive analysis was performed using t-tests for continuous variables and Chi-square for categorical variables. Continuous variables are shown using mean and standard deviation; categorical variables using count and percentage. Wilcoxon rank-sum tests were used for non-normally distributed continuous variables. Survival analysis was performed using Kaplan-Meier analysis. Logistic regression was applied to clinically significant variables. Statistical analysis was performed using Prism software version 7.03 (La Jolla, CA, USA) and SAS version 9.4. A p value of <0.05 was considered significant.

3. Results

3.1. Postoperative Outcomes

Of the 511 grafts that were included in this analysis, 40 were found to have moderate (>30%) macrovesicular steatosis. The average steatosis percentage was 41.1% ± 15.8% in the moderate group, compared to 3.8% ± 5.8% in the non-steatotic group ($p < 0.001$) (Table 1, Figure 1A,B). For the entire cohort, the incidence of post-LT AKI was 19.6% ($n = 100$). In assessing clinical risk factors for kidney disease, 12.5% ($n = 64$) of LT recipients were diabetic, 12.7% ($n = 65$) had hypertension, and 13.5% ($n = 69$) were both diabetic and hypertensive. The distribution of diabetes and hypertension did not vary between the steatotic and non-steatotic grafts ($p = 0.95$). There were no differences in age ($p = 0.39$), sex ($p = 0.18$), ethnicity ($p = 0.72$), race ($p = 0.57$), the biologic Model for End-Stage Liver Disease (MELD) ($p = 0.14$) or indications for liver transplant ($p = 0.16$) between the recipients receiving moderately steatotic and non-steatotic grafts (Table 1).

Table 1. Pre- and Post-Liver Transplant Recipient Demographics.

	Steatotic Grafts (n = 40)	Non-Steatotic Grafts (n = 471)	p Value
Pre-Liver Transplant			
Steatosis (%)	41.1 ± 15.8	3.8 ± 5.8	<0.0001
Recipient Age (years)	57. 4 ± 9.7	56.0 ± 10.3	0.39
Biologic MELD	18.0 ± 8.3	16.1 ± 7.0	0.14
Female	9 (22.5%)	155 (32.9%)	0.18
Indication for LT			0.16
Hepatitis C (HCV)	6 (22.5%)	55 (11.6%)	
Cholestatic	5 (12.5%)	53 (11.3%)	
Hepatocellular Carcinoma (HCC)/Other MELD Exception	11 (27.5%)	223 (47.3%)	
Alcohol-Related Liver Disease (ALD)	8 (20.0%)	46 (9.8%)	
Nonalcoholic Steatohepatitis (NASH)	6 (15.0%)	49 (10.4%)	
Other	4 (10.0%)	45 (9.6%)	
Pre-LT Creatinine (mg/dL)	1.0 ± 0.3	0.9 ± 0.9	0.14
Pre-LT eGFR	57.7 ± 6.3	57.7 ± 6.6	0.97
Post-Liver Transplant			
Post-LT AKI	21 (52.5%)	79 (16.8%)	<0.0001
Post-LT Temporary Dialysis	4 (10.0%)	5 (1.1%)	0.003
ICU LOS (days)	2.0 ± 1.8	1.8 ± 2.6	0.62
Total Hospital LOS (days)	9.1 ± 10.3	9.9 ± 10.9	0.67
One-Year Post-Liver Transplant			
Creatinine (mg/dL)	1.3 ± 0.3	1.3 ± 0.7	0.97
eGFR (mL/min)	53.1 ± 7.9	53.5 ± 10.1	0.70
New Chronic Post-LT Dialysis	0 (0.0%)	2 (0.4%)	>0.99

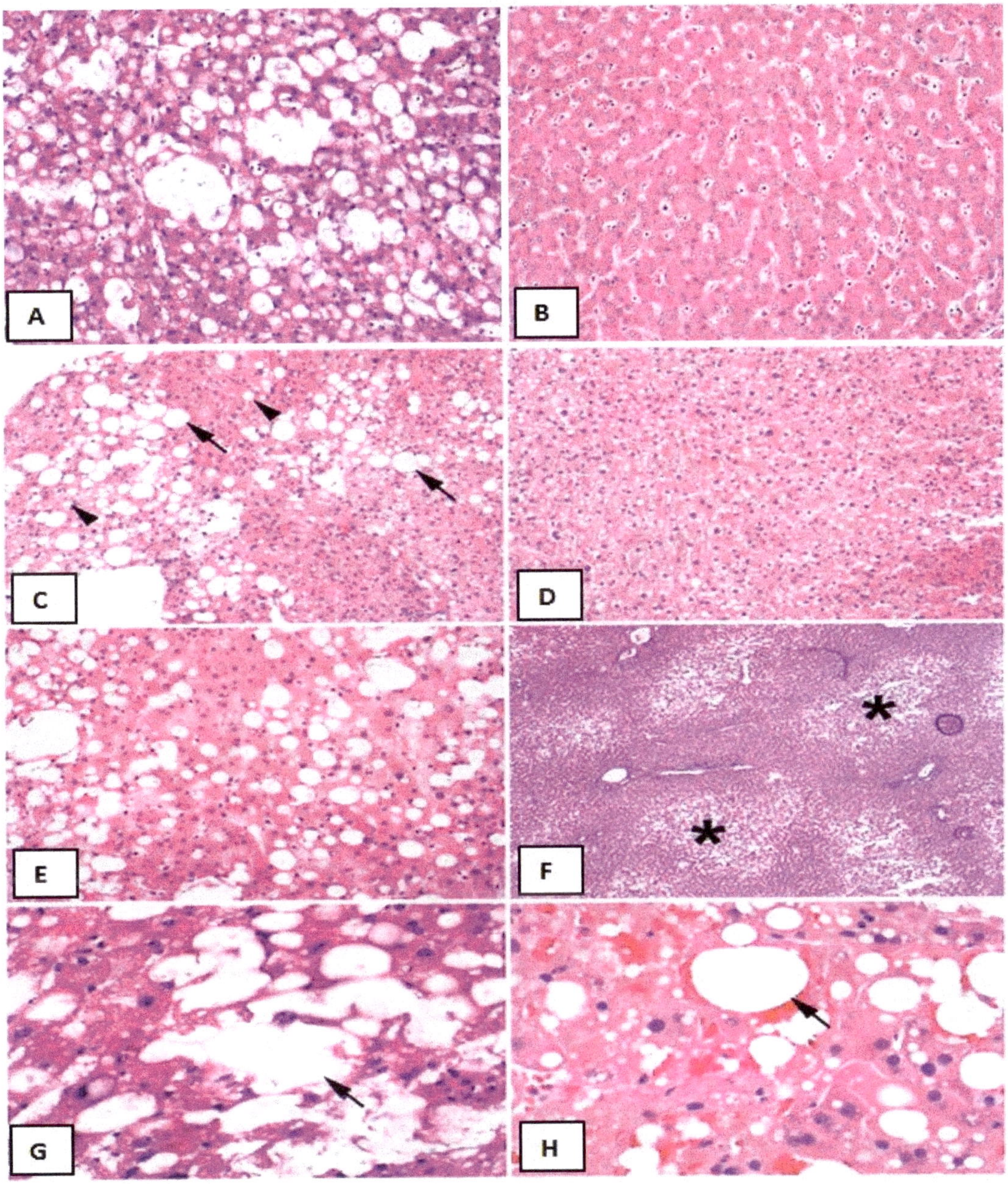

Figure 1. Liver Graft Biopsy Findings Liver Biopsy Findings. (**A**) Representative biopsy of a >30% macrovesicular steatotic allograft. (**B**) Representative biopsy of a non-steatotic allograft. (**C**) Approximately 30% macrovesicular steatosis with a mixture of large (arrows) and small (arrowheads) droplet fat (hematoxylin and eosin (H&E), 200×). (**D**) Microvesicular steatosis characterized by diffuse deposition of fat droplets in the hepatocyte cytoplasm without any macrovesicular steatosis (H&E, 200×). (**E**) Approximately 40% macrovesicular steatosis seen on a pre-implantation biopsy (H&E frozen section, 400×). (**F**) Zonal distribution of macrovesicular steatosis with fat deposition accentuated in zone three (asterisks) around the central veins (H&E, frozen section, 100×). (**G**), Lipopeliosis characterized by the rupture of hepatocytes with coalescence of fat droplets (arrow) in the sinusoidal spaces (H&E, frozen section, 600×). (**H**), Lipopeliosis (arrow) in post-reperfusion biopsy (H&E, 600×).

Post-LT AKI was observed in 52.5% of patients receiving moderately steatotic grafts versus 16.8% in the non-steatotic cohort ($p < 0.0001$). No patients in the entire cohort had liver allograft primary non-function. Patients transplanted with moderately steatotic grafts had significantly more early allograft dysfunction immediately following surgery (AST: 3212 ± 2413 U/L vs. 1118 ± 1473 U/L,

$p < 0.0001$). The rise in AST was four-fold higher for recipients of steatotic grafts that went on to develop post-LT AKI ($p < 0.0001$). There was a greater need for newly initiated temporary post-LT dialysis in the moderately steatotic group (10.0% vs. 1.1%, $p = 0.003$). There were no differences in intensive care unit (ICU) length of stay (2.0 ± 1.8 vs. 1.8 ± 2.6, $p = 0.62$) or total hospital length of stay (9.1 ± 10.3 vs. 9.9 ± 10.9, $p = 0.67$). At one-year post-LT, there were no observed differences in the need for new chronic (ongoing) post-LT dialysis ($p > 0.99$), serum creatinine (1.3 ± 0.3 vs. 1.3 ± 0.7, $p = 0.97$), or eGFR (53.1 ± 7.9 vs. 53.5 ± 10.1, $p = 0.70$) (Table 1).

3.2. Moderately Steatotic Graft Subgroup Analysis

In order to investigate postoperative outcomes in moderately steatotic livers allografts in further detail, we reviewed the characteristics of the 40 patients who were transplanted with such grafts (Table 2). In this cohort, there were no differences in age ($p = 0.61$), sex ($p = 0.43$), ethnicity ($p = 0.60$), race ($p = 0.64$), or indication for transplant ($p = 0.53$) among those who developed AKI versus those who did not (Table 2). Of those receiving steatotic grafts, 52.5% went on to develop AKI; the other 47.5% maintained normal renal function post-transplant. Recipients of steatotic grafts that went on to develop post-LT AKI had a higher biologic MELD (20.5 ± 8.9 vs. 15.3 ± 6.9, $p = 0.04$) (Table 2). There were no differences in pre-LT creatinine ($p = 0.21$) or eGFR ($p = 0.88$).

Table 2. Moderately Steatotic Graft Subgroup Analysis.

	Post-LT AKI (n = 21)	**No AKI (n = 19)**	***p* Value**
Pre-Liver Transplant			
Macrovesicular Steatosis (%)	41.9 ± 15.7	40.3 ± 16.2	0.75
Recipient Age (years)	56.7 ± 8.3	58.3 ± 11.3	0.61
Biologic MELD	20.5 ± 8.9	15.3 ± 6.9	0.04
Female	3 (14.3%)	6 (31.6%)	0.43
Indication for LT			0.53
HCV	4 (19.0%)	2 (10.5%)	
Cholestatic	1 (4.8%)	4 (21.1%)	
HCC/Other MELD Exception	5 (23.8%)	6 (31.6%)	
ALD	4 (19.0%)	4 (21.1%)	
NASH	4 (19.0%)	2 (10.5%)	
Other	3 (14.3%)	1 (5.3%)	
Total Hospital LOS (median)	10.4 ± 13.5 (7.0)	7.1 ± 4.1 (6.0)	0.32
One-Year Post-LT			
Creatinine (mg/dL)	1.3 ± 0.2	1.2 ± 0.4	0.27
eGFR (mL/min)	52.7 ± 6.9	53.6 ± 9.1	0.74

Recipients of moderately steatotic grafts were all noted to have early allograft dysfunction as demonstrated through a significantly elevated AST immediately following surgery (Figure 2). This occurred regardless of whether or not they developed AKI. The rise in AST was four-fold higher for recipients of steatotic grafts that went on to develop post-LT AKI as compared to non-steatotic grafts (40001.0 ± 2471.0 U/L vs. 1118.0 ± 1473.0, $p < 0.0001$). The rise in AST was also two-fold higher when comparing steatotic grafts of recipients with and without post-LT AKI (40001.0 ± 2471.0 U/L vs. 2339.0 ± 2074.0, $p < 0.0001$). There were no differences between the post-LT AKI and no AKI groups with regards to graft type (i.e., donation after brain death, DBD, vs. donation after cardiac death, DCD) (19.0% vs. 10.5%, $p = 0.66$), sex (female: 42.9% vs. 47.4%, $p = 0.38$), or BMI (32.8 ± 5.9 kg/m^2 vs. 32.6 ± 9.4 kg/m^2, $p = 0.92$). Donor age was yonger (43.2 ± 12.6 vs. 52.8 ± 14.9%, $p = 0.03$) in steatotic grafts that went on to develop AKI. In addition, there were no differences in allograft cold ischemia time (CIT) ($p = 0.28$) or estimated operative blood loss (EBL) ($p = 0.49$) (Table 3).

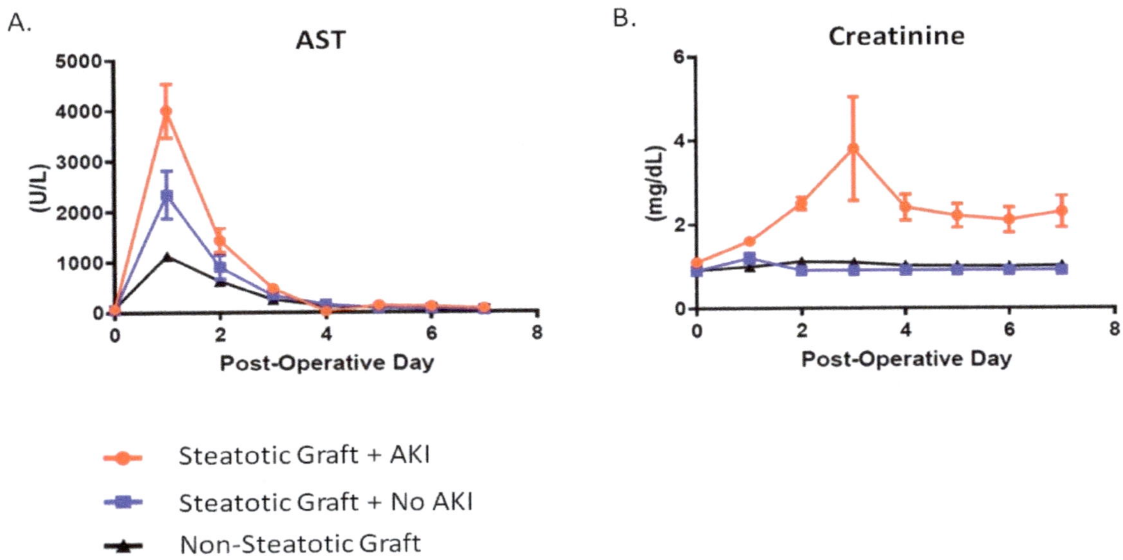

Figure 2. Post-Liver Transplant Patterns in Steatotic and Non-Steatotic Grafts. (**A**) Post-LT aspartate aminotransferase (AST) levels. Compared to non-steatotic graft, AST levels were 2-times higher in steatotic grafts without post-LT AKI and 4-times higher for steatotic grafts with AKI. (**B**) Post-LT creatinine levels.

Table 3. Steatotic Graft Recipient Operative Variables.

	Post-LT AKI (n = 21)	No AKI (n = 19)	p Value
CIT (h)	6.8 ± 2.1	6.1 ± 1.7	0.28
EBL (mL)	2157 ± 1649	1821 ± 1405	0.49
Pre-Anhepatic			
SBP (mmHg)	111.2 ± 21.8	104.2 ± 14.5	0.25
MAP	75.1 ± 13.3	73.8 ± 13.6	0.76
Inotrope Score	4.1 ± 11.9	1.7 ± 6.9	0.45
Anhepatic			
SBP (mmHg)	106.5 ± 15.4	104.4 ± 15.1	0.67
MAP	75.4 ± 11.0	76.7 ± 9.6	0.71
Inotrope Score	4.3 ± 11.9	2.6 ± 6.8	0.58
Post Reperfusion			
SBP (mmHg)	95.6 ± 13.8	96.2 ± 7.9	0.87
MAP	67.0 ± 11.8	65.5 ± 9.8	0.69
Inotrope Score	19.5 ± 20.0	3.8 ± 4.4	0.03

When operative hemodynamics of AKI and non-AKI recipients receiving moderately steatotic grafts were compared, there were no differences observed in inotrope requirements ($p = 0.45$), systolic blood pressure (SBP) ($p = 0.25$) or mean arterial pressure (MAP) ($p = 0.76$) during the pre-anhepatic phase or anhepatic phase (inotrope score $p = 0.58$; SBP $p = 0.67$; MAP $p = 0.71$) of the operation (Table 3). Post-reperfusion, SBP ($p = 0.87$) and MAP ($p = 0.69$) were similar in patients who went on to develop post-LT AKI versus those who did not suggesting appropriate perfusion parameters were able to be maintained. The post-reperfusion inotrope requirements, however, were significantly higher in the post-LT AKI group (19.5 ± 20.0 vs. 3.8 ± 4.4, $p = 0.03$). Ten percent of the patients in the steatotic post-LT AKI group ($n = 4$) required initiation of new dialysis post-LT ($p = 0.003$) (Table 2). There were no differences in ICU length of stay ($p = 0.62$) and total hospital length of stay ($p = 0.67$) between steatotic AKI and no AKI groups.

At one-year post-LT, there were no observed differences between those receiving steatotic grafts that developed AKI versus those who did not with regards to serum creatinine (1.3 ± 0.2 vs. 1.2 ± 0.4,

$p = 0.27$) and eGFR (52.7 ± 6.9 vs. 53.6 ± 9.1, $p = 0.74$) (Table 2). At five years, there were no differences for AKI vs. no AKI patient survival (HR 0.95, 95% CI 0.08–10.6, $p = 0.95$) or allograft survival (HR 1.73, 95% CI 0.23–13.23, $p = 0.59$) for those using steatotic grafts (Figure 3).

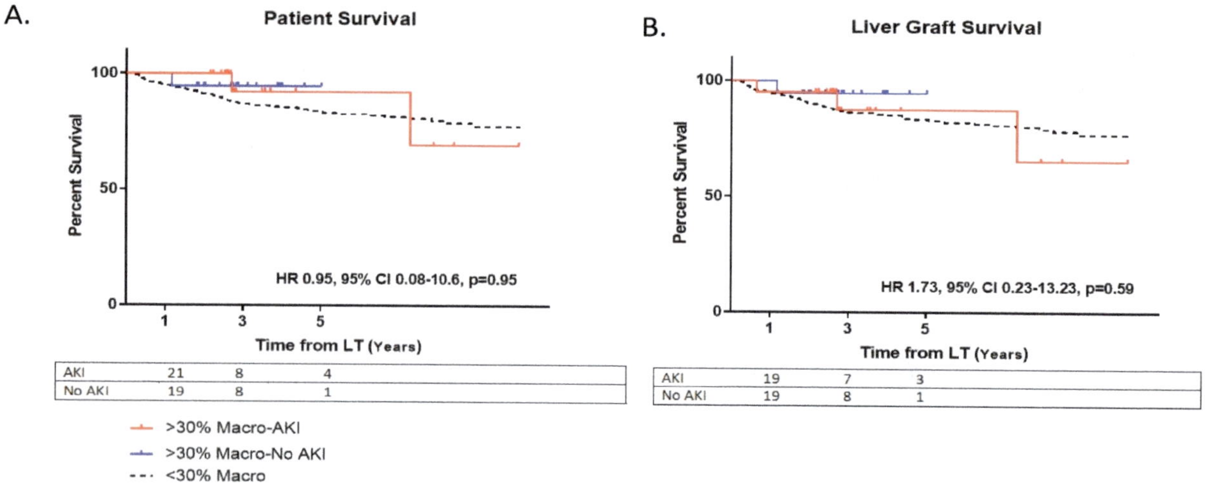

Figure 3. Survival. (**A**) Patient survival post-LT. Hazard ratio (HR); Confidence Interval (CI). (**B**) Liver allograft survival post-transplant. Moderately steatotic grafts with AKI (>30% Macro-AKI); Moderately steatotic grafts without AKI (>30% Macro-No AKI); Non-steatotic grafts (<30% Macro).

3.3. *Liver Graft Biopsy Findings*

In prospectively re-reviewing biopsies of all liver allografts with moderate (>30%) macrovesicular steatosis, the majority of the steatosis was found to be large droplet (Table 4) (Figure 1C,E). When comparing biopsies in patients with and without post-LT AKI, no differences were observed with regard to large droplet versus small droplet percentage composition (Figure 1C) ($p = 0.41$). Although microvesicular steatosis was minimal in both groups (Figure 1D) (0.0% vs. 21.1%), a higher frequency was observed in the no AKI group ($n = 4$, $p = 0.04$) (Table 4). No significant differences were observed in the histologic distribution of the steatosis (zonation) in the allograft ($p = 0.75$) (Figure 1F), inflammation ($p = 0.73$), ballooning ($p = 0.65$), or Mallory hyaline (Table 4). A larger percentage of biopsies in the post-LT AKI group contained lipopeliosis (61% vs. 31.6%, $p = 0.04$) (Figure 1G–H). When plotted against MELD at the time of transplant, recipients of moderately steatotic grafts with lipopeliosis with a MELD ≥ 20 were found to more likely to develop AKI (88.9%) than recipients of such grafts with MELD < 20 (40.0%; $p = 0.04$) (Figure 4). In using logistic regression, variables predictive of post-LT AKI included the finding of lipopeliosis on liver biopsy and donor age (Table 5).

Table 4. Steatotic Liver Graft Biopsy Findings.

	Post-LT AKI ($n = 21$)	**No AKI ($n = 19$)**	***p* Value**
Macrovesicular Steatosis			
Large Droplet (%)	69.2 ± 16.1	64.7 ± 16.9	0.41
Small Droplet (%)	30.8 ± 16.1	35.3 ± 16.9	
Microvesicular Steatosis	0 (0.0%)	4 (21.1%)	0.04
Zonation	14 (66.7%)	11 (57.9%)	0.75
Inflammation	5 (23.8%)	6 (31.5%)	0.73
Ballooning	2 (9.5%)	3 (15.8%)	0.65
Mallory Hyaline	0 (0.0%)	0 (0.0%)	-
Lipopeliosis	13 (61.9%)	6 (31.6%)	0.03

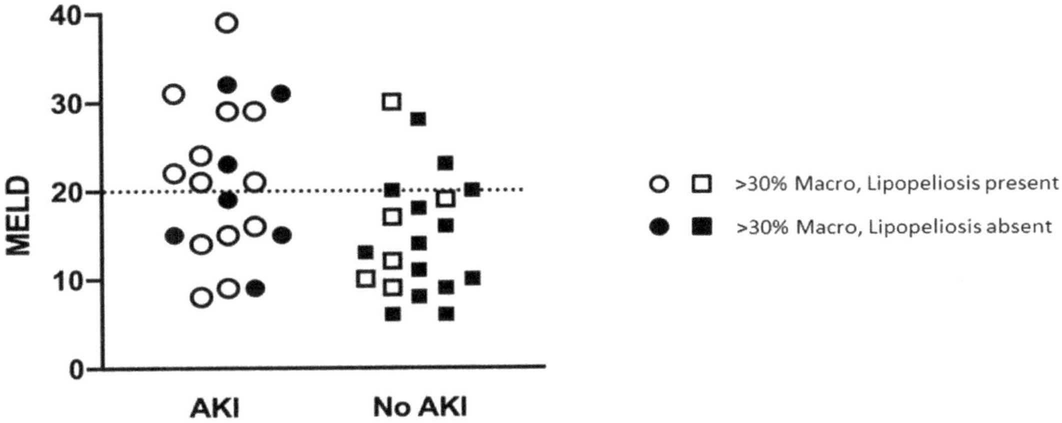

Figure 4. Relationship between MELD, Lipopeliosis and Post-LT AKI.

Table 5. Predictors of AKI in Steatotic Grafts—Logistic Regression.

Effect	Odds Ratio	95% CI		*p* Value
Donor Age	0.93	0.87	0.99	0.02
Lipopeliosis	6.04	1.05	34.61	0.04
Post-Reperfusion Systolic BP	1.01	0.95	1.08	0.75

4. Discussion

Primary nonfunction, poor early graft function, and decreased patient and allograft survival have all been associated with the use of steatotic liver allografts for transplantation [1–3,5]. This, combined with inaccurate and inconsistent reporting of liver allograft biopsies, has led to a high discard rate of grafts with moderate (>30%) steatosis [11]. While the risk of adverse events with severely steatotic liver allografts (>60%) remains well recognized, the use of moderately steatotic grafts (30%–60%) has been increasing [7].

It has been our experience that steatotic grafts almost universally exhibit early allograft dysfunction and require additional resource utilization postoperatively specific to the development of post-LT AKI and the need to initiate new dialysis [7,12–15]. In this study, the occurrence of AKI post-LT was noted to be markedly increased at 52.5% compared to 19.6% observed in the general liver transplant recipient pool. Although early allograft dysfunction, best demonstrated by significantly elevated transaminases, was common to all steatotic grafts, not all recipients developed post-LT AKI (Figure 2). We have clinically observed this divergent pattern; however, it remains difficult to quantify why some steatotic grafts behave in this manner while others do not. In this study, patients receiving steatotic grafts that developed post-LT AKI were noted to have higher inotrope requirements post-reperfusion. Despite having higher inotrope requirements, no differences were observed in hemodynamic parameters (systolic blood pressure and MAP) between the patients with and without post-LT AKI, suggesting that variables other than hemodynamics influence the development of AKI. Not surprisingly, a higher MELD score was associated with an increased risk of post-LT AKI. This association was particularly strong when steatotic grafts with lipopeliosis on biopsy were transplanted to patients with MELD scores of 20 or above (Tables 2 and 5) (Figure 4).

Proper classification of graft steatosis remains challenging even within the transplant community [9]. Historically, steatosis was classified as microvesicular or macrovesicular, based on hepatocyte fat droplet size and nucleus displacement. Although often reported, true microvesicular steatosis is rare and manifests histologically as diffuse deposition of small lipid droplets in the hepatocyte cytoplasm with a resulting foamy appearance (Figure 1D). Two types of fat droplets are seen in the setting of macrovesicular steatosis: small droplets and large droplets (Figure 1C). Fat droplets in small droplet steatosis are not large enough to displace the nucleus; this finding is often inaccurately reported as being microvesicular steatosis on biopsy. Although both small and large droplet steatosis contribute to overall macrovesicular steatosis, historically small droplet macrovesicular steatosis and microvesicular steatosis were used synonymously, resulting in ongoing confusion [3]. We hypothesize that some of the observed differences in post-LT AKI between otherwise similarly-appearing steatotic grafts might be related to this histological variation.

The term lipopeliosis was first identified in the early days of hepatic transplantation and describes the coalescence of fat droplets from ruptured hepatocytes into larger droplets of fat in the sinusoidal space [16]. Due to the universal finding of preservation-related injury in these biopsies, lipopeliosis was presumed to not be of clinical significance [17]. In our experience, however, the histologic finding of lipopeliosis is, by far, more common in patients who develop post-LT AKI and, in our experience, has been associated with inferior post-transplant outcomes [18].

Although the current study was not designed to elucidate the mechanisms of AKI post-LT, we have previously shown that fat droplets, through the process of lipopeliosis, embolize to the pulmonary vasculature following reperfusion with resulting respiratory failure [18]. This mechanism is likely similar to that seen after long bone traumatic injuries, where fat droplets are released into the venous system and migrate to the pulmonary capillary beds [19,20]. Microvascular lodging results in ischemia, inflammation, and release of inflammatory mediators. The breakdown of fat emboli by pneumocytes can results in release of free fatty acids that, in turn, enter systemic circulation and result in multisystem dysfunction [21]. The finding of fat droplets in the urine under these circumstances correlates with the development of AKI and a systemic process triggered by fat embolization [22]. Whether lipopeliosis in steatotic liver graft biopsies can be used to predict clinical instability and the development of post-LT AKI will need to be validated in a larger prospective study. Limitations to this study include its overall small cohort size. The results also represent the experience of only two centers. Patients with pre-LT AKI were also excluded in this study to better assess post-LT outcomes specific to AKI development. The impact of steatosis on renal function in patients with preexisting AKI remains uncertain.

In conclusion, utilization of moderately steatotic grafts is associated with a significantly higher risk for developing post-LT AKI. This risk appears to be independent of pre-reperfusion operative hemodynamics. In utilizing these grafts, laboratory abnormalities persist 2 to 3 months post-LT, but there does not appear to be an impact on long-term renal function, patient, or graft survival. The risk for AKI in this setting appears increased when the MELD score is greater than 20 and lipopeliosis is histologically present on biopsy. These outcomes are more favorable as compared to older studies, and suggest that, with lower MELD recipients, satisfactory outcomes can be achieved with the use of these grafts [5].

Author Contributions: For research articles with several authors, a short paragraph specifying their individual contributions must be provided. The following statements should be used "Conceptualization, C.J. and T.T.; methodology, C.J. and T.T.; software, C.J. and M.N.; validation, C.J., M.N. and T.T.; formal analysis, C.J., M.S., M.N., S.M., D.A., K.R., A.M., B.A., T.T.; investigation, C.J., M.S., T.T.; resources, C.J.; data curation, C.J., M.S., M.N., S.M, D.A. and T.T.; writing—original draft preparation, C.J., M.S., M.N., S.M., D.A., K.R., A.M., B.A., T.T.; writing—review and editing, C.J., M.S., M.N., S.M., D.A., K.R., A.M., B.A., T.T.; visualization, C.J. and T.T.; supervision, T.T.; project administration, C.J.; funding acquisition, Not applicable. All authors have read and agreed to the published version of the manuscript.

References

1. Verran, D.; Kusyk, T.; Painter, D.; Fisher, J.; Koorey, D.; Strasser, S.; Stewart, G.; McCaughan, G. Clinical experience gained from the use of 120 steatotic donor livers for orthotopic liver transplantation. *Liver Transpl.* **2003**, *9*, 500–505. [CrossRef]
2. Selzner, M.; Clavien, P.A. Fatty liver in liver transplantation and surgery. *Semin. Liver Dis.* **2001**, *21*, 105–113. [CrossRef] [PubMed]
3. Wu, C.; Lu, C.; Xu, C. Short-term and long-term outcomes of liver transplantation using moderately and severely steatotic donor livers: A systemic review. *Medicine (Baltimore)* **2018**, *97*, e12026. [CrossRef] [PubMed]

4. Spitzer, A.L.; Lao, O.B.; Dick, A.A.; Bakthavatsalam, R.; Halldorson, J.B.; Yeh, M.M.; Upton, M.P.; Reyes, J.D.; Perkins, J.D. The biopsied donor liver: Incorporating macrosteatosis into high-risk donor assessment. *Liver Transpl.* **2010**, *16*, 874–884. [CrossRef] [PubMed]
5. Wadei, H.M.; Lee, D.D.; Croome, K.P.; Mai, M.L.; Golan, E.; Brotman, R.; Keaveny, A.P.; Taner, C.B. Early Allograft Dysfunction After Liver Transplantation Is Associated With Short- and Long-Term Kidney Function Impairment. *Am. J. Transplant.* **2016**, *16*, 850–859. [CrossRef]
6. Fishbein, T.M.; Fiel, M.I.; Emre, S.; Cubukcu, O.; Guy, S.R.; Schwartz, M.E.; Miller, C.M.; Sheiner, P.A. Use of livers with microvesicular fat safely expands the donor pool. *Transplantation* **1997**, *64*, 248–251. [CrossRef]
7. Croome, K.P.; Lee, D.D.; Croome, S.; Chadha, R.; Livingston, D.; Abader, P.; Keaveny, A.P.; Taner, C.B. The impact of postreperfusion syndrome during liver transplantation using livers with significant macrosteatosis. *Am. J. Transpl.* **2019**, *19*, 2550–2559. [CrossRef]
8. McCormack, L.; Dutkowski, P.; El-Badry, A.M.; Clavien, P.A. Liver transplantation using fatty livers: Always feasible? *J. Hepatol.* **2011**, *54*, 1055–1062. [CrossRef]
9. Hall, A.R.; Dhillon, A.P.; Green, A.C.; Ferrell, L.; Crawford, J.M.; Alves, V.; Balabaud, C.; Bhathal, P.; Bioulac-Sage, P.; Guido, M.; et al. Hepatic steatosis estimated microscopically versus digital image analysis. *Liver Int.* **2013**, *33*, 926–935. [CrossRef] [PubMed]
10. Kobashigawa, J.; Zuckermann, A.; Macdonald, P.; Leprince, P.; Esmailian, F.; Luu, M.; Mancini, D.; Patel, J.; Razi, R.; Reichenspurner, H.; et al. Report from a consensus conference on primary graft dysfunction after cardiac transplantation. *J. Heart Lung Transpl.* **2014**, *33*, 327–340. [CrossRef]
11. Doyle, M.M.; Vachharajani, N.; Wellen, J.R.; Anderson, C.D.; Lowell, J.A.; Shenoy, S.; Brunt, E.M.; Chapman, W.C. Short- and long-term outcomes after steatotic liver transplantation. *Arch Surg.* **2010**, *145*, 653–660. [CrossRef]
12. Leithead, J.A.; Rajoriya, N.; Gunson, B.K.; Muiesan, P.; Ferguson, J.W. The evolving use of higher risk grafts is associated with an increased incidence of acute kidney injury after liver transplantation. *J. Hepatol.* **2014**, *60*, 1180–1186. [CrossRef] [PubMed]
13. Cabezuelo, J.B.; Ramirez, P.; Acosta, F.; Bueno, F.S.; Robles, R.; Pons, J.A.; Miras, M.; Munitiz, V.; Fernandez, J.A.; Lujan, J.; et al. Prognostic factors of early acute renal failure in liver transplantation. *Transpl. Proc.* **2002**, *34*, 254–255. [CrossRef]
14. O'Riordan, A.; Wong, V.; McQuillan, R.; McCormick, P.A.; Hegarty, J.E.; Watson, A.J. Acute renal disease, as defined by the RIFLE criteria, post-liver transplantation. *Am. J. Transpl.* **2007**, *7*, 168–176. [CrossRef] [PubMed]
15. Leithead, J.A.; Armstrong, M.J.; Corbett, C.; Andrew, M.; Kothari, C.; Gunson, B.K.; Muiesan, P.; Ferguson, J.W. Hepatic ischemia reperfusion injury is associated with acute kidney injury following donation after brain death liver transplantation. *Transpl. Int.* **2013**, *26*, 1116–1125. [CrossRef]
16. Ferrell, L.; Bass, N.; Roberts, J.; Ascher, N. Lipopeliosis: Fat induced sinusoidal dilation in transplanted liver mimicking peliosis hepatitis. *J. Clin. Pathol.* **1992**, *45*, 1109–1110. [CrossRef] [PubMed]
17. Cha, I.; Bass, N.; Ferrell, L.D. Lipopeliosis: An Immunohistochemical and Clinicopathologic Study of Five Cases. *Am. J. Surg. Pathol.* **1994**, *18*, 789–795. [CrossRef] [PubMed]
18. Rosenfeld, D.M.; Smith, M.L.; Seamans, D.P.; Giorgakis, E.; Gaitan, B.D.; Khurmi, N.; Aqel, B.A.; Reddy, K.S. Fatal diffuse pulmonary fat microemboli following reperfusion in orthotopic liver transplantation with the use of marginal steatotic allografts. *Am. J. Transpl.* **2019**, *19*, 2640–2645. [CrossRef]
19. Shaikh, N. Emergency management of fat embolism syndrome. *J. Emergencies Trauma Shock* **2009**, *2*, 29–33. [CrossRef]
20. Glossing, H.R.; Pellegrini, V.D. Fat embolism syndrome: A review of pathology and physiological basis of treatment. *Clin. Orthop. Relat. Res.* **1982**, *165*, 68–82.
21. Baker, P.L.; Paxel, J.A.; Pettier, L.F. Free fatty acids, catecholamine and arterial hypoxia in patients with fat embolism. *J. Trauma* **1971**, *11*, 1026–1030. [CrossRef] [PubMed]
22. Evarts, C.M. Diagnosis and treatment of fat embolism. *JAMA* **1965**, *194*, 899–901. [CrossRef] [PubMed]

9

Erythropoietin, Fibroblast Growth Factor 23, and Death After Kidney Transplantation

Michele F. Eisenga [1,*], Maarten A. De Jong [1], David E. Leaf [2], Ilja M. Nolte [3], Martin H. De Borst [1], Stephan J. L. Bakker [1] and Carlo A. J. M. Gaillard [1,4]

1 Division of Nephrology, Department of Internal Medicine, University of Groningen, University Medical Center Groningen, 9700 RB Groningen, The Netherlands; m.a.de.jong03@umcg.nl (M.A.D.J.); m.h.de.borst@umcg.nl (M.H.D.B.); s.j.l.bakker@umcg.nl (S.J.L.B.)

2 Division of Renal Medicine, Brigham and Women's Hospital, Harvard Medical School, Boston, MA 02215, USA; deleaf@bwh.harvard.edu

3 Department of Epidemiology, University of Groningen, University Medical Center Groningen, 9700 RB Groningen, The Netherlands; i.m.nolte@umcg.nl

4 Department of Internal Medicine and Dermatology, University of Utrecht, University Medical Center Utrecht, 3508 GA Utrecht, The Netherlands; C.A.J.M.Gaillard@umcutrecht.nl

* Correspondence: m.f.eisenga@umcg.nl

Abstract: Elevated levels of erythropoietin (EPO) are associated with an increased risk of death in renal transplant recipients (RTRs), but the underlying mechanisms remain unclear. Emerging data suggest that EPO stimulates production of the phosphaturic hormone fibroblast growth factor 23 (FGF23), another strong risk factor for death in RTRs. We hypothesized that the hitherto unexplained association between EPO levels and adverse outcomes may be attributable to increased levels of FGF23. We included 579 RTRs (age 51 ± 12 years, 55% males) from the TransplantLines Insulin Resistance and Inflammation Cohort study (NCT03272854). During a follow-up of 7.0 years, 121 RTRs died, of which 62 were due to cardiovascular cause. In multivariable Cox regression analysis, EPO was independently associated with all-cause (HR, 1.66; 95% CI 1.16–2.36; $P = 0.005$) and cardiovascular death (HR, 1.87; 95% CI 1.14–3.06; $P = 0.01$). However, the associations were abrogated following adjustment for FGF23 (HR, 1.28; 95% CI 0.87–1.88; $P = 0.20$, and HR, 1.45; 95% CI 0.84–2.48; $P = 0.18$, respectively). In subsequent mediation analysis, FGF23 mediated 72% and 50% of the association between EPO and all-cause and cardiovascular death, respectively. Our results underline the strong relationship between EPO and FGF23 physiology, and provide a potential mechanism underlying the relationship between increased EPO levels and adverse outcomes in RTRs.

Keywords: erythropoietin; fibroblast growth factor 23; death; kidney transplantation

1. Introduction

Renal transplant recipients (RTRs) have a high residual risk of all-cause and cardiovascular death, compared to the general population [1]. Previous studies demonstrated an independent association between higher circulating endogenous erythropoietin (EPO) levels and risk of all-cause and cardiovascular death among RTRs, similar to other patient populations such as chronic heart failure patients and the elderly [2–4]. In addition, administration of exogenous EPO may increase the risk of cardiovascular events in patients with chronic kidney disease (CKD) and end stage renal disease (ESRD) [5,6]. However, the underlying mechanisms responsible for the link between endogenous and exogenous EPO and adverse outcomes are unknown.

Studies from our group and others suggest that EPO is prominently involved in fibroblast growth factor-23 (FGF23) physiology [7–10]. FGF23 is an osteocyte-derived hormone that plays an essential role in regulating phosphate and vitamin D metabolism. In RTRs, increased FGF23 levels post-transplant are independently associated with an increased risk of graft failure and death [11,12]. Hypoxia, the main stimulus for EPO synthesis, stabilizes hypoxia-inducible factor (HIF)-1α, which is a heterodimeric transcription factor that regulates oxygen homeostasis [13,14]. Subsequently, stabilized HIF1-α upregulates FGF23 production while concomitantly increasing FGF23 cleavage into inactive fragments, resulting in elevated total FGF23 levels but normal levels of intact, bioactive FGF23 [15–18].

In the current study, we hypothesized that the previously established, but hitherto unexplained association between EPO levels and adverse outcomes may be attributable to increased levels of total FGF23. Therefore, we investigated the associations between EPO and total FGF23 levels and prospective outcomes in our RTRs cohort.

2. Methods

2.1. Patient Population

All RTRs (aged $\geq$ 18 years) who were at least 1-year post-transplantation were approached for participation in the current study during outpatient clinic visits between 2001 and 2003. All RTRs were transplanted in the University Medical Center Groningen (Groningen, the Netherlands). The study has been described in detail previously [19]. Among 847 RTRs approached for participation, 606 RTRs agreed to participate and were included. All patients provided written informed consent and the study protocol was approved by the local medical ethical committee (METc 2001/039). The study protocol adhered to principles of the Declaration of Helsinki and the Declaration of Istanbul. The co-primary endpoints of the study were all-cause and cardiovascular death. Cause of death was obtained by linking the number of the death certificate to the primary cause of death as coded by a physician from the Central Bureau of Statistics according to the International Classification of Diseases, 9th revision (ICD-9; https://icd.codes/icd9cm). CV death was defined as deaths in which the principal cause of death was cardiovascular in nature, using ICD-9 codes 410 to 447. Secondary endpoint constituted death-censored graft failure (DCGF). DCGF was defined as return to dialysis or re-transplantation. For the current analyses, we excluded RTRs who did not have plasma samples available for measuring EPO levels (n = 14) and RTRs who used exogenous EPO (n = 13) due to positive interference in EPO measurement, resulting in 579 RTRs eligible for analyses. Median follow-up time from inclusion to endpoint was 7.0 (interquartile range (IQR), 6.2 to 7.4) years. Data on the co-primary and secondary endpoints were available in all 579 participants. There was no loss-to-follow-up in the current study.

2.2. Data Collection

Relevant donor, recipient, and transplant characteristics at baseline were extracted from the Groningen Renal Transplant Database, as described in detail previously [19]. Information on medical history and medication use was obtained from patient records. Participants' height and weight were measured with participants wearing light indoor clothing without shoes. Blood pressure was measured according to a strict protocol as previously described [19]. Alcohol consumption and smoking behavior were recorded using a self-reported questionnaire. Smoking behavior was classified as never, former, or current smoker.

2.3. Laboratory Procedures

Blood samples were drawn during the next outpatient clinic visit after agreeing to participate. Blood was drawn in the morning after an 8–12 h overnight fast, and all measurements were performed in samples of the same timepoint. In plasma EDTA samples frozen at −80°C, we measured plasma EPO levels using an immunoassay based on chemiluminescence (Immulite, Los Angeles, CA) [20]. We measured plasma total FGF23 levels with a human FGF23 (C-terminal) enzyme-linked immunosorbent assay (ELISA; Quidel Corp., San Diego, CA, USA) with intra-assay and interassay coefficients (CVs) of variation of <5% and <16% in blinded replicated samples, respectively [21].

The total FGF23 immunometric assay uses two antibodies directed against different epitopes within the C-terminal part of FGF23, and as such the assay detects both the intact hormone as well as C-terminal cleavage products, and therefore measures total FGF23 levels. We measured plasma ferritin levels using an electrochemiluminescence immunoassay (Modular analytics E170, Roche diagnostics, Mannheim, Germany). Renal function was determined by estimating GFR by applying the Chronic Kidney Disease Epidemiology Collaboration equation [22]. Proteinuria was defined as urinary protein excretion ≥ 0.5 g/24 h in 24-h urine collection. Serum cholesterol was measured using standard laboratory procedures. Serum creatinine was assessed using a modified version of the Jaffé method (MEGA AU 510; Merck Diagnostica, Darmstadt, Germany). Erythrocytosis was defined as hemoglobin level higher than 16.0 g/dL for women, and higher than 16.5 g/dL for men [23].

2.4. Statistical Analyses

Data were analyzed using IBM SPSS software, version 23.0 (SPSS Inc., Chicago, IL), R version 3.2.3 (Vienna, Austria) and STATA 14.1 (STATA Corp., College Station, TX). Data are expressed as mean ± standard deviation [SD] for normally distributed variables and as median (25th–75th interquartile range (IQR)) for variables with a skewed distribution. Categorical data are expressed as numbers (percentages). Co-linearity was tested by means of variance inflation factor (VIF) calculation, with a VIF score of lower than 5 indicating no evidence for co-linearity. We used Cox proportional hazards regression analysis to investigate the association between EPO levels and prospective outcomes. Assumptions of proportionality in Cox regression analyses were checked using Schoenfeld residuals plots and checking nonsignificance of covariates and with the global test (Model 1; EPO with death and CV death; $P > 0.30$ for global test). In these Cox regression analyses, we adjusted for potential confounders based on univariable associations or for factors of known biologic importance. We adjusted for age, sex, body surface area (BSA), eGFR, proteinuria, time since transplantation, presence of diabetes, systolic blood pressure (SBP), total cholesterol, and use of calcineurin inhibitors, proliferation inhibitors, and angiotensin-converting enzyme (ACE)-inhibitors and angiotensin II-receptor blockers (ARBs) (Model 1). We subsequently adjusted for potential mediators in the pathway between EPO and death, i.e., hemoglobin levels (Model 2); for ferritin (Model 3), high-sensitive C-reactive protein (hs-CRP) (Model 4), and finally for total FGF23 (Model 5). Due to skewed distribution, EPO, ferritin, hs-CRP, and total FGF23 were natural log-transformed. We repeated the Cox regression analyses between EPO and outcomes with EPO levels being divided in quartiles. Furthermore, we generated Kaplan–Meier curves to visually show the effect of increased risk of death and cardiovascular death while being in the highest EPO quartile. A log-rank test for trend was used to compare rates of death across quartiles. We also assessed the association between FGF23 levels and prospective outcomes adjusting for all potential confounders according to Model 1 and including EPO. To reflect the contribution of covariates in the different Cox regression models, we generated Supplementary Tables S1–S4 showing the strength of covariates in univariable and multivariable models. To allow comparability between the hazard ratios (HR) of covariates, HR of continuous variables in Supplementary Tables S1–S4 are shown as expressed per SD. As sensitivity analysis, we assessed the prevalence of different etiologies of CKD in total cohort and across EPO quartiles, and we adjusted the association between EPO and all-cause and cardiovascular death for etiology of CKD. Subsequently, we calculated the percentage of change in HR before and after adjustment for FGF23. Percentage change in HR was calculated as—(HR without adjustment − HR with adjustment)/(HR without adjustment − 1) × 100% [24]. Hereafter, we performed mediation analyses with the methods as previously described by Preacher and Hayes, which are based on logistic regression [25,26]. These analyses allow for testing significance and magnitude of mediation on the association between EPO and outcomes [25,26]. Overall, 0.4% of demographic data were missing and these data were imputed using regressive switching [27]. Five datasets were multiply-imputed, and results were pooled and analyzed according to Rubin's rules [28]. In all analyses, a two-sided p-value < 0.05 was considered significant.

3. Results

3.1. Baseline Characteristics

We included 579 RTRs (mean age of 51 ± 12 years; 55% male) at a median of 6.0 (2.6–11.6) years after transplantation. Erythrocytosis was present in 27 (5%) of the included RTRs. Further demographics and clinical baseline characteristics across quartiles of EPO are shown in Table 1.

Table 1. Baseline characteristics of the included 579 renal transplant recipients (RTRs) across erythropoietin (EPO) quartiles.

	All Patients (n = 579)	Quartiles of EPO (IU/L) Q1 (n = 146) [4.0–11.9]	Q2 (n = 143) [12.0–17.2]	Q33 (n = 145) [17.3–23.9]	Q4 (n = 145) [24.2–182.0]	P-value
Age (years)	51 ± 12	47 ± 13	50 ± 12	53 ± 11	54 ± 11	<0.001
Male sex (n, %)	317 (55)	92 (63)	78 (55)	73 (50)	74 (51)	0.11
Body surface area, m^2	1.87 ± 0.19	1.86 ± 0.19	1.86 ± 0.20	1.87 ± 0.18	1.88 ± 0.20	0.81
Alcohol use (n, %)	290 (50)	77 (52)	73 (51)	64 (44)	76 (52)	0.35
Smoking status						0.29
Never smoker (n, %)	205 (35)	47 (32)	49 (34)	59 (41)	50 (35)	
Former smoker (n, %)	246 (43)	64 (44)	68 (48)	59 (41)	55 (38)	
Current smoker (n, %)	126 (22)	35 (24)	25 (18)	27 (19)	39 (27)	
Time since Tx (yrs)	6.0 (2.6–11.6)	4.6 (2.1–9.2)	5.7 (3.1–11.2)	6.5 (3.3–12.4)	7.0 (2.8–13.7)	0.007
Diabetes mellitus (n, %)	102 (18)	25 (17)	21 (15)	27 (19)	29 (20)	0.67
SBP (mmHg)	153 ± 23	150 ± 20	151 ± 21	153 ± 22	157 ± 26	0.05
DBP (mmHg)	90 ± 10	90 ± 9	90 ± 9	90 ± 10	90 ± 11	0.91
Laboratory measurements						
FGF23 (RU/mL)	137 (94–212)	115 (81–168)	125 (88–184)	138 (95–212)	195 (115–363)	<0.001
Hemoglobin (g/dL)	13.9 ± 1.5	14.2 ± 1.5	14.0 ± 1.5	13.8 ± 1.5	13.5 ± 1.5	0.001
Erythrocytosis (n, %)‡	27 (5)	11 (8)	8 (6)	5 (3)	3 (2)	0.13
MCV (fL)	91 ± 6	89 ± 4	91 ± 6	92 ± 6	92 ± 8	<0.001
Ferritin (μg/L)	154 (76–282)	154 (76–320)	164 (100–305)	159 (89–283)	118 (61–240)	0.02
Total cholesterol (mmol/L)	5.6 ± 1.1	5.7 ± 0.9	5.7 ± 1.3	5.6 ± 1.0	5.6 ± 1.1	0.78
Phosphate (mmol/L)	1.1 ± 0.2	1.05 ± 0.21	1.07 ± 0.21	1.05 ± 0.19	1.07 ± 0.22	0.85
Calcium (mmol/L)	2.39 ± 0.16	2.39 ± 0.14	2.38 ± 0.16	2.39 ± 0.18	2.41 ± 0.15	0.51
Vit. 25(OH) D, nmol/l *	53 ± 23	52 ± 24	51 ± 21	57 ± 21	53 ± 25	0.33
Vit. 1,25$(OH)_2$ D, pmol/L*	109 ± 46	106 ± 50	112 ± 46	107 ± 40	110 ± 47	0.80
PTH (pmol/L)	9.1 (6.0–13.4)	8.8 (6.2–13.2)	9.6 (5.8–13.9)	9.2 (6.0–13.7)	8.9 (6.0–14.0)	0.93
eGFR (ml/min/1.73m^2)	48 ± 15	50 ± 16	48 ± 14	47 ± 15	46 ± 16	0.16
Creatinine (μmol/L)	144 ± 52	145 ± 51	139 ± 40	142 ± 51	148 ± 62	0.50
Proteinuria (>0.5g) (n, %)	155 (27)	34 (23)	32 (22)	39 (27)	50 (35)	0.07
hs-CRP (mg/L)	2.0 (0.8–4.8)	1.4 (0.6–3.8)	2.0 (0.7–4.1)	2.1 (1.0–4.2)	3.2 (1.2–7.2)	<0.001
Treatment						
ACE-i/AII-antagonists (n, %)	190 (33)	65 (45)	50 (35)	37 (26)	38 (26)	0.001
ACE-I (n, %)	154 (27)	53 (36)	37 (26)	31 (24)	33 (23)	
AII-antagonists (n,%)	36 (6)	12 (8)	13 (9)	6 (4)	5 (3)	
Bèta-blocker (n, %)	356 (62)	88 (63)	96 (67)	81 (56)	91 (63)	0.26
Ca^{2+} channel blockers (n, %)	220 (39)	56 (38)	52 (36)	51 (35)	61 (42)	0.45
Diuretic use (n, %)	250 (43)	52 (36)	62 (43)	60 (41)	76 (52)	0.04
Proliferation inhibitor (n, %)	428 (74)	95 (65)	99 (69)	115 (79)	119 (82)	0.002
Azathioprine (n, %)	187 (32)	18 (12)	42 (29)	55 (38)	72 (50)	
Mycophenolic acid (n, %)	241 (42)	77 (53)	57 (40)	60 (41)	47 (32)	
Calcineurin inhibitor (n, %)	457 (79)	131 (90)	120 (84)	103 (71)	103 (71)	<0.001
Ciclosporin (n,%)	376 (65)	108 (78)	101 (71)	81 (56)	86 (59)	
Tacrolimus (n, %)	81 (14)	23 (16)	19 (13)	22 (15)	17 (12)	

‡ Erythrocytosis defined as hemoglobin level >16 g/dL (F) and >16.5 g/dL (M) * Only available in a subset cohort of 415 RTRs. Values are means ± standard deviation, medians (interquartile range) or proportions (%). Diabetes mellitus was defined as serum glucose > 7 mmol/L or the use of antidiabetic drugs. Abbreviations—ACE-i, angiotensin converting enzyme inhibitors; DBP, diastolic blood pressure; eGFR, estimated glomerular filtration rate; FGF23, fibroblast growth factor 23; hs-CRP, high-sensitivity C-reactive protein; MCV, mean corpuscular volume; SBP, systolic blood pressure; Tx, transplantation.

Median plasma EPO levels were 17.4 (11.9–24.2) IU/L and median FGF23 levels were 137 (94–212) RU/mL. Increased FGF23 levels were noted across EPO quartiles (115 (81–168) RU/mL; 125 (88–184) RU/mL; 138 (95–212) RU/mL; and 195 (115–363) RU/mL respectively, P < 0.001). FGF23 levels were positively correlated with EPO levels (r = 0.28, P < 0.001), with a VIF of 1.15, indicating very minimal co-linearity.

3.2. EPO, FGF23, and Death

During a median follow-up of 7.0 (6.2–7.4) years, 121 RTRs died. Of the 121 deceased RTRs, 62 RTRs (51%) died from cardiovascular causes. Other causes of death were infection (18%), malignancy (24%), and miscellaneous causes (8%).

In univariable Cox regression analyses, higher EPO levels were associated with an increased risk of all-cause death (HR per 1 ln IU/L increase, 1.74; 95% confidence interval (CI), 1.29–2.34; $P < 0.001$). A full list of HRs for covariates univariably with death are described in Supplementary Table S1.

In multivariable Cox regression analyses, the association between EPO and all-cause death remained significant (HR, 1.66; 95% CI, 1.16-2.36; P=0.005) independent of adjustment for age, sex, BSA, eGFR, proteinuria, time since transplantation, presence of diabetes, SBP, total cholesterol, use of calcineurin inhibitors, proliferation inhibitors, ACE-inhibitors or ARB (Model 1). Further adjustment for hemoglobin, ferritin, or hs-CRP levels did not materially alter the results. However, further adjustment for FGF23 levels attenuated the association between EPO and all-cause death such that the association no longer remained significant (HR, 1.28; 95% CI, 0.87–1.88; $P = 0.20$) (Table 2). A full list of HRs for covariates in the multivariable model can be found in Supplementary Table S2.

Table 2. Association between erythropoietin levels and risk of all-cause and cardiovascular death.

	EPO (IU/L)	
All–cause death	**HR (95% CI) ***	***P*-value**
Univariable	1.74 (1.29–2.34)	<0.001
Model 1	1.66 (1.16–2.36)	0.005
Model 2	1.72 (1.21–2.46)	0.003
Model 3	1.80 (1.25–2.60)	0.002
Model 4	1.60 (1.12–2.29)	0.01
Model 5	1.28 (0.87–1.88)	0.20
Cardiovascular death	**HR (95% CI) ***	***P*-value**
Univariable	1.70 (1.12–2.58)	0.01
Model 1	1.87 (1.14–3.06)	0.01
Model 2	1.90 (1.16–3.12)	0.01
Model 3	2.05 (1.22–3.44)	0.006
Model 4	1.87 (1.14–3.06)	0.01
Model 5	1.45 (0.84–2.48)	0.18

* Hazard ratios are shown per 1 ln IU/L increase in EPO levels; Model 1: Adjusted for age, sex, body surface area, eGFR, proteinuria, time since transplantation, presence of diabetes, systolic blood pressure, total cholesterol, use of calcineurin inhibitors, proliferation inhibitors, and ACE-inhibitors or ARB; Model 2: Model 1 + adjustment for hemoglobin; Model 3: Model 1 + adjustment for ferritin; Model 4: Model 1 + adjustment for hs-CRP; Model 5: Model 1 + adjustment for FGF23. Ferritin, hs-CRP, and FGF23 were naturally log transformed before adding to the Cox regression analysis due to skewed distribution. Abbreviations—ACE, angiotensin-converting enzyme; ARB, angiotensin-receptor blockers; FGF23, fibroblast growth factor 23; CI, confidence interval; eGFR, estimated glomerular filtration rate; HR, hazard ratio; hs-CRP, high-sensitive C-reactive protein.

We identified similar results when subdividing EPO levels into quartiles (Table 3; Figure 1 with Kaplan–Meier curves showing the univariably increased risk of death across EPO quartiles).

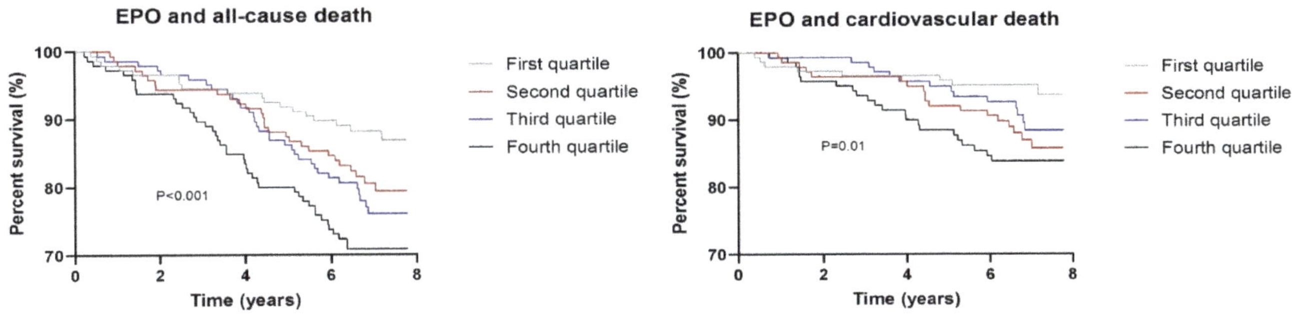

Figure 1. Kaplan–Meier Curves depicting the association between EPO quartiles and risk of all-cause (left panel) and cardiovascular death (right panel). Reported p-values have been calculated with the log-rank test for trend.

Table 3. Association between erythropoietin quartiles and risk of all-cause and cardiovascular death.

	Quartiles of EPO (IU/L)			
	Q1	Q2	Q3	Q4
All–cause death	**Ref**	**HR (95% CI)**	**HR (95% CI)**	**HR (95% CI)**
Univariable	1.00	1.64 (0.91–2.97)	1.93 (1.08–3.42)	2.62 (1.51–4.55)
Model 1	1.00	1.57 (0.85–2.89)	1.47 (0.81–2.69)	2.11 (1.15–3.86)
Model 2	1.00	1.54 (0.83–2.84)	1.51 (0.83–2.75)	2.19 (1.19–4.05)
Model 3	1.00	1.65 (0.88–3.11)	1.57 (0.84–2.93)	2.29 (1.21–4.31)
Model 4	1.00	1.55 (0.85–2.85)	1.42 (0.78–2.58)	1.99 (1.09–3.65)
Model 5	1.00	1.63 (0.89–3.01)	1.41 (0.77–2.57)	1.55 (0.82–2.91)
Cardiovascular Death	**Ref**	**HR (95% CI)**	**HR (95% CI)**	**HR (95% CI)**
Univariable	1.00	2.38 (1.04–5.48)	1.85 (0.78–4.40)	3.08 (1.37–6.92)
Model 1	1.00	2.73 (1.15–6.45)	1.69 (0.68–4.18)	3.34 (1.36–8.20)
Model 2	1.00	2.58 (1.08–6.16)	1.71 (0.69–4.25)	3.41 (1.31–8.47)
Model 3	1.00	2.91 (1.17–7.23)	1.77 (0.68–4.59)	3.57 (1.39–9.20)
Model 4	1.00	2.65 (1.12–6.25)	1.60 (0.65–3.95)	3.10 (1.27–7.60)
Model 5	1.00	2.90 (1.22–6.91)	1.65 (0.66–4.08)	2.47 (0.97–6.31)

Model 1: Adjusted for age, sex, body surface area, eGFR, proteinuria, time since transplantation, presence of diabetes, systolic blood pressure, total cholesterol, use of calcineurin inhibitors, proliferation inhibitors, and ACE-inhibitors or ARB. Model 2: Model 1 + adjustment for hemoglobin; Model 3: Model 1 + adjustment for ferritin; Model 4: Model 1 + adjustment for hs-CRP; Model 5: Model 1 + adjustment for FGF23. Ferritin, hs-CRP, and FGF23 were naturally log transformed before adding to the Cox regression analysis due to skewed distribution. Abbreviations—ACE, angiotensin-converting enzyme; ARB, angiotensin-receptor blockers; FGF23, fibroblast growth factor 23; CI, confidence interval; eGFR, estimated glomerular filtration rate; HR, hazard ratio; hs-CRP, high-sensitive C-reactive protein.

In multivariable Cox regression analysis, RTRs in the upper quartile of EPO had a more than two times higher risk of death (HR, 2.11; 95% CI, 1.15–3.86), when compared to RTRs in the lowest quartile, independent of potential confounders. In line with the association between EPO as continuous variable and death, further adjustment for FGF23 levels attenuated the association between the upper EPO quartile and risk of death (HR, 1.55; 95% CI, 0.82–2.91; Table 3; Figure 2A). A full list of HRs for covariates in the multivariable model for EPO divided in quartiles can be found in Supplementary Table S3.

When we assessed the associations between EPO and cardiovascular death, we found similar findings. Higher EPO levels were associated with an increased risk of cardiovascular death in univariable analyses (Figure 1) and in all subsequent models (Table 2). However, the association no longer remained significant, both as a continuous variable and as divided in quartiles, after further adjustment for FGF23 (Tables 2 and 3; Figure 2B).

In contrast, FGF23 levels per se were strongly associated with all-cause death independent of adjustment for potential confounders including EPO (HR per RU/mL, 1.76; 95% CI, 1.33–2.34; $P < 0.001$). Likewise, FGF23 levels per se were also strongly associated with cardiovascular death independent of adjustment for potential confounders including EPO (HR, 1.84; 95% CI, 1.23–2.76; $P = 0.003$). A full list of HRs for covariates can be found in Supplementary Table S4.

As sensitivity analysis, we assessed the prevalence of different etiologies of CKD in the total cohort and across quartiles of EPO (Supplementary Table S5). The most prevalent etiologies of CKD were primary glomerular disease (28%), polycystic disease (18%), and tubulo-interstitial disease (16%). Following adjustment for etiology of CKD additive to model 1, the association between EPO and all-cause death (HR, 1.57; 95% CI, 1.09–2.26; $P = 0.02$) and between EPO and cardiovascular death (HR, 1.75; 95% CI, 1.05–2.90; $P = 0.03$) remained materially unchanged.

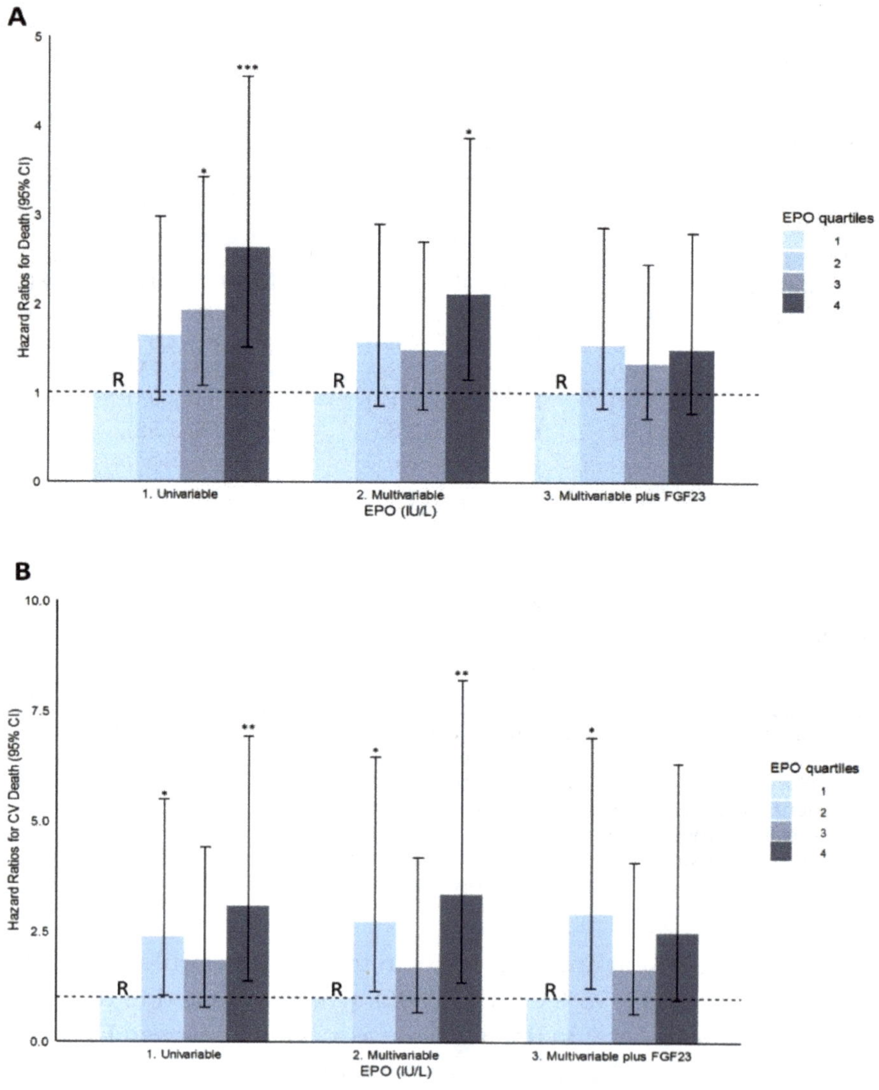

Figure 2. Hazard ratios and corresponding 95% confidence intervals are depicted for risk of death, both all-cause (**A**) and cardiovascular death (**B**), according to quartiles of erythropoietin levels. First, the univariate association is shown. Second, the multivariable adjustment is performed with adjustment for age, sex, body surface area (BSA), eGFR, proteinuria, time since transplantation, presence of diabetes, systolic blood pressure (SBP), total cholesterol, and use of calcineurin inhibitors, proliferation inhibitors, and angiotensin-converting enzyme (ACE)-inhibitors and angiotensin II-receptor blockers (ARBs). Third, adjustment for FGF23 is performed following the multivariable adjustment. The first quartile was chosen as a reference group in all analyses. Significance levels are indicated by numbers of asterisks, i.e., *** <0.001, ** <0.01, * <0.05; Abbreviations—BSA, body surface area; CI, confidence interval; eGFR, estimated glomerular filtration rate.

3.3. EPO, FGF23, and Graft Failure

During a median follow-up of 6.9 (6.1–7.4) years, 46 RTRs developed DCGF. When we assessed the associations between EPO and DCGF, we did not find an association (HR, 0.82; 95% CI, 0.48–1.41; $P = 0.48$). Further adjustment for potential confounders did not ameliorate the association between EPO and DCGF. In contrast, FGF23 levels were univariately associated with DCGF (HR, 3.07; 95% CI, 2.22–4.24; $P < 0.001$). However, after adjustment for potential confounders including EPO, FGF23 was no longer associated with DCGF (HR, 1.57; 95% CI, 0.94–2.64; $P = 0.09$).

3.4. Percentage Change HR and Mediation Analyses

Adjustment for FGF23 caused a large reduction in HR in the Cox Regression analysis in the association between EPO and all-cause and cardiovascular death (58% reduction in HR between EPO and all-cause death; and 48% reduction in HR between EPO and cardiovascular death). In subsequent mediation analyses, we identified that FGF23 was a significant mediator of the association between EPO and all-cause death (P value for indirect effect <0.05; 72% of the association was explained by FGF23; Table 4). Similarly, FGF23 explained 50% of the association between EPO and cardiovascular death (P value for indirect effect <0.05; Table 4).

Table 4. Mediation analysis of FGF23 on the association between EPO and all-cause and cardiovascular death in renal transplant recipients.

Potential Mediator	Outcome	Effect (path) *	Multivariable Model **	
			Coefficient (95% CI, bc) †	Proportion Mediated ***
FGF23	All-cause death	Indirect effect (ab path)	0.090 (0.044; 0.139)	72%
		Total effect (ab + c′ path)	0.124 (−0.011; 0.255)	
		Unstandardized total effect ‡	0.120 (−0.385; 0.624)	
FGF23	Cardiovascular death	Indirect effect (ab path)	0.065 (0.015; 0.122)	50%
		Total effect (ab + c′ path)	0.129 (−0.040; 0.290)	
		Unstandardized total effect ‡	0.218 (−0.405; 0.840)	

* The coefficients of the indirect *ab* path and the total *ab + c′* path are standardized for the standard deviations of EPO, FGF23, all-cause and cardiovascular death. **All coefficients are adjusted for age, sex, body surface area, eGFR, proteinuria, time since transplantation, presence of diabetes, systolic blood pressure, total cholesterol, use of calcineurin inhibitors, proliferation inhibitors, ACE-inhibitors or ARB. *** The size of the significant mediated effect is calculated as the standardized indirect effect divided by the standardized total effect multiplied by 100, e.g., 0.090 divided by 0.124 multiplied by 100 constitutes 72% as percentage of mediation ‡ Odds ratios for risk of outcomes can be calculated by taking the exponent of the unstandardized total effect. For example, the unstandardized coefficient of the direct effect of EPO on all-cause death while adjusting for FGF23 is 0.120, which can be calculated to an OR by taking the exponent of this regression coefficient, i.e., $e^{0.120}=1.12$, which corresponds to the HR of 1.28 (see Table 2). The discrepancy between the ratios is due to taking into account time-to-event with HR in contrast to OR. †95% CIs for the indirect and total effects were bias-corrected confidence intervals after running 2000 bootstrap samples. Abbreviations—ACE, angiotensin converting enzyme; ARB, angiotensin receptor blockers; Bc, bias corrected; CI, confidence interval; eGFR, estimated glomerular filtration rate; FGF23, fibroblast growth factor 23.

4. Discussion

In this study, we show that higher endogenous EPO levels are associated with an increased risk of all-cause and cardiovascular death in RTRs, and that these associations are largely explained by variation in FGF23 levels. This study confirms recent studies about the essential role of EPO in FGF23 physiology in experimental and human models [7–10], extends these findings to RTRs, and support the notion that FGF23 is an important mediator in the association between EPO and risk of death.

EPO, a hormone mainly produced in the kidney in response to hypoxia, is essential for erythropoiesis [29]. EPO controls proliferation, maturation, and also survival of erythroid progenitor cells [30]. Previously, it has been shown that high endogenous EPO levels were associated with an increased risk of all-cause and cardiovascular death in RTRs [2,3]. Similarly, in the setting of CKD and ESRD, correction of anemia with recombinant EPO led an increased risk of cardiovascular morbidity and death [5,6]. The mechanisms responsible for these adverse effects of both endogenous as exogenous EPO are unknown. In the Correction of Hemoglobin and Outcomes in Renal Insufficiency (CHOIR) trial, the highest risk of cardiovascular death was seen in patients with the highest EPO dose, suggesting that EPO resistance through inflammation and/or functional iron deficiency might be a possible link [6]. However, in the current study, the association between endogenous EPO levels and death was independent of adjustment for inflammation as well as independent of iron parameters, renal function, and standard classical cardiovascular risk factors including systolic blood pressure and cholesterol levels. Although there was a difference in prevalence of use of calcineurin and proliferation inhibitors across EPO quartiles, the association between EPO and death remained independent of adjustment for calcineurin and proliferation inhibitors. In contrast, adjustment for FGF23 markedly attenuated the association between EPO and death.

Elevated total FGF23 levels have previously been shown to be associated with increased risk of death in RTRs, as well as in various other patient groups including postoperative acute kidney injury, nondialysis CKD, and ESRD [31–35]. FGF23 regulation is determined by a complex interplay between parathyroid hormone, 1,25-dihydroxyvitamin D, klotho, glucocorticoids, calcium, and phosphate [36,37]. In recent years, iron deficiency has been identified as an important regulator of FGF23 [38–40]. In addition, recent studies demonstrated that EPO stimulates murine and human FGF23 [7,8]. Clinkenbeard and colleagues reported increased FGF23 mRNA expression in vitro, ex vivo, and in vivo due to EPO treatment in UMR-106 cells, in isolated bone marrow cells, and in marrow from mice, respectively [7]. In addition, Rabadi et al. showed in experimental animal models that an acute loss of 10% blood volume led to an increase in total FGF23 and EPO levels within six hours. Furthermore, exogenous administration of EPO resulted in an acute increase in plasma total FGF23 levels similar to those seen in acute blood loss [8]. Similarly, Flamme et al. described in animal models an increase in plasma total FGF23 both after injection of recombinant human EPO and after HIF-proline hydroxylase inhibitor [41]. The present findings in our study underscore these observations and emphasize the important role of EPO in FGF23 physiology. Importantly, the current study is the first to show that prospective associations between EPO and adverse outcomes in RTRs seem to be, at least to large extent, related to increased levels of total FGF23.

The mechanisms through which EPO, as reflection of tissue hypoxia, lead to increased bone marrow FGF23 transcription are currently unknown and require additional investigation. The previously performed studies showed that EPO acutely increases total FGF23 levels out of proportion to intact FGF23 (iFGF23), suggesting an upregulated FGF23 production with concomitantly increased cleavage, with as a result an increase in C-terminal FGF23 fragments. To date, it remains incompletely understood how EPO increases post-translational cleavage. Results from our group and collaborators found previously in EPO-overexpressing mice a decreased GalNT3 bone marrow mRNA expression, without differences in Fam20C or furin expression, implying that a decreased GalNT3 might play a possible role [9]. However, more investigation is imperative to unravel this mechanistic link.

The downstream consequences of elevated levels of FGF23 and the subsequent excess risk of death have not been fully elucidated yet. Several previous reports have shown that iFGF23 has biologic activity through binding to several FGF23 receptors. Besides the well-known functions of iFGF23 in the regulation of renal phosphate handling and vitamin D metabolism, recent studies have shown a myriad "off-target" effects of iFGF23 on the heart and other organs. Preclinical studies demonstrated that FGF23 can lead to left ventricular hypertrophy in cardiac myocytes, and promote endothelial dysfunction [42,43]. In addition, FGF23 stimulates renal fibrosis [44], exerts pro-inflammatory effects [45], and disrupts normal immune function [46]. Most likely, the increased death risk due to elevated levels of FGF23 is attributable to a combination of these effects. Although the biologic activity of iFGF23 has unequivocally been demonstrated, the biologic activity of C-terminal FGF23 fragments remains uncertain. Previously, it has been shown that C-terminal FGF23 may function as an iFGF23 antagonist, by competing with iFGF23 for binding to its receptor, which may reduce phosphaturia and aggravate soft tissue calcification [47]. In addition, Courbabaisse et al. has shown, at least in vitro, that C-terminal FGF23 increases adult rat ventricular cardiomyocyte size by stimulation of FGF receptor

4 in the absence of co-stimulatory factor alpha-klotho, and in sickle cell disease patients that elevated cleaved FGF23 levels were associated with heart hypertrophy [48].

Our study has multiple strengths as well as limitations. The major strength of the current study is the large prospective cohort of stable RTRs with detailed clinical and laboratory data available, including EPO, FGF23, hs-CRP, and ferritin levels. Additionally, no participants were lost to follow-up with respect to the endpoints, despite a considerable follow-up period. Limitations of the current study include that, due to the observational status of our single center study, we cannot exclude the possibility of residual confounding, and conclusions about causality cannot be drawn. Furthermore, we were unable to measure iFGF23 levels, since samples were not stored with protease inhibitors, and iFGF23 has been shown to be susceptible to degradation with long-term storage [49]. This precludes us to discern whether the elevated total FGF23 levels are the result of increased iFGF23 levels or due to an increase in allegedly assumed inactive C-terminal fragments. Another limitation of the study is that we only used CRP levels as inflammatory parameter, other markers of inflammation (e.g., cytokines, cell subtypes) were not available, but could possibly have contributed to the results. In addition, another limitation of current study is the use of single-time measurements hampering the possibility to track the levels of EPO and FGF23 over time with respect to each other and with respect to risk of death. However, it should be realized that most epidemiological studies use a single baseline measurement to investigate associations of variables with outcomes, which adversely affects the strength and significance of the association of these variables with outcomes. If intraindividual variability of variables is taken into account, this results in strengthening of associations that also existed for single measurements of these variables [50,51]. Finally, we want to emphasize that the mediation analyses that we performed are plain straightforward mediation analyses. Although based on literature, we have strong evidence that FGF23 is a mediator in the association of EPO with risk of death, we cannot exclude that an unmeasured cause of mortality or alternative potential mediators has influenced the currently identified results.

In conclusion, we identified that elevated levels of EPO were independently associated with an increased risk of death in RTRs, and that this association was to a large extent explained by variation in FGF23 levels. Further research is needed to fully elucidate the mechanism through which this ensues and to unravel whether the currently identified results can be extrapolated to exogenous EPO in RTRs.

Supplementary Materials:
Supplementary Table S1: Univariable associations of variables with prospective outcomes (i.e., all-cause death and cardiovascular death), Supplementary Table S2: Reporting of all hazard ratios of all covariates included in the Cox Regression Analyses for the association between erythropoietin as continuous variable and risk of all-cause and cardiovascular death (according to model 5 [including FGF23]), Supplementary Table S3: Reporting of all hazard ratios of all covariates included in the Cox Regression Analyses for the association between quartiles of erythropoietin and risk of all-cause and cardiovascular death (according to model 5 [including FGF23]), Supplementary Table S4: Reporting of all hazard ratios of all covariates included in the Cox Regression Analyses for the association between FGF23 as continuous variable and risk of all-cause and cardiovascular death (multivariable excluding erythropoietin [Supplementary Table S2 includes erythropoietin]), Supplementary Table S5: Prevalence of the different etiologies of CKD described in the total cohort of 579 RTRs and across the quartiles of erythropoietin levels.

Author Contributions: Conceptualization, M.F.E.; Data curation, M.H.D.B. and S.J.L.B.; Formal analysis, M.F.E., M.A.D.J., D.E.L. and I.M.N.; Investigation, S.J.L.B.; Methodology, M.F.E., M.H.D.B., S.J.L.B. and C.A.J.M.G.; Supervision, S.J.L.B. and C.A.J.M.G.; Visualization, M.F.E.; Writing—original draft, M.F.E.; Writing—review and editing, M.A.D.J., D.E.L., I.M.N., M.H.D.B., S.J.L.B. and C.A.J.M.G. All authors have read and agreed to the published version of the manuscript.

Acknowledgments: The current study was based on TransplantLines Insulin Resistance and Inflammation (TxL-IRI) Cohort Study (NCT03272854).

References

1. Jardine, A.; Gaston, R.S.; Fellström, B.C.; Holdaas, H. Prevention of cardiovascular disease in adult recipients of kidney transplants. *Lancet* **2011**, *378*, 1419–1427. [CrossRef]
2. Sinkeler, S.J.; Zelle, D.M.; van der Heide, J.J.H.; Gans, R.; Navis, G.; Bakker, S.J.L. Endogenous plasma erythropoietin, cardiovascular mortality and all-cause mortality in renal transplant recipients. *Arab. Archaeol. Epigr.* **2011**, *12*, 485–491. [CrossRef] [PubMed]
3. Molnar, M.Z.; Tabak, A.G.; Alam, A.; Czira, M.E.; Rudas, A.; Ujszaszi, A.; Beko, G.; Novak, M.; Kalantar-Zadeh, K.; Kovesdy, C.P.; et al. Serum erythropoietin level and mortality in kidney transplant recipients. *Clin. J. Am. Soc. Nephrol.* **2011**, *6*, 2879–2886. [CrossRef] [PubMed]
4. Den Elzen, W.P.; Willems, J.M.; Westendorp, R.G.; de Craen, A.J.; Blauw, G.J.; Ferrucci, L.; Assendelft, W.J.; Gussekloo, J. Effect of erythropoietin levels on mortality in old age: The leiden 85-plus study. *Can. Med. Assoc. J.* **2010**, *182*, 1953–1958. [CrossRef]
5. Pfeffer, M.A.; Burdmann, E.; Chen, C.-Y.; E Cooper, M.; de Zeeuw, D.; Eckardt, K.-U.; Ivanovich, P.; KewalRamani, R.; Levey, A.S.; Lewis, E.F.; et al. Baseline characteristics in the trial to reduce cardiovascular events with aranesp therapy (TREAT). *Am. J. Kidney Dis.* **2009**, *54*, 59–69. [CrossRef] [PubMed]
6. Singh, A.K.; Szczech, L.; Tang, K.L.; Barnhart, H.; Sapp, S.; Wolfson, M.; Reddan, D.; CHOIR Investigators. Correction of anemia with epoetin alfa in chronic kidney disease. *New Engl. J. Med.* **2006**, *355*, 2085–2098. [CrossRef]
7. Clinkenbeard, E.L.; Hanudel, M.R.; Stayrook, K.R.; Appaiah, H.N.; Farrow, E.G.; Cass, T.A.; Summers, L.J.; Ip, C.S.; Hum, J.M.; Thomas, J.C.; et al. Erythropoietin stimulates murine and human fibroblast growth factor-23, revealing novel roles for bone and bone marrow. *Haematologica* **2017**, *102*, e427–e430. [CrossRef]
8. Rabadi, S.; Udo, I.; Leaf, D.E.; Waikar, S.S.; Christov, M. Acute blood loss stimulates fibroblast growth factor 23 production. *Am. J. Physiol. Ren. Physiol.* **2017**, *314*, F132–F139. [CrossRef]
9. Hanudel, M.R.; Eisenga, M.; Rappaport, M.; Chua, K.; Qiao, B.; Jung, G.; Gabayan, V.; Gales, B.; Ramos, G.; A De Jong, M.; et al. Effects of erythropoietin on fibroblast growth factor 23 in mice and humans. *Nephrol. Dial. Transpl.* **2018**, *34*, 2057–2065. [CrossRef]
10. Toro, L.; Barrientos, V.; León, P.; Rojas, M.; González, M.; González-Ibáñez, A.; Illanes, S.; Sugikawa, K.; Abarzúa, N.; Bascuñán, C.; et al. Erythropoietin induces bone marrow and plasma fibroblast growth factor 23 during acute kidney injury. *Kidney Int.* **2018**, *93*, 1131–1141. [CrossRef]
11. Baia, L.C.; Humalda, J.K.; Vervloet, M.G.; Navis, G.; Bakker, S.J.; De Borst, M.H. Fibroblast growth factor 23 and cardiovascular mortality after kidney transplantation. *Clin. J. Am. Soc. Nephrol.* **2013**, *8*, 1968–1978. [CrossRef] [PubMed]
12. Wolf, M.; Molnar, M.Z.; Amaral, A.P.; Czira, M.E.; Rudas, A.; Ujszaszi, A.; Kiss, I.; Rosivall, L.; Kosa, J.; Lakatos, P.; et al. Elevated fibroblast growth factor 23 is a risk factor for kidney transplant loss and mortality. *J. Am. Soc. Nephrol.* **2011**, *22*, 956–966. [CrossRef]
13. Stockmann, C.; Fandrey, J. Hypoxia-Induced erythropoietin production: A paradigm for oxygen-regulated gene expression. *Clin. Exp. Pharmacol. Physiol.* **2006**, *33*, 968–979. [CrossRef] [PubMed]
14. Ziello, J.E.; Jovin, I.S.; Huang, Y. Hypoxia-Inducible factor (HIF)-1 regulatory pathway and its potential for therapeutic intervention in malignancy and ischemia. *Yale J. Boil. Med.* **2007**, *80*, 51–60.
15. Hamrick, S.E.G.; McQuillen, P.S.; Jiang, X.; Mu, D.; Madan, A.; Ferriero, D.M. A role for hypoxia-inducible factor-1α in desferoxamine neuroprotection. *Neurosci. Lett.* **2005**, *379*, 96–100. [CrossRef] [PubMed]
16. McMahon, S.; Grondin, F.; McDonald, P.P.; Richard, D.E.; Dubois, C.M. Hypoxia-enhanced expression of the proprotein convertase furin is mediated by hypoxia-inducible factor-1: Impact on the bioactivation of proproteins. *J. Biol. Chem.* **2005**, *280*, 6561–6569. [CrossRef] [PubMed]
17. Wolf, M.; White, K.E. Coupling fibroblast growth factor 23 production and cleavage. *Curr. Opin. Nephrol. Hypertens.* **2014**, *23*, 411–419. [CrossRef]
18. Hanudel, M.R.; Wesseling-Perry, K.; Gales, B.; Ramos, G.; Campbell, V.; Ethridge, K.; Scotti, M.; Elashoff, D.A.; Alejos, J.; Reemtsen, B.; et al. Effects of acute kidney injury and chronic hypoxemia on fibroblast growth factor 23 levels in pediatric cardiac surgery patients. *Pediatr. Nephrol.* **2015**, *31*, 661–669. [CrossRef]
19. De Vries, A.; Bakker, S.J.L.; van Son, W.J.; van der Heide, J.J.H.; Ploeg, R.J.; The, H.T.; de Jong, P.E.; Gans, R.O.B. Metabolic syndrome is associated with impaired long-term renal allograft function; Not all component criteria contribute equally. *Arab. Archaeol. Epigr.* **2004**, *4*, 1675–1683. [CrossRef]

20. Benson, E.W.; Hardy, R.; Chaffin, C.; Robinson, C.A.; Konrad, R.J. New automated chemiluminescent assay for erythropoietin. *J. Clin. Lab. Anal.* **2000**, *14*, 271–273. [CrossRef]
21. Heijboer, A.C.; Levitus, M.; Vervloet, M.; Lips, P.; Wee, P.M.T.; Dijstelbloem, H.M.; Blankenstein, M. Determination of fibroblast growth factor 23. *Ann. Clin. Biochem. Int. J. Lab. Med.* **2009**, *46*, 338–340. [CrossRef] [PubMed]
22. Levey, A.S.; Stevens, L.A.; Schmid, C.H.; Zhang, Y.L.; Castro, A.F., 3rd; Feldman, H.I.; Kusek, J.W.; Eggers, P.; Van Lente, F.; Greene, T.; et al. A new equation to estimate glomerular filtration rate. *Ann. Intern. Med.* **2009**, *150*, 604–612. [CrossRef] [PubMed]
23. Arber, D.A.; Orazi, A.; Hasserjian, R.; Thiele, J.; Borowitz, M.J.; Beau, M.M.L.; Bloomfield, C.D.; Cazzola, M.; Vardiman, J.W. The 2016 revision to the World Health Organization classification of myeloid neoplasms and acute leukemia. *Blood* **2016**, *127*, 2391–2405. [CrossRef] [PubMed]
24. Oterdoom, L.H.; de Vries, A.; van Ree, R.M.; Gansevoort, R.T.; van Son, W.J.; van der Heide, J.J.H.; Navis, G.; de Jong, P.E.; Gans, R.O.; Bakker, S.J. N-Terminal Pro-B-Type natriuretic peptide and mortality in renal transplant recipients versus the general population. *Transplantation* **2009**, *87*, 1562–1570. [CrossRef]
25. Preacher, K.J.; Hayes, A.F. SPSS and SAS procedures for estimating indirect effects in simple mediation models. *Behav. Res. Methods Instrum. Comput.* **2004**, *36*, 717–731. [CrossRef]
26. Hayes, A.F. Beyond baron and kenny: Statistical mediation analysis in the new millennium. *Commun. Monogr.* **2009**, *76*, 408–420. [CrossRef]
27. White, I.R.; Wood, A.M.; Royston, P. Multiple imputation using chained equations: Issues and guidance for practice. *Stat. Med.* **2010**, *30*, 377–399. [CrossRef]
28. Rubin, D.B. *Multiple Imputation for Nonresponse in Surveys*; Wiley: New York, NY, USA, 1987.
29. Jelkmann, W. Regulation of erythropoietin production. *J. Physiol.* **2010**, *589*, 1251–1258. [CrossRef]
30. Rossert, J.; Eckardt, K.-U. Erythropoietin receptors: Their role beyond erythropoiesis. *Nephrol. Dial. Transpl.* **2005**, *20*, 1025–1028. [CrossRef]
31. Gutierrez, O.M.; Mannstadt, M.; Isakova, T.; Rauh-Hain, J.A.; Tamez, H.; Shah, A.; Smith, K.; Lee, H.; Thadhani, R.; Jüppner, H.; et al. Fibroblast growth factor 23 and mortality among patients undergoing hemodialysis. *New Engl. J. Med.* **2008**, *359*, 584–592. [CrossRef]
32. Isakova, T.; Xie, H.; Yang, W.; Xie, D.; Anderson, A.H.; Scialla, J.; Wahl, P.; Gutierrez, O.M.; Steigerwalt, S.; He, J.; et al. Chronic renal insufficiency cohort (CRIC) study group fibroblast growth factor 23 and risks of mortality and end-stage renal disease in patients with chronic kidney disease. *J. Am. Med. Assoc.* **2011**, *305*, 2432–2439. [CrossRef] [PubMed]
33. Leaf, D.E.; Christov, M.; Jüppner, H.; Siew, E.; Ikizler, T.A.; Bian, A.; Chen, G.; Sabbisetti, V.S.; Bonventre, J.V.; Cai, X.; et al. Fibroblast growth factor 23 levels are elevated and associated with severe acute kidney injury and death following cardiac surgery. *Kidney Int.* **2016**, *89*, 939–948. [CrossRef] [PubMed]
34. Kendrick, J.; Cheung, A.K.; Kaufman, J.S.; Greene, T.; Roberts, W.L.; Smits, G.; Chonchol, M.; HOST Investigators. FGF-23 associates with death, cardiovascular events, and initiation of chronic dialysis. *J. Am. Soc. Nephrol.* **2011**, *22*, 1913–1922. [CrossRef] [PubMed]
35. Mendoza, J.M.; Isakova, T.; Cai, X.; Bayes, L.Y.; Faul, C.; Scialla, J.J.; Lash, J.P.; Chen, J.; He, J.; Navaneethan, S.; et al. CRIC study investigators inflammation and elevated levels of fibroblast growth factor 23 are independent risk factors for death in chronic kidney disease. *Kidney Int.* **2017**, *91*, 711–719. [CrossRef]
36. Nguyen-Yamamoto, L.; Karaplis, A.C.; St–Arnaud, R.; Goltzman, D. Fibroblast growth factor 23 regulation by systemic and local osteoblast-synthesized 1,25-Dihydroxyvitamin D. *J. Am. Soc. Nephrol.* **2016**, *28*, 586–597. [CrossRef]
37. Kovesdy, C.P.; Quarles, L.D. Fibroblast growth factor-23: What we know, what we don't know, and what we need to know. *Nephrol. Dial. Transpl.* **2013**, *28*, 2228–2236. [CrossRef]
38. Eisenga, M.; van Londen, M.; Leaf, D.E.; Nolte, I.M.; Navis, G.; Bakker, S.J.; De Borst, M.H.; Gaillard, C.A. C-Terminal fibroblast growth factor 23, iron deficiency, and mortality in renal transplant recipients. *J. Am. Soc. Nephrol.* **2017**, *28*, 3639–3646. [CrossRef]
39. Wolf, M.; Koch, T.A.; Bregman, D.B. Effects of iron deficiency anemia and its treatment on fibroblast growth factor 23 and phosphate homeostasis in women. *J. Bone Miner. Res.* **2013**, *28*, 1793–1803. [CrossRef]
40. David, V.; Martin, A.; Isakova, T.; Spaulding, C.; Qi, L.; Ramirez, V.; Zumbrennen-Bullough, K.B.; Sun, C.C.; Lin, H.Y.; Babitt, J.L.; et al. Inflammation and functional iron deficiency regulate fibroblast growth factor 23 production. *Kidney Int.* **2016**, *89*, 135–146. [CrossRef]

41. Flamme, I.; Ellinghaus, P.; Urrego, D.; Krüger, T. FGF23 expression in rodents is directly induced via erythropoietin after inhibition of hypoxia inducible factor proline hydroxylase. *PLoS ONE* **2017**, *12*, e0186979. [CrossRef]
42. Silswal, N.; Touchberry, C.; Daniel, D.R.; McCarthy, D.L.; Zhang, S.; Andresen, J.; Stubbs, J.R.; Wacker, M.J. FGF23 directly impairs endothelium-dependent vasorelaxation by increasing superoxide levels and reducing nitric oxide bioavailability. *Am. J. Physiol. Metab.* **2014**, *307*, E426–E436. [CrossRef]
43. Faul, C.; Amaral, A.P.; Oskouei, B.; Hu, M.-C.; Sloan, A.; Isakova, T.; Gutierrez, O.M.; Aguillon-Prada, R.; Lincoln, J.; Hare, J.M.; et al. FGF23 induces left ventricular hypertrophy. *J. Clin. Investig.* **2011**, *121*, 4393–4408. [CrossRef]
44. Smith, E.R.; Tan, S.-J.; Holt, S.G.; Hewitson, T. FGF23 is synthesised locally by renal tubules and activates injury-primed fibroblasts. *Sci. Rep.* **2017**, *7*, 3345. [CrossRef] [PubMed]
45. Singh, S.; Grabner, A.; Yanucil, C.; Schramm, K.; Czaya, B.; Krick, S.; Czaja, M.J.; Bartz, R.; Abraham, R.; Marco, G.S.D.; et al. Fibroblast growth factor 23 directly targets hepatocytes to promote inflammation in chronic kidney disease. *Kidney Int.* **2016**, *90*, 985–996. [CrossRef] [PubMed]
46. Rossaint, J.; Oehmichen, J.; van Aken, H.; Reuter, S.; Pavenstädt, H.J.; Meersch, M.; Unruh, M.L.; Zarbock, A. FGF23 signaling impairs neutrophil recruitment and host defense during CKD. *J. Clin. Investig.* **2016**, *126*, 962–974. [CrossRef] [PubMed]
47. Goetz, R.; Nakada, Y.; Hu, M.C.; Kurosu, H.; Wang, L.; Nakatani, T.; Shi, M.; Eliseenkova, A.V.; Razzaque, M.S.; Moe, O.W.; et al. Isolated C-terminal tail of FGF23 alleviates hypophosphatemia by inhibiting FGF23-FGFR-Klotho complex formation. *Proc. Natl. Acad. Sci. USA* **2009**, *107*, 407–412. [CrossRef]
48. Courbebaisse, M.; Mehel, H.; Petit-Hoang, C.; Ribeil, J.-A.; Sabbah, L.; Tuloup-Minguez, V.; Bergerat, D.; Arlet, J.-B.; Stanislas, A.; Souberbielle, J.-C.; et al. Carboxy-terminal fragment of fibroblast growth factor 23 induces heart hypertrophy in sickle cell disease. *Haematologica* **2016**, *102*, e33–e35. [CrossRef]
49. El-Maouche, D.; Dumitrescu, C.E.; Andreopoulou, P.; Gafni, R.I.; Brillante, B.A.; Bhattacharyya, N.; Fedarko, N.S.; Collins, M.T. Stability and degradation of fibroblast growth factor 23 (FGF23): The effect of time and temperature and assay type. *Osteoporos. Int.* **2016**, *27*, 2345–2353. [CrossRef]
50. Koenig, W.; Sund, M.; Fröhlich, M.; Löwel, H.; Hutchinson, W.L.; Pepys, M.B. Refinement of the association of serum C-reactive protein concentration and coronary heart disease risk by correction for within-subject variation over time: The MONICA Augsburg studies, 1984 and 1987. *Am. J. Epidemiol.* **2003**, *158*, 357–364. [CrossRef]
51. Danesh, J.; Wheeler, J.G.; Hirschfield, G.; Eda, S.; Eiriksdottir, G.; Rumley, A.; Lowe, G.; Pepys, M.B.; Gudnason, V. C-Reactive protein and other circulating markers of inflammation in the prediction of coronary heart disease. *New Engl. J. Med.* **2004**, *350*, 1387–1397. [CrossRef] [PubMed]

10

The Effect of Proton Pump Inhibitor Use on Renal Function in Kidney Transplanted Patients

Dominik J. G. Flothow, Barbara Suwelack, Hermann Pavenstädt, Katharina Schütte-Nütgen † and Stefan Reuter *,†

Department of Medicine D, University Hospital of Muenster, 48149 Münster, Germany; d_flot01@uni-muenster.de (D.J.G.F.); barbara.suwelack@ukmuenster.de (B.S.); hermann.pavenstaedt@ukmuenster.de (H.P.); Katharina.schuette-nuetgen@ukmuenster.de (K.S.-N.)

* Correspondence: sreuter@uni-muenster.de

† These authors contributed to this work equally.

Abstract: Recently, proton pump inhibitor (PPI) intake has been linked to acute kidney injury and chronic kidney disease. The objective of this study was to assess the effect of PPIs on renal function and rejection rate in kidney transplant patients. We performed a single center, retrospective analysis of 455 patients who received a kidney transplant between May 2010 and July 2015. Median follow-up time was 3.3 years. PPI prescription was assessed in half-year intervals. Primary outcome parameters were the estimated glomerular filtration rate (eGFR), change in the eGFR, and >30% and >50% eGFR decline for different time periods (up to four years post-transplantation). Our secondary outcome parameter was occurrence of biopsy proven acute rejection (BPAR) in the first two years after transplantation. Except for >30% eGFR decline from half a year to two years post-transplantation ($p = 0.044$) and change in the eGFR, >30% and >50% eGFR decline showed no association with PPI intake in our patient cohort ($p > 0.05$). Similarly, by analyzing 158 rejection episodes, BPAR showed no correspondence with mean daily PPI intake. We conclude that prolonged PPI intake has no relevant adverse effect on kidney transplant function or rejection rates. Polypharmacy, however, remains a problem in renal transplant recipients and it is thus advisable to question the necessity of PPI prescriptions when clear indications are missing.

Keywords: proton pump inhibitor; kidney transplantation; transplant rejection; GFR

---

1. Introduction

With only a single transplanted kidney and oftentimes reduced renal filtration rates, kidney transplant (KTx) recipients are particularly vulnerable to the nephrotoxic adverse effects of drugs. Care is taken to avoid such drugs that could further impair kidney function. For this reason, recent epidemiological studies that have observed a relationship between acute kidney injury (AKI), chronic kidney disease (CKD) and proton pump inhibitor (PPI) intake have been of special interest for practitioners involved in the care of KTx patients [1–5].

Furthermore, in the setting of KTx, two medication interactions of possible relevance are the interaction between PPIs and mycophenolate mofetil (MMF) and between PPIs and tacrolimus. The first may lead to decreased blood levels of the active metabolites of MMF [6–12], which may result in increased rejection rates [13–16]. Tacrolimus is known to be nephrotoxic and it is thought that interactions with PPIs may change its uptake and/or metabolism [17–19], potentially increasing tacrolimus blood concentration. This could be detrimental to kidney transplant function.

In the face of surgical stress and long-term polypharmacy, upper gastrointestinal symptoms are frequent in KTx patients [20]. Even in those patients receiving acid suppressive therapy, the risk of ulcer disease is still elevated [20]. Gastrointestinal complications have also been associated with decreased graft survival [21]. As PPIs are a very effective form of acid suppression, they are frequently given as prophylaxes among transplant recipients [20,22,23]. In our center, they are the standard of care for KTx patients.

In light of the mentioned studies and the possibility of adverse drug interactions between PPIs and mycophenolate mofetil or tacrolimus, we carried out this study. Previous PPI studies in KTx patients have focused on the possible interaction of MMF with PPIs [22,24,25] or the occurrence of other PPI intake related adverse events [23]. We retrospectively evaluated if a relationship between PPI intake and renal function could be found. We analyzed follow-up data of up to four years after transplantation. To our knowledge, no study exists to date that has specifically analyzed the changes in renal function after KTx with regard to PPI intake over a comparable time frame. Additionally, we compared rejection rates, as these may be of relevance regarding MMF and PPI interactions.

2. Patients and Methods

2.1. Patients

Prior to analysis, the data of all patients was anonymized. The local ethics committee (Ethik Kommission der Ärztekammer Westfalen-Lippe und der Medizinischen Fakultät der Westfälischen Wilhelms-Universität, No. 2014-381-f-N) approved the study. Methods in this study were carried out in accordance with the current transplantation guidelines and the Declarations of Istanbul and Helsinki. Written informed consent was given by all participants at the time of transplantation for recording their clinical data.

We herein performed an explorative, retrospective, single-center cohort study. We enrolled all patients receiving a KTx between May 2010 and July 2015 at the University Hospital Muenster. Inclusion criteria were patient age ≥18 years and PPI therapy at primary hospital discharge post-transplantation (pTx). Patients receiving multiple organ transplants remained included. The recipient and donor data was collected from the patients' electronic files. The following data was collected and used: recipient and donor age and sex; recipient body mass index (BMI); prior renal transplants; transplant under European Senior Program; donor type (living or deceased); delayed graft function (DGF; dialysis within the first week pTx); cold ischemia time; pre-transplant time dialyzed; pre-transplant arterial hypertension; pre-transplant diabetes; presence of peripheral arterial occlusive disease; cerebral arterial occlusive disease or stroke; coronary heart disease or myocardial infarction; anticoagulant prescription; antiplatelet drug prescription (including acetylsalicylic acid (ASA)); statin prescription; MMF dosage at primary discharge and two years pTx; cortisone intake at primary discharge and one year pTx; tacrolimus dose and blood level three months pTx; prior smoking history; continuation of smoking after KTx; number of human leukocyte antigen (HLA) mismatches; ABO incompatibility of transplant; induction therapy; pre-transplant donor specific antibody (DSA) occurrence; panel reactive antibodies; transplant rejection occurrence and type according to Banff criteria; eGFR from half a year to four years pTx; and data on PPI prescription. At primary discharge, none of the patients had any non-steroidal anti-inflammatory drug prescriptions, except for ASA. To improve adjustment for confounding through comorbidities, additional data was collected to calculate the Charlson comorbidity index [26] at transplantation [27].

The induction therapy was chosen according to the immunological risks of the patients. One gram of mycophenolate mofetil was given twice a day; the dosage was reduced in case of adverse events. Prednisolone was started at 500 mg intravenously (i.v.) before KTx, followed by 100 mg for three days; then reduced by 20 mg/day. A dosage of 20 mg/day was maintained until day 30 and then slowly reduced to 5 mg/day. Immunosuppressive maintenance therapy usually consisted of a calcineurin inhibitor (tacrolimus or cyclosporine A), mycophenolate sodium or mycophenolate mofetil and prednisolone.

2.2. Proton Pump Inhibitors—Data Collection

Data on the prescription of PPIs (agent and dose prescribed) were collected in half year intervals for all patients starting at primary discharge. PPI intake was assumed according to this prescription until the next interval. If data was not present for a certain interval, the prescription from the preceding interval was assumed.

Due to the favorable drug interaction profile of pantoprazole in comparison to other PPIs [28], pantoprazole is used as the PPI of choice at our center. Therefore, it has also been used as the standard PPI in this study. In order to also use data from different PPIs, equivalent doses were calculated for the two other agents (omeprazole and esomeprazole) used. We used the ratio: 40 mg pantoprazole $\hat{=}$ 20 mg omeprazole $\hat{=}$ 20 mg esomeprazole [29,30].

At our center, patients are instructed to ingest tacrolimus and MMF on an empty stomach one hour before intake of PPIs. Both tacrolimus and MMF are usually taken twice daily, while PPIs are mostly taken once per day.

2.3. Group Formation

Based on PPI intake (n = 363) and non-intake (n = 82) at half a year pTx, two patient groups were formed. These were used for a direct comparison of GFR and change thereof.

For the outcome measures >30% and >50% eGFR decline and the number of rejections, the groups 0 mg, 1–20 mg, 21–40 mg and >40 mg mean daily PPI intake were compared. The standard dose at our center is 40 mg pantoprazole, 20 mg is the common reduced dose, and above >40 mg (often 80 mg) is an elevated dose (rationale for the group formation).

2.4. Outcome Measures

Primary outcome measures were: the eGFR (at six months, one year, two years, three years and four years), change in the eGFR (from six months pTx to one year, two years, three years and four years), eGFR decline >30% and eGFR decline >50% (from six months to two years and two years to four years). All eGFR-values were calculated using the CKD-EPI (Chronic Kidney Disease Epidemiology Collaboration) equation [31].

Our secondary outcome was biopsy proven acute rejection (BPAR) in months one to six, seven to twelve and in the second year pTx. For each time period, every patient with a rejection was counted (not only a patient's first rejection). The usual indication for biopsy in our center is a rise in creatinine with no apparent cause.

2.5. Statistical Analysis

Statistical analysis was performed using IBM SPSS® Statistics 24 for Windows (IBM Corporation, Somers, NY, USA). Microsoft Excel was used for data collection, simple calculations, and graphing.

This is an explorative study and no adjustment was made for multiple testing. p-values ≤ 0.05 were regarded as statistically noticeable. Normally distributed continuous variables are displayed as mean ± standard deviation (SD), non-normally distributed as median and interquartile range (IQR), and categorial variables as frequencies and percentage of total. Pairwise comparisons of independent samples were performed using student's t-test or Welch's unequal variance t-test for normally distributed data and the Mann–Whitney U test was used for non-normally distributed data. For categorial variables, groups were compared using Fisher's exact test.

For the group comparison of the eGFR and change in the eGFR, the Mann–Whitney U test and multivariable linear regression were performed. Further information on model building and the included variables is found in Supplementary Materials 2A.

A possible relationship between >30% and >50% eGFR decline endpoints and mean daily PPI intake was investigated using Fischer's exact test and multivariable logistic regression analysis. Mean daily PPI intake was calculated by averaging the prescribed PPI dose at half year intervals up to half a year before the final relevant eGFR value. Information on model building and the herein included variables can be found in Supplementary Materials 2B.

Correlation of BPAR in months one to six, seven to twelve and in the second year pTx with mean daily PPI intake, respectively, was investigated univariably using Fischer's exact test and multivariably using logistic regression analysis with forward selection of confounders (same procedure as for >30% and >50% eGFR decline endpoints). A list of the variables included and further information on the testing can be found in Supplementary Materials 2C.

3. Results

3.1. Patients

A total of 511 patients were transplanted in the study period. The following exclusions were made: 37 patients as they were <18 years of age, 13 as they did not receive PPIs at primary discharge, five due to non-onset of graft function after transplantation and one due to death before primary discharge. A final number of 455 patients were included; the median follow-up time was 3.3 years (IQR, 2.2–4.9). In our cohort, 12 patients died and 10 experienced graft loss within the first year; seven died and eight graft losses occurred within the second year pTx. Most patients (96%) initially received pantoprazole as their PPI agent. Patient and donor characteristics are displayed in Table 1 (and Supplementary Materials 1).

Table 1. Patient characteristics at primary hospital discharge post-transplantation (additional information included in Supplementary Materials 1).

Patient Characteristic	All Patients (n = 455)	PPI Group (n = 363)	No PPI Group (n = 82)	p-Value of Group Comparison
Recipient age, mean ± SD (years)	52.6 ± 14.2	53.1 ± 13.9	49.3 ± 14.5	0.026
Recipient male gender, n (%)	279 (61.3)	219 (60.3)	52 (63.4)	0.707
Recipient BMI, mean ± SD (kg/m^2)	25.9 ± 4.4	26.0 ± 4.3	24.9 ± 4.5	0.053
Prior renal transplantation, n (%)	64 (14.1)	45 (12.4)	16 (19.5)	0.109
Age of donor, mean ± SD (years)	53.1 ± 14.0	53.3 ± 14.4	51.4 ± 11.9	0.204
Living donor, n (%)	153 (33.6)	112 (30.9)	41 (50.0)	0.001
Male donor, n (%)	208 (45.7)	170 (46.8)	33 (40.2)	0.326
Delayed graft function, n (%)	79 (17.4)	59 (16.3)	11 (13.4)	0.616
European Senior Program, n (%)	76 (16.7)	62 (17.1)	10 (12.2)	0.322
Cold ischemia time (hours), median (IQR)	7.8 (2.5–11.6)	7.8 (2.7–11.7)	5.2 (2.3–11.1)	0.053
Pre-Tx time dialyzed (months), median (IQR)	45.3 (21.0–86.0)	48.2 (23.2–88.5)	32.4 (8.6–67.2)	0.002
Tacrolimus therapy at primary discharge, n (%)	432 (94.9)	347 (95.6)	76 (92.7)	0.265
Cyclosporin therapy at primary discharge, n (%)	23 (5.1)	16 (4.4)	6 (7.3)	0.265
MPS therapy at primary discharge, n (%)	76 (16.7)	57 (15.7)	18 (22.0)	0.191
MMF therapy at primary discharge, n (%)	341 (74.9)	278 (76.6)	57 (69.5)	0.200
MMF mean daily dosage (mg), median (IQR)	1000 (500–1000)	1000 (500–1000)	1000 (0–1063)	0.851
Cortisone intake at primary discharge, n (%)	444 (97.6)	353 (97.2)	81 (98.8)	0.698
CCI, median (IQR)	2 (2–4)	3 (2–4)	2 (2–3)	<0.001
HLA mismatch on A, B and DR, mean ± SD	2.9 ± 1.7	2.9 ± 1.7	2.9 ± 1.7	0.875
Basiliximab induction, n (%)	363 (79.8)	293 (80.7)	61 (74.4)	0.272
ATG induction, n (%)	14 (3.1)	13 (3.6)	1 (1.2)	0.482
ABO blood type incompatible transplant, n (%)	37 (8.1)	26 (7.2)	11 (13.4)	0.077
PRA >20%, n (%)	60 (13.2)	48 (13.2)	10 (12.2)	1.000

The two compared groups were formed based on PPI (proton pump inhibitor) intake (PPI Group) or non-intake (No PPI Group) at half a year post-transplantation. Results are presented as mean ± standard deviation (SD), median and interquartile range (IQR) or as absolute and relative frequencies. Abbreviations: BMI, body mass index; Tx, transplantation; MPS, enteric-coated mycophenolate sodium; MMF, mycophenolate mofetil; CCI, Charlson comorbidity index; HLA, human leukocyte antigen; ATG, Antithymocyte globulin; PRA, panel reactive antibodies. Along with HLA mismatch (n = 3) and Basiliximab induction (n = 7), four other variables have one patient with missing values.

Lost to follow-up rates in the PPI group and no PPI group were 16/363 (4.4%) and 2/82 (2.4%) at one year, 64/363 (17.6%) and 6/82 (7.3%) at two years, 152/363 (41.9%) and 28/82 (34.1%) at three years, 229/363 (63.1%) and 54/82 (65.9%) at four years, respectively.

3.2. Group Comparison

The two groups differed noticeably regarding recipient age, donor type (living or deceased), time dialyzed before transplantation, active smoking, smoking history, cerebral artery occlusive disease or stroke, coronary artery disease or myocardial infarction and Charlson index at the time of transplantation. These characteristics were favorable for the no PPI group. A noticeable difference was also found in the number of fast tacrolimus metabolizers three months pTx. (Table 1 and Supplementary Materials 1).

The PPI group showed significantly lower eGFR compared to the no PPI group at half a year, one year and two years pTx ($p < 0.05$) (multivariable). For the third and fourth year, the difference was not statistically significant (Supplementary Materials 3). The trend in the mean eGFR can be seen in Figure 1.

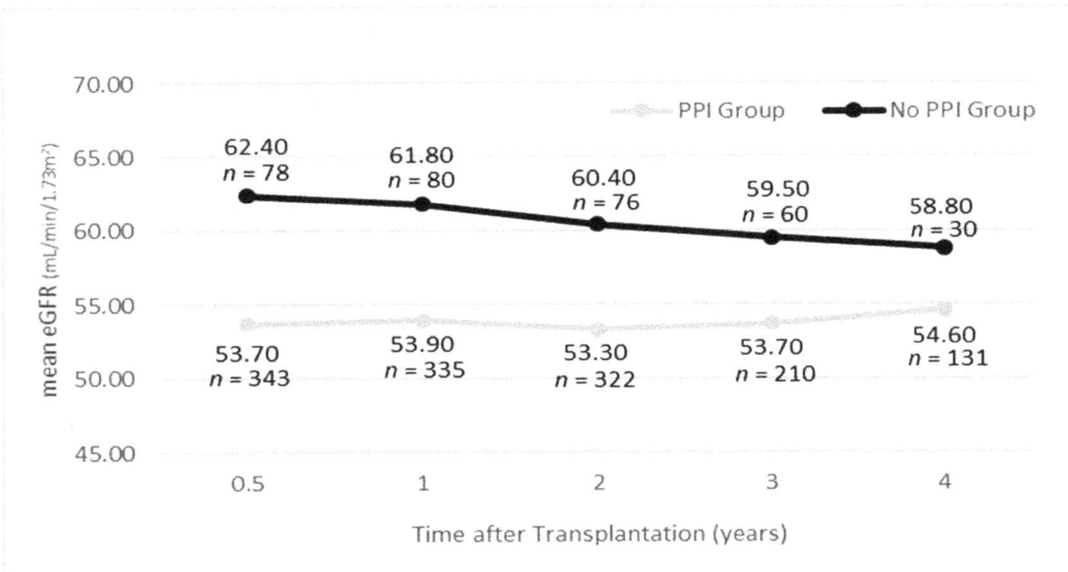

Figure 1. Trend in mean estimated glomerular filtration rate (eGFR). Mean eGFR is plotted against time in the two patient groups. Grouping is according to PPI intake or non-intake at half a year post-transplantation.

Regarding the change in the eGFR, both groups were similar over all time periods (Table 2).

Table 2. Results of the PPI group comparison of change in the eGFR.

Time Period of Analyzed eGFR Change	Groups 1 = PPI 0 = No PPI	*n*	Mean Change in the eGFR ± SD (mL/min/1.73 m²)	Median (IQR) Change in the eGFR	*p*-Value in Univariable Analysis	*p*-Value (CI) in Multivariable Linear Regression Model
0.5–1 year	1	323	−0.6 ± 12.0	1.0 (−6.0–6.5)	0.488	0.498 (−1.9–3.8)
	0	78	−0.5 ± 8.3	−0.5 (−5.6–4.4)		
0.5–2 years	1	310	−1.6 ± 14.2	0.2 (−9.0–7.5)	0.274	0.542 (−2.3–4.5)
	0	74	−2.4 ± 10.2	−1.5 (−9.2–5.2)		
0.5–3 years	1	202	−0.8 ± 15.1	0.35 (−8.0–8.4)	0.331	0.452 (−2.6–5.8)
	0	58	−2.5 ± 11.0	−1.3 (−7.0–5.4)		
0.5–4 years	1	125	−0.1 ± 14.5	−0.1 (−7.3–8.6)	0.101	0.228 (−2.2–9.1)
	0	28	−4.2 ± 9.1	−1.7 (−10.5–2.9)		

Results of the comparison of the change in the eGFR, values between groups. The eGFR value measured at half a year is always used as the reference value and was subtracted from that of the later date. Groups were formed based on PPI intake or non-intake at half a year pTx (post-transplantation). For the linear regression models, the patient number is slightly reduced (<3 patients difference per test) due to missing covariables in a few patients. Abbreviation: CI, confidence interval.

3.3. >30% and >50% eGFR Decline

Multivariable logistic regression was only carried out for the outcome >30% eGFR decline from half a year to two years pTx. In all others, only univariable analysis was performed (due to the low number of events). eGFR decline >30% from half a year to two years showed statistical correlation with higher PPI doses in multivariable logistic regression ($p = 0.044$). All other eGFR decline endpoints showed no relation to mean daily PPI intake. eGFR decline >50% from two to four years showed some tendency in the same direction ($p = 0.056$). However, here, only three events occurred. Tables with the results can be viewed in Supplementary Materials 4A–D.

3.4. Secondary Outcomes

BPAR occurred in 96 patients in months one to six, in 32 patients in months seven to twelve and in 36 patients in the second year pTx. For the rejection analysis, patients who did not complete a follow up of at least 5/6 of the analyzed time points were excluded from analysis. Those with death or transplant loss with prior rejection, however, were included. Twelve patients were excluded from multivariable analyses due to missing data. The results of the analysis are presented in Figure 2A–C. Regarding rejection types, mean daily PPI intake only showed a correlation with antibody mediated rejections (AMR) in the second year pTx in univariable analysis ($p = 0.027$); multivariable (logistic regression) analysis was not feasible in this case due to zero events in one group. All other tests did not show any association.

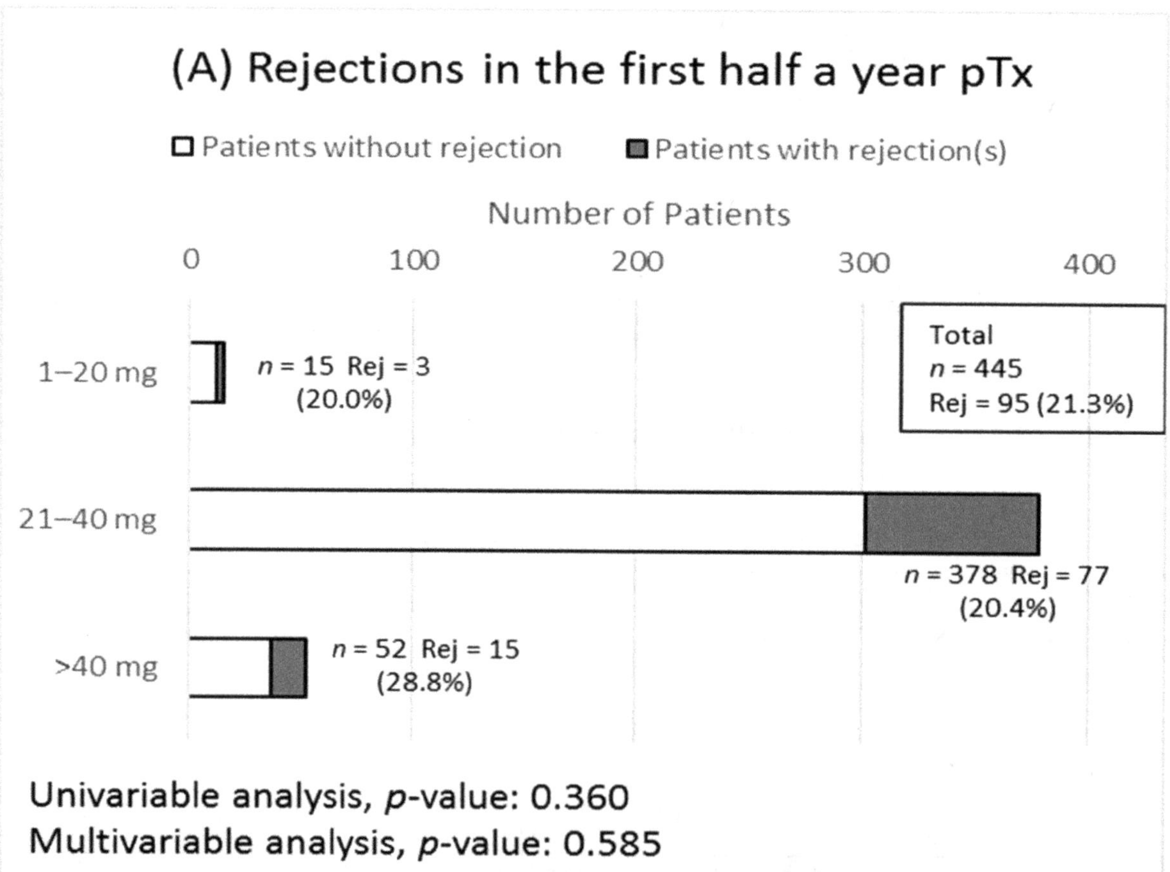

Figure 2. *Cont.*

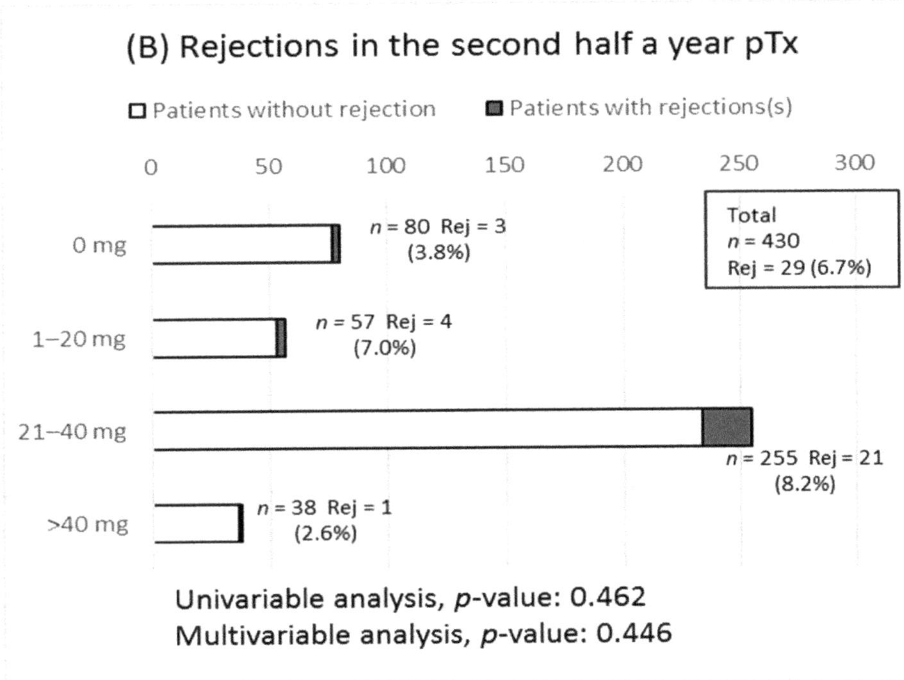

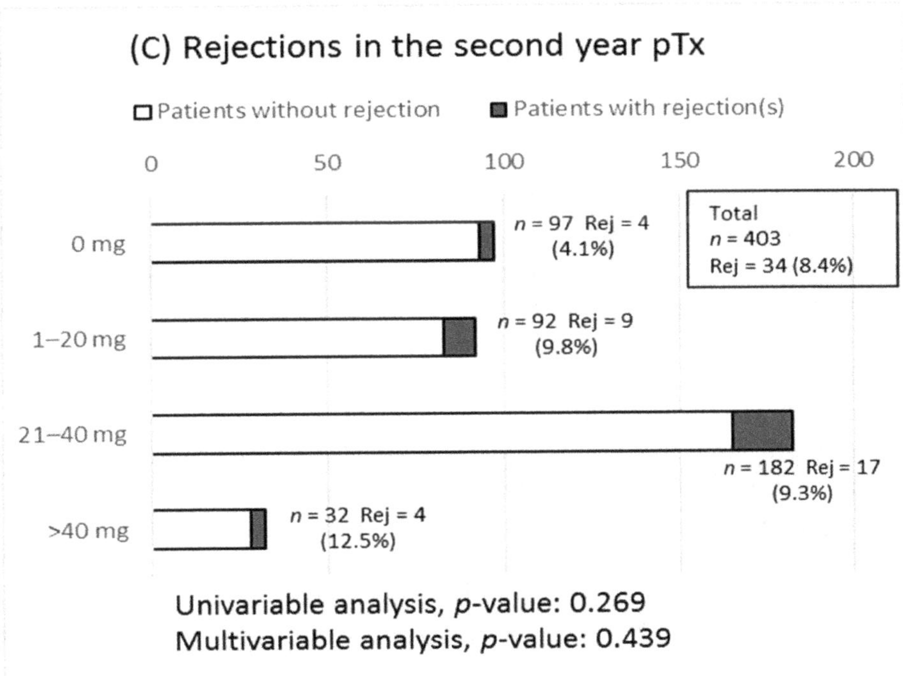

Figure 2. Results of the biopsy proven rejection analyses are shown. Grouping is according to PPI intake (pantoprazole equivalent) in the relevant time period. Rejection prevalence is shown as absolute number and as percentage of patients in the group. The dark part of each bar represents the number of patients with rejections. Abbreviations: n, total number of patients in the group; Rej, number of patients who experienced a graft rejection; pTx, post transplantation. (**A**) Analysis of rejections in months 1–6 pTx. (**B**) Analysis of rejections in months 7–12 pTx. (**C**) Analysis of rejections months 13–24 pTx.

As the possible drug interaction of MMF with PPIs was of special interest, all rejection analyses were repeated, analyzing the data of patients who had MMF at primary discharge only. None of these tests showed any significant association.

4. Discussion

Our results demonstrate that prolonged PPI intake after KTx does not lead to any meaningful decline in kidney function within the first four years after transplantation. Additionally, our analyses of rejection rates are in line with recent studies showing no relevant association between rejection rates and PPI-intake after KTx [22,24,25].

Several large epidemiological studies observed a relationship between AKI, CKD, and PPI intake [1–5]. From case studies, an association between PPI intake and interstitial nephritis was previously assumed [32]. Estimates of the impact of this finding have not been around as long [33–35]. However, the relevance and the stake of interstitial nephritis for AKI in PPI observational studies still remains unclear [35,36]. As AKI can lead to CKD, it was not surprising that an association between CKD and PPI intake was recently proposed [1]. Nevertheless, Xie and colleagues provided evidence that PPI-associated CKD even occurred in the absence of AKI [3]. The pathomechanism, however, remains unknown. Proposed mechanisms include elevation of plasma asymmetric dimethylarginine levels [37], microinflammation due to gut microbe dysbiosis [38], endothelial senescence [39] and PPI-induced hypomagnesemia [40]. In addition to hypomagnesemia, PPI intake was recently associated to be dose-dependently linked to iron deficiency and hypomagnesemia in a kidney transplant cohort from the Netherlands [41,42]. The authors speculated that the effects were associated with reduced intestinal absorption of both elements under PPI therapy. However, our center's policy is to monitor the iron status and to replace magnesium after KTx, because iron-deficiency is common and calcineurin inhibitors frequently lead to magnesium loss. Considering these findings, our results may relieve unwarranted fear when prescribing PPIs in KTx patients.

Following the Kidney Disease Improving Global Outcomes (KDIGO) guideline, a form of mycophenolate acid (MPA) together with the calcineurin inhibitor tacrolimus and low dose corticosteroid therapy is the preferred maintenance therapy after KTx at our center (Table 1 and Supplementary Materials 1) [43]. The tacrolimus target level in our center was 6–10 ng/mL from months one to three and 4–8 ng/mL for the following time.

Tacrolimus and PPI potentially interfere e.g., at the cytochrome P450 system (CYP3A) [17,18]. Another mechanism proposed is that PPI can increase the uptake of tacrolimus in the small intestine [19,44]. Both mechanisms could increase blood tacrolimus levels. Usually, these interactions are not clinically noticeable as several factors have a more profound effect on tacrolimus metabolism and exposure [45]. However, as tacrolimus can be nephrotoxic, slight increases in exposure may be relevant in the course of time [18,46]. Although analysis of tacrolimus blood levels was not the goal of this study, it is interesting to note that tacrolimus blood levels at three months pTx showed a tendency ($p = 0.07$) to be higher in the PPI group (Supplementary Materials 1). Furthermore, significantly more fast tacrolimus metabolizers were found in the no PPI group ($p = 0.035$). However, the previously mentioned Dutch KTx magnesium study found no relevant interaction between PPI and tacrolimus in their observational study [42]. Thus, these interesting findings may warrant further investigation.

It may also be worth mentioning that we did not investigate a possible effect of PPIs on the intrapatient variability of tacrolimus. It has been shown that the intrapatient variability of tacrolimus correlates with poor long-term outcomes in kidney transplant recipients [47]. It may be assumed that any drug with the possibility of interfering with tacrolimus pharmacokinetics may potentially change the intrapatient variability of tacrolimus [48]. To our knowledge, no study exists which has directly investigated a potential relationship between PPI intake and increased intrapatient variability in kidney transplant recipients. However, we suspect this effect to be minimal when adherence to our center's instruction of ingesting tacrolimus on an empty stomach is followed. As we did not see any differences regarding the eGFR changes between the groups, a clinically relevant effect of PPIs on transplant function does not seem to exist.

Mycophenolate mofetil is a prodrug that is hydrolyzed to the active metabolite MPA. It acts as a selective uncompetitive inhibitor of inosine monophosphate dehydrogenase (IMPDH) and thus inhibits de novo guanosine synthesis [6]. Pharmacokinetic studies have shown that PPIs may reduce

MPA exposure in patients receiving concomitant MMF and PPI treatment, whereas the alternative drug enteric-coated mycophenolate sodium is not affected [6–12]. Decreased MPA exposure can increase rejection rates [13–16]. However, in a recent pharmacokinetic blinded cross-over study [49], this mentioned interaction was not found. In line with this and with previously published observational studies, rejection rates in our cohort were comparable between groups [22,24,25].

Previous PPI studies in KTx patients relevant to our investigation have focused on the possible interaction of MMF with PPIs. Van Boeckel and colleagues compared 125 patients taking pantoprazole with 77 patients using ranitidine [22]. The primary outcome was BPAR and secondary outcomes were creatinine and the eGFR at three months pTx. No significant differences were found in any of the outcomes. Knorr and colleagues [24] came to similar results in their comparative study of 213 patients receiving PPIs, and 390 with ranitidine. The primary outcome was BPAR in the first year pTx. Both groups had comparable rejection rates and eGFRs. Notably, in the subgroup of African American recipients (predominantly fast tacrolimus metabolizers), PPI intake and rejection rates correlated. The recent study by Patel and colleagues [25] compared rejection rates in 183 patients taking PPIs and 339 using histamine-2 receptor antagonists. The primary outcome was the incidence of acute rejection within one year pTx, but eGFR values at one month and one year were also compared between the two groups. None of these parameters showed a significant difference.

Our study adds to the existing literature as we extended the analyses of the eGFR and changes thereof to a longer time period (half a year to four years) than previous studies (analyzing three to twelve months).

A simple comparison of the eGFR reflected differences in patient characteristics (Table 1 and Supplementary Materials 1). These differences were not a result of PPI therapy as is shown by comparable changes in the eGFR in both groups during follow-up (Table 2).

Moreover, similar rejection rates in the groups taking different doses of PPI, namely 0 mg, 1–20 mg, 21–40 mg and >40 mg pantoprazole equivalent, led us to conclude that the relevance of PPI intake for MMF efficacy is at best minimal. This is in line with the previously mentioned observational studies that used different methodologies. Correction for various potentially relevant confounders did not change the results with regards to kidney function or rejection rates. In line with our observations is a recently published meta-analysis that evaluated the data of 6786 KTx patients. The authors found that PPI use was linked to hypomagnesemia, but not associated with acute rejection, graft loss, or one-year mortality [40].

One limitation of our study is the retrospective study design analyzing a limited number of patients from one center. For part of the rejection analysis and >30% and >50% eGFR decline, the inclusion of covariables in the multivariable logistic regression analyses was limited due to the low number of events. Confounding by indication proved a serious difficulty in this study. Patients with longer, higher PPI intake showed a tendency to higher comorbidity and risk factors (Table 1 and Supplementary Material 1). To cope with this, we included information on the Charlson comorbidity index. PPI therapy post-transplant is the standard of care at our center. Discontinuance of PPI medication was assumedly due to clinical evaluation or patient choice, not by standard procedure.

For the statistically observed relation of second year AMRs and >30% eGFR decline (from half a year to two years) with PPI average intake, we presume residual confounding to be the reason because in a post-hoc comparison of the groups used for the >30% eGFR decline analysis, we found significant differences for the following patient characteristics: recipient age and BMI, pre-transplant dialysis time, prior renal transplant, donor type (living or deceased), pre-transplant diabetes, ABO transplant incompatibility, cerebral arterial occlusive disease or stroke, coronary heart disease or myocardial infarction, statins, prior smoking history, continuation of smoking after KTx, and Charlson comorbidity index. All of these, apart from prior renal transplant and ABO incompatibility, showed an unfavorable tendency with higher PPI intake.

5. Conclusions

We conclude from our data that prolonged PPI therapy is safe in regard to KTx function. However, further studies into a possible interaction between PPIs and tacrolimus may be of interest. In addition, our findings highlight the importance of examining changes in the eGFR rather than single eGFR measurements in similar studies. Polypharmacy is a relevant problem in the transplant population [50] and it is always advisable to question unnecessary medication [51]. This may include PPI therapy.

Author Contributions: D.J.G.F., K.S.-N., S.R. and conceived and designed the study, D.J.G.F. and K.S.-N. collected the data. D.J.G.F. and K.S.-N. analyzed the data. H.P. and B.S. supervised the project and discussed the data, D.J.G.F., K.S.-N. and S.R. wrote the main manuscript text. All authors have read and agreed to the published version of the manuscript.

Acknowledgments: We are grateful to René Schmidt for his statistical advice during the course of the project. We also acknowledge support by the Open Access Publication Fund of the University of Münster.

References

1. Lazarus, B.; Chen, Y.; Wilson, F.P.; Sang, Y.; Chang, A.R.; Coresh, J.; Grams, M.E. Proton Pump Inhibitor Use and the Risk of Chronic Kidney Disease. *JAMA Intern. Med.* **2016**, *176*, 238–246. [CrossRef] [PubMed]
2. Xie, Y.; Bowe, B.; Li, T.; Xian, H.; Balasubramanian, S.; Al-Aly, Z. Proton Pump Inhibitors and Risk of Incident CKD and Progression to ESRD. *J. Am. Soc. Nephrol.* **2016**, *27*, 3153–3163. [CrossRef] [PubMed]
3. Xie, Y.; Bowe, B.; Li, T.; Xian, H.; Yan, Y.; Al-Aly, Z. Long-term kidney outcomes among users of proton pump inhibitors without intervening acute kidney injury. *Kidney Int.* **2017**, *91*, 1482–1494. [CrossRef] [PubMed]
4. Klatte, D.C.F.; Gasparini, A.; Xu, H.; de Deco, P.; Trevisan, M.; Johansson, A.L.; Wettermark, B.; Ärnlöv, J.; Janmaat, C.J.; Dekker, F.W.; et al. Association between Proton Pump Inhibitor Use and Risk of Progression of Chronic Kidney Disease. *Gastroenterology* **2017**, *153*, 702–710. [CrossRef] [PubMed]
5. Arora, P.; Gupta, A.; Golzy, M.; Patel, N.; Carter, R.L.; Jalal, K.; Lohr, J.W. Proton pump inhibitors are associated with increased risk of development of chronic kidney disease. *BMC Nephrol.* **2016**, *17*, 112. [CrossRef]
6. *Product Monograph: CellCept, Mycophenolate Mofetil*; Hoffmann-La Roche Ltd.: Mississauga, ON, Canada, 2017; Available online: https://www.rochecanada.com/PMs/CellCept/CellCept_PM_E.pdf (accessed on 5 May 2018).
7. Schaier, M.; Scholl, C.; Scharpf, D.; Hug, F.; Bönisch-Schmidt, S.; Dikow, R.; Schmitt, W.H.; Schwenger, V.; Zeier, M.; Sommerer, C. Proton pump inhibitors interfere with the immunosuppressive potency of mycophenolate mofetil. *Rheumatology* **2010**, *49*, 2061–2067. [CrossRef]
8. Rupprecht, K.; Schmidt, C.; Raspé, A.; Schweda, F.; Shipkova, M.; Fischer, W.; Bucher, M.; Kees, F.; Faerber, L. Bioavailability of mycophenolate mofetil and enteric-coated mycophenolate sodium is differentially affected by pantoprazole in healthy volunteers. *J. Clin. Pharmacol.* **2009**, *49*, 1196–1201. [CrossRef]
9. Kofler, S.; Shvets, N.; Bigdeli, A.K.; König, M.A.; Kaczmarek, P.; Deutsch, M.A.; Vogeser, M.; Steinbeck, G.; Reichart, B.; Kaczmarek, I. Proton pump inhibitors reduce mycophenolate exposure in heart transplant recipients: A prospective case-controlled study. *Am. J. Transplant.* **2009**, *9*, 1650–1656. [CrossRef]
10. Miura, M.; Satoh, S.; Inoue, K.; Kagaya, H.; Saito, M.; Suzuki, T.; Habuchi, T. Influence of lansoprazole and rabeprazole on mycophenolic acid pharmacokinetics one year after renal transplantation. *Ther. Drug Monit.* **2008**, *30*, 46–51. [CrossRef]
11. Kofler, S.; Wolf, C.; Shvets, N.; Sisic, Z.; Müller, T.; Behr, J.; Sohn, H.-Y.; Vogeser, M.; Shipkova, M.; Steinbeck, G.; et al. The proton pump inhibitor pantoprazole and its interaction with enteric-coated mycophenolate sodium in transplant recipients. *J. Heart Lung Transplant.* **2011**, *30*, 565–571. [CrossRef]
12. Xu, L.; Cai, M.; Shi, B.-Y.; Li, Z.-L.; Li, X.; Jin, H.-L. A prospective analysis of the effects of enteric-coated mycophenolate sodium and mycophenolate mofetil co-medicated with a proton pump inhibitor in kidney transplant recipients at a single institute in China. *Transplant. Proc.* **2014**, *46*, 1362–1365. [CrossRef] [PubMed]

13. van Gelder, T.; Hilbrands, L.B.; Vanrenterghem, Y.; Weimar, W.; De Fijter, J.W.; Squifflet, J.P.; Hené, R.J.; Verpooten, G.A.; Navarro, M.T.; Nicholls, A.J.; et al. A randomized double-blind, multicenter plasma concentration controlled study of the safety and efficacy of oral mycophenolate mofetil for the prevention of acute rejection after kidney transplantation. *Transplantation* **1999**, *68*, 261–266. [CrossRef] [PubMed]
14. Langone, A.; Doria, C.; Greenstein, S.; Narayanan, M.; Ueda, K.; Sankari, B.; Pankewycz, O.; Shihab, F.; Chan, L. Does reduction in mycophenolic acid dose compromise efficacy regardless of tacrolimus exposure level? An analysis of prospective data from the Mycophenolic Renal Transplant (MORE) Registry. *Clin. Transplant.* **2013**, *27*, 15–24. [CrossRef] [PubMed]
15. Cooper, M.; Deering, K.L.; Slakey, D.P.; Harshaw, Q.; Arcona, S.; McCann, E.L.; Rasetto, F.A.; Florman, S.S. Comparing outcomes associated with dose manipulations of enteric-coated mycophenolate sodium versus mycophenolate mofetil in renal transplant recipients. *Transplantation* **2009**, *88*, 514–520. [CrossRef] [PubMed]
16. Knoll, G.A.; Macdonald, I.; Khan, A.; van Walraven, C. Mycophenolate Mofetil Dose Reduction and the Risk of Acute Rejection after Renal Transplantation. *J. Am. Soc. Nephrol.* **2003**, *14*, 2381–2386. [CrossRef] [PubMed]
17. Itagaki, F.; Homma, M.; Yuzawa, K.; Nishimura, M.; Naito, S.; Ueda, N.; Ohkohchi, N.; Kohda, Y. Effect of lansoprazole and rabeprazole on tacrolimus pharmacokinetics in healthy volunteers with CYP2C19 mutations. *J. Pharm. Pharmacol.* **2004**, *56*, 1055–1059. [CrossRef] [PubMed]
18. *Product Monograph: Sandoz Tacrolimus*; Sandoz Canada Inc.: Boucherville, QC, Canada, 2016; Available online: https://www.sandoz.ca/sites/www.sandoz.ca/files/Tacrolimus%20Cap%20Product%20Monograph.pdf (accessed on 12 April 2018).
19. Miura, M.; Niioka, T.; Kagaya, H.; Saito, M.; Hayakari, M.; Habuchi, T.; Satoh, S. Pharmacogenetic determinants for interindividual difference of tacrolimus pharmacokinetics 1 year after renal transplantation. *J. Clin. Pharm. Ther.* **2011**, *36*, 208–216. [CrossRef]
20. Telkes, G.; Peter, A.; Tulassay, Z.; Asderakis, A. High frequency of ulcers, not associated with Helicobacter pylori, in the stomach in the first year after kidney transplantation. *Nephrol. Dial. Transplant.* **2011**, *26*, 727–732. [CrossRef]
21. Hardinger, K.L.; Brennan, D.C.; Lowell, J.; Schnitzler, M.A. Long-term outcome of gastrointestinal complications in renal transplant patients treated with mycophenolate mofetil. *Transpl. Int.* **2004**, *17*, 609–616. [CrossRef]
22. van Boekel, G.A.J.; Kerkhofs, C.H.H.; van de Logt, F.; Hilbrands, L.B. Proton pump inhibitors do not increase the risk of acute rejection. *Neth. J. Med.* **2014**, *72*, 86–90.
23. Courson, A.Y.; Lee, J.R.; Aull, M.J.; Lee, J.H.; Kapur, S.; McDermott, J.K. Routine prophylaxis with proton pump inhibitors and post-transplant complications in kidney transplant recipients undergoing early corticosteroid withdrawal. *Clin. Transplant.* **2016**, *30*, 694–702. [CrossRef] [PubMed]
24. Knorr, J.P.; Sjeime, M.; Braitman, L.E.; Jawa, P.; Zaki, R.; Ortiz, J. Concomitant proton pump inhibitors with mycophenolate mofetil and the risk of rejection in kidney transplant recipients. *Transplantation* **2014**, *97*, 518–524. [CrossRef] [PubMed]
25. Patel, K.S.; Stephany, B.R.; Barnes, J.F.; Bauer, S.R.; Spinner, M.L. Renal Transplant Acute Rejection with Lower Mycophenolate Mofetil Dosing and Proton Pump Inhibitors or Histamine-2 Receptor Antagonists. *Pharmacotherapy* **2017**, *37*, 1507–1515. [CrossRef] [PubMed]
26. Charlson, M.E.; Pompei, P.; Ales, K.L.; MacKenzie, C.R. A new method of classifying prognostic comorbidity in longitudinal studies: Development and validation. *J. Chronic Dis.* **1987**, *40*, 373–383. [CrossRef]
27. Wu, C.; Evans, I.; Joseph, R.; Shapiro, R.; Tan, H.; Basu, A.; Smetanka, C.; Khan, A.; McCauley, J.; Unruh, M. Comorbid conditions in kidney transplantation: Association with graft and patient survival. *J. Am. Soc. Nephrol.* **2005**, *16*, 3437–3444. [CrossRef] [PubMed]
28. Wedemeyer, R.-S.; Blume, H. Pharmacokinetic drug interaction profiles of proton pump inhibitors: An update. *Drug Saf.* **2014**, *37*, 201–211. [CrossRef]
29. McAuley, D. Drug Comparisons—Proton Pump Inhibitors: Equivalent Dosages [Internet]. 2017. Available online: http://www.globalrph.com/proton_pump_inhibitors.htm (accessed on 25 July 2017).

30. Abbreviated Drug Class Review: Proton Pump Inhibitors VHA Pharmacy Benefits Management Strategic Healthcare Group and the Medical Advisory Panel. 2006. Available online: https://www.pbm.va.gov/PBM/clinicalguidance/drugclassreviews/ProtonPumpInhibitorsAbbreviatedDrugClassReview.pdf (accessed on 6 February 2018).
31. Levey, A.S.; Stevens, L.A.; Schmid, C.H.; Zhang, Y.L.; Castro, A.F.; Feldman, H.I.; Coresh, J. A New Equation to Estimate Glomerular Filtration Rate. *Ann. Intern. Med.* **2009**, *150*, 604. [CrossRef]
32. Sierra, F.; Suarez, M.; Rey, M.; Vela, M.F. Systematic review: Proton pump inhibitor-associated acute interstitial nephritis. *Aliment. Pharmacol. Ther.* **2007**, *26*, 545–553. [CrossRef]
33. Leonard, C.E.; Freeman, C.P.; Newcomb, C.W.; Reese, P.P.; Herlim, M.; Bilker, W.B.; Hennessy, S.; Strom, B.L. Proton pump inhibitors and traditional nonsteroidal anti-inflammatory drugs and the risk of acute interstitial nephritis and acute kidney injury. *Pharmacoepidemiol. Drug Saf.* **2012**, *21*, 1155–1172. [CrossRef]
34. Blank, M.-L.; Parkin, L.; Paul, C.; Herbison, P. A nationwide nested case-control study indicates an increased risk of acute interstitial nephritis with proton pump inhibitor use. *Kidney Int.* **2014**, *86*, 837–844. [CrossRef]
35. Antoniou, T.; Macdonald, E.M.; Hollands, S.; Gomes, T.; Mamdani, M.M.; Garg, A.X.; Paterson, J.M.; Juurlink, D.N. Proton pump inhibitors and the risk of acute kidney injury in older patients: A population-based cohort study. *CMAJ Open* **2015**, *3*, E166–E171. [CrossRef] [PubMed]
36. Klepser, D.G.; Collier, D.S.; Cochran, G.L. Proton pump inhibitors and acute kidney injury: A nested case-control study. *BMC Nephrol.* **2013**, *14*, 150. [CrossRef] [PubMed]
37. Ghebremariam, Y.T.; LePendu, P.; Lee, J.C.; Erlanson, D.A.; Slaviero, A.; Shah, N.H.; Leiper, J.; Cooke, J.P. Unexpected effect of proton pump inhibitors: Elevation of the cardiovascular risk factor asymmetric dimethylarginine. *Circulation* **2013**, *128*, 845–853. [CrossRef] [PubMed]
38. Ramezani, A.; Raj, D.S. The gut microbiome, kidney disease, and targeted interventions. *J. Am. Soc. Nephrol.* **2014**, *25*, 657–670. [CrossRef] [PubMed]
39. Yepuri, G.; Sukhovershin, R.; Nazari-Shafti, T.Z.; Petrascheck, M.; Ghebre, Y.T.; Cooke, J.P. Proton Pump Inhibitors Accelerate Endothelial Senescence. *Circ. Res.* **2016**, *118*, e36–e42. [CrossRef] [PubMed]
40. Boonpheng, B.; Thongprayoon, C.; Bathini, T.; Sharma, K.; Mao, M.A.; Cheungpasitporn, W. Proton pump inhibitors and adverse effects in kidney transplant recipients: A meta-analysis. *World J. Transplant.* **2019**, *9*, 35–47. [CrossRef]
41. Douwes, R.M.; Gomes-Neto, A.W.; Eisenga, M.F.; Vinke, J.S.J.; de Borst, M.H.; van den Berg, E.; Berger, S.P.; Touw, D.J.; Hak, E.; Navis, G.; et al. Chronic Use of Proton-Pump Inhibitors and Iron Status in Renal Transplant Recipients. *J Clin. Med.* **2019**, *8*, 1382. [CrossRef]
42. Douwes, R.M.; Gomes-Neto, A.W.; Schutten, J.C.; van den Berg, E.; de Borst, M.H.; Berger, S.P.; Touw, D.J.; Hak, E.; Blokzijl, H.; Bakker, S.J.; et al. Proton-Pump Inhibitors and Hypomagnesaemia in Kidney Transplant Recipients. *J Clin. Med.* **2019**, *8*, 2162. [CrossRef]
43. Kidney Disease: Improving Global Outcomes (KDIGO) Transplant Work Group. KDIGO clinical practice guideline for the care of kidney transplant recipients. *Am. J. Transplant.* **2009**, *9*, S1–S157. [CrossRef]
44. Peloso, L.J.; Faria, P.N.; Bossolani, M.V.; Oliveira, H.B.; Filho Sebastiao, R.F. The Serum Concentration of Tacrolimus after Ingesting Omeprazole: A Pilot Study. *Transplantation* **2014**, *98*, e63–e64. [CrossRef]
45. Schütte-Nütgen, K.; Thölking, G.; Suwelack, B.; Reuter, S. Tacrolimus—Pharmacokinetic Considerations for Clinicians. *Curr. Drug Metab.* **2018**, *19*, 342–350. [CrossRef] [PubMed]
46. Jacobson, P.A.; Schladt, D.; Israni, A.; Oetting, W.S.; Lin, Y.C.; Leduc, R.; Guan, W.; Lamba, V.; Matas, A.J. Genetic and clinical determinants of early, acute calcineurin inhibitor-related nephrotoxicity: Results from a kidney transplant consortium. *Transplantation* **2012**, *93*, 624–631. [CrossRef] [PubMed]
47. Mo, H.; Kim, S.-Y.; Min, S.; Han, A.; Ahn, S.; Min, S.K.; Lee, H.; Ahn, C.; Kim, Y.; Ha, J. Association of Intrapatient Variability of Tacrolimus Concentration with Early Deterioration of Chronic Histologic Lesions in Kidney Transplantation. *Transplant. Direct* **2019**, *5*, e455. [CrossRef] [PubMed]
48. Shuker, N.; van Gelder, T.; Hesselink, D.A. Intra-patient variability in tacrolimus exposure: Causes, consequences for clinical management. *Transplant. Rev.* **2015**, *29*, 78–84. [CrossRef] [PubMed]
49. Rissling, O.; Glander, P.; Hambach, P.; Mai, M.; Brakemeier, S.; Klonower, D.; Halleck, F.; Singer, E.; Schrezenmeier, E.-V.; Neumayer, H.H.; et al. No relevant pharmacokinetic interaction between pantoprazole and mycophenolate in renal transplant patients: A randomized crossover study. *Br. J. Clin. Pharmacol.* **2015**, *80*, 1086–1096. [CrossRef] [PubMed]

50. Bril, F.; Castro, V.; Centurion, G.I.; Espinosa, J.; Keller, A.G.; Gonzalez, D.C.; Soler, R.M.; Saubidet, L.C.; Di Girolamo, D.G.; Pujol, S.G.; et al. A Systematic Approach to Assess the Burden of Drug Interactions in Adult Kidney Transplant Patients. *Curr. Drug Saf.* **2016**, *11*, 156–163. [CrossRef]
51. Polypharmacy and Medicines Optimisation: Making It Safe and Sound. The King's Fund: London, UK, 2013. Available online: https://www.kingsfund.org.uk/sites/default/files/field/field_publication_file/polypharmacy-and-medicines-optimisation-kingsfund-nov13.pdf (accessed on 17 January 2020).

11

Artificial Intelligence in Acute Kidney Injury Risk Prediction

Joana Gameiro [1,*], Tiago Branco [2] and José António Lopes [1]

[1] Division of Nephrology and Renal Transplantation, Department of Medicine, Centro Hospitalar Lisboa Norte, EPE, Av. Prof. Egas Moniz, 1649-035 Lisboa, Portugal; jalopes93@hotmail.com
[2] Department of Medicine, Centro Hospitalar Lisboa Norte, EPE, Av. Prof. Egas Moniz, 1649-035 Lisboa, Portugal; tiagobranco.md@gmail.com
* Correspondence: joana.estrelagameiro@gmail.com

Abstract: Acute kidney injury (AKI) is a frequent complication in hospitalized patients, which is associated with worse short and long-term outcomes. It is crucial to develop methods to identify patients at risk for AKI and to diagnose subclinical AKI in order to improve patient outcomes. The advances in clinical informatics and the increasing availability of electronic medical records have allowed for the development of artificial intelligence predictive models of risk estimation in AKI. In this review, we discussed the progress of AKI risk prediction from risk scores to electronic alerts to machine learning methods.

Keywords: acute kidney injury; risk prediction; artificial intelligence

---

1. Introduction

Acute kidney injury (AKI) is a complex syndrome caused by multiple etiologies and characterized by a sudden decrease in kidney function, defined by an increase in serum creatinine or a decrease in urine output [1,2]. AKI is a frequent complication in hospitalized patients, which is associated with worse short and long-term outcomes, namely, increased length of hospital stay, increased health care costs, increased risk of in-hospital and long-term mortality, long-term progression to chronic kidney disease, and long-term risk of cardiovascular events [3–7].

The incidence of AKI has increased in the past decades due to the population aging and rising incidence of comorbidities, such as chronic kidney disease, diabetes, and hypertension [2,8–10]. Furthermore, the development of a standardized definition for AKI and the acknowledgment of the impact of AKI on patient outcomes are also responsible for the increased recognition of this syndrome [2]. Despite the decrease in mortality rates associated with AKI, these remain significant, ranging from 15% among hospitalized patients to more than 50% in critically ill patients [11–13].

Considering the impact of AKI on short and long-term outcomes, it is of high importance to develop methods to identify patients at risk for AKI and to diagnose subclinical AKI in order to improve patient outcomes [4]. The advances in clinical informatics and the increasing availability of electronic medical records (EMR) have allowed for the development of predictive models of risk estimation in AKI [14].

In this review, we discussed the progress of AKI risk prediction from risk scores to electronic alerts to machine learning (ML) methods.

2. AKI Definition and Biomarkers

The Kidney Disease Improving Global Outcomes workgroup defines AKI as an increase in serum creatinine (SCr) of at least 0.3 mg/dL within 48 h, or an increase in SCr to more than 1.5 times of baseline level, which is known or presumed to have occurred within the prior 7 days, or a urine output (UO) decrease to less than 0.5 mL/kg/h for 6 h [15].

Despite the importance of the development and use of this standardized classification in the epidemiology of AKI, SCr and UO are insensitive and unspecific markers of AKI, which do not account for the duration or cause of AKI [16]. Values of SCr are influenced by age, gender, muscle mass, fluid balance, and medications, which limit its secretion, and values of UO are influenced by patient volemic status and diuretic use. Baseline SCr is frequently unknown, and UO assessment is complex without a urinary catheter.

Novel biomarkers have been investigated in multiple settings to increase diagnostic accuracy, which so far include cystatin C (Cys-C), neutrophil gelatinase-associated lipocalin (NGAL), N-acetyl-glucosaminidase (NAG), kidney injury molecule 1 (KIM-1), interleukin-6 (IL-6), interleukin-8 (IL-8), interleukin 18 (IL-18), liver-type fatty acid-binding protein (L-FABP), calprotectin, urine angiotensinogen (AGT), urine microRNAs, insulin-like growth factor-binding protein 7 (IGFBP7), and tissue inhibitor of metalloproteinases-2 (TIMP-2) [17–27].

Important weaknesses have limited the generalization of the use of these biomarkers in clinical practice [19]. These have not consistently distinguished pre-renal from renal AKI; several patient characteristics and comorbidities can produce range variations that limit their validity; cost-effectiveness is limited due to the increased costs associated with these biomarkers and need for multiple assessments, and evidence of outcome improvement is still lacking [28,29]. Given the complexity of AKI, perhaps the use of a panel of several biomarkers covering different stages of the syndrome could provide a better understanding of its pathophysiology and identify future treatment targets [29,30].

3. AKI Risk Factors

Several investigators have focused on determining significant risk factors for AKI [31–33]. Both patient susceptibilities and exposures are important risk factors for AKI. Patient age is an important non-modifiable risk factor [34–36]. The loss of renal reserve and physiologic decline of glomerular filtration rate (GFR) may place older patients at risk for AKI [37,38].

Chronic kidney disease (CKD) is another major risk factor for AKI [38] The loss of autoregulation, abnormal vasodilation, susceptibility to antihypertensive agents and nephrotoxins, and the side effects of medication contribute to the development of AKI in CKD patients [38].

Patient comorbidities, such as diabetes mellitus, hypertension, cardiovascular disease, chronic liver disease, and chronic obstructive pulmonary disease, have also been identified as important AKI predictors [15,31–33,36,39,40]. It is also important to note that HIV infection is a risk factor, predisposing patients to AKI, given the increasing incidence of HIV-infected patients in the past decades. Furthermore, AKI remains an important predictor of mortality in these patients despite the decrease in the incidence of AKI with the widespread use of antiretroviral therapy [41,42].

Exposure to sepsis, surgery, nephrotoxins, and shock are specific modifiable factors, which contribute to AKI [8,15]. Large cohort studies focusing on critically ill patients report that the two most important causes of AKI are sepsis and surgery [9,10,43–45].

More recent research has reported that hyperuricemia, hypoalbuminemia, obesity, anemia, and hyperglycemia may be new predictors of AKI [36].

Uric acid can contribute to AKI in several settings due to intratubular crystal precipitation, but also by inducing renal vasoconstriction and impairing autoregulation, and due to proinflammatory and antiangiogenic effects [46–49].

Hypoalbuminemia has been used as a nonspecific marker of patient nutrition, inflammation, hepatic function, and catabolic state and has been reported as an independent predictor of AKI in multiple settings [50–54].

The increasing incidence of obesity has raised the interest to study its association with AKI. Although the exact mechanisms are still uncertain, there is substantial evidence that obesity is an independent predictor of AKI in multiple medical and surgical settings [55–58].

Anemia has been associated with increased AKI risk, mainly in the surgical setting [59,60]. Furthermore, transfusions of red blood cells are also associated with increased risk of AKI [61,62]. The mechanisms are likely multifactorial, including reduced renal oxygen delivery, worsening oxidative stress, systemic inflammation, and impaired hemostasis [36,59,63]. Stored red blood cells have an impaired ability to carry oxygen and proinflammatory effects, associated with the direct toxic effect of by-products of red blood cell storage, contributing to organ failure in critically ill patients [59,64].

Hyperglycemia is another novel risk factor, which has been associated with increased AKI development [65–70]. However, the target level of glucose to decrease AKI risk has not been determined. The exact mechanism is still uncertain, but hyperglycemia might contribute to AKI through stimulation of oxidative stress, vasoconstriction and reduced renal oxygen delivery, and volume depletion due to osmotic diuresis [68,70].

4. AKI Risk Scores

A precise risk prediction score should be able to identify at-risk patients and guide clinicians on performing further diagnostic tests and prompting preventive and/or treatment measures. A risk score is produced by the combination of independent predictors of AKI and assigning relative impact, ideally with external validation analysis [14].

Risk prediction scores for AKI have been reported in several clinical settings, mostly in critical care, surgery, and contrast-induced nephropathy [71–77]. Still, most AKI cases are reported in general hospital wards, and risk scores in this setting are scarce [78–81].

Most models include age, gender, baseline kidney function, comorbidities, such as chronic kidney disease, diabetes, liver failure, and heart failure, medication history, namely, diuretics, angiotensin-converting-enzyme inhibitors and angiotensin-receptor blockers, and intra-procedure data to predict the risk of AKI [76,82]. An ideal risk prediction score for AKI should include a combination of demographic, clinical, and biological factors, along with biomarkers [76,77].

Malhotra et al. developed an easily calculated risk prediction score for AKI in critical care patients [77]. This risk score combines chronic kidney disease, chronic liver disease, congestive heart failure, hypertension, atherosclerotic coronary vascular disease, acidemia, nephrotoxin exposure, sepsis, mechanical ventilation, and anemia and has demonstrated good calibration in the test and external validation cohorts [77].

Flechet et al. developed four prediction scores, which can be used successively, based on the clinical information available [83]. The variables included in the baseline risk score are age, baseline SCr, surgical or medical category, diabetes, and planned admission. For the admission risk score, it includes blood glucose, suspected sepsis, hemodynamic support, and previous risk score variables. On day 1, the risk score includes SCr, Acute Physiology And Chronic Health Evaluation (APACHE) II score, maximum lactate, bilirubin, hours of ICU stay, and previous risk score variables. The risk score to be used after the first day includes the previous risk score variables and the total amount of urine, urine slope, mean arterial pressure, and hemodynamic support. One of the main strong points of this study is the availability of the online calculator of this risk score, which enhances its use in clinical practice and promotes further validation [83].

The most widely validated risk prediction score for AKI in cardiac surgery was developed by Thakar et al. and comprises 13 pre-operative variables, namely, gender, heart failure, left ventricular ejection fraction, preoperative use of intra-aortic balloon pump, chronic obstructive pulmonary disease, diabetes, previous cardiac surgery, emergency setting, type of surgery, and pre-operative SCr [84].

The clinical application of these risk prediction scores has been limited by the lack of external validation of several studies, the use of heterogeneous definitions of AKI, the difficulty in assessing baseline renal function, and importantly the lack of impact analysis studies and lack of evidence of clinical use [14,76].

5. Automated Electronic Alerts

The use of automated electronic alerts (E-alerts) has received considerable consideration in the past years [85]. E-alerts consist of algorithms configured from patients' EMRs and clinical information to notify early or imminent AKI, prompting an earlier clinical evaluation and prompt prevention and treatment strategies [86,87].

Theoretically, this would prompt early treatment and improve patient outcomes. Nevertheless, a recent systematic review of randomized AKI E-alert trials pooled data from six studies and 10,165 patients and found that these did not reduce mortality (OR 1.05; 95% CI, 0.84–1.31), need for renal replacement therapy (OR 1.20; 95% CI, 0.91–1.57), or change patient care practices (OR 2.18; 95% CI, 0.46–10.31) [88]. In these studies, E-alerts were issued within one hour, following the detection of changes in SCr; however, there was significant variability in study design, alert format, and targeted providers [88].

Beyond the limitations of SCr as a marker of AKI, other important challenges of the use of E-alerts are the distinction of community and hospital-acquired AKI cases, the presence of multiple alerts per patient, the assessment of significance of small SCr changes in patients with CKD, and the limitations on cases without baseline renal function [14].

A care bundle is a group of evidence-based and easily applicable interventions that have a better outcome when performed together than if performed individually [14]. There is no current specific treatment for AKI, and the most recent guidelines suggest supportive management, including treatment of sepsis, shock, and hypovolemia, avoidance of nephrotoxins, appropriate investigations, and referral to specialists when indicated [15].

Kolhe et al. demonstrated that implementing a care bundle with E-alerts improved outcomes in patients with AKI in two cohort studies. The care bundle consists of standardized investigations and interventions, namely, Assessment of history and examination, Urinalysis, establishing a clinical Diagnosis of AKI, plan Investigations, and Treatment and Seeking advice from a nephrologist (AUDITS) [89,90].

These findings were also reported in a study by Chandrasekar et al., in which an E-alert was combined with a care bundle consisting of treatment of Acute complications, Blood pressure control, Catheterization, review Drug prescription, Investigate the cause, and Treat the underlying cause (ABCD-IT) [91]. The authors reported a decrease in mortality and length of stay [91].

A recent study by Hodgson et al. evaluated the impact of combining care bundles to a risk prediction score and to E-alerts. This study demonstrated a decrease in hospital-acquired AKI and a decrease in AKI-associated mortality [92].

Therefore, it may not be enough to merely alert for the presence of AKI but important to initiate appropriate care to lead to improved outcomes [14].

We believe that it is essential to incorporate these scientific advances in daily clinical practice in the near future.

6. The Era of Artificial Intelligence

The past decade has seen significant development of electronic technology in medicine, namely, in EMR, data registries and management, and analytic methodologies [93].

Indeed, a new era of AKI prediction and detection has started with the increasing use of risk prediction scores and E-alerts [93]. More recently, artificial intelligence (AI), namely, ML techniques, has been reported to identify AKI predictors [94].

AI is a branch of engineering, generally defined as the ability of a machine to reason, communicate, and function with the minimal human intervention [95]. In the medical field, AI can be applied as two branches: physical or virtual [95]. The physical branch includes medical devices and sophisticated robots, which contribute to the delivery of care [95]. The virtual branch refers to ML, which includes the algorithms and statistical models that learn from data from which they are able to recognize and deduce patterns [95].

There are numerous types of ML algorithms, which have the ability to find patterns, to classify and predict algorithms based on previous examples, and to create a strategy for prediction by sequences of rewards and punishments [94–98]. The dynamic ability of these algorithms is key to identify and integrate variables from numerous electronic data [94]. Thus, ML techniques can be used alone or combined to analyze datasets and determine AKI predictors. The description of each available ML algorithm is out of the scope of this review.

Currently, logistic regression is the most frequently used statistical algorithm of multivariate analysis to determine risk predictors in the short-term [99]. In complex settings in which clinical features and outcomes have a non-linear relationship and for big data analysis, many investigators support the use of more advanced ML algorithms in detriment of logistic regression to develop predictive models [100].

Considering that AKI can be determined from the calculation of SCr levels and the increasing integration of the available EMRs, ML algorithms are promising in the development of AKI risk prediction models.

The development of risk prediction models has flourished in recent years. However, inefficient statistical methods, the use of small samples, missing data, and lack of validation are common faults, which limit the use of these models [99]. The development of risk prediction models should include internal validation within the original study sample to quantify the predictive ability of the model and should preferably also include external validation to evaluate the predictive ability of the model in other participant data [99]. To improve the quality of reporting of published prediction model studies, the Transparent Reporting of a multivariable prediction model for Individual Prognosis or Diagnosis (TRIPOD) Statement produced a checklist of items to include in studies developing or validating a multivariable prediction model [99].

Furthermore, it is important to consider the specificity and sensitivity of these models, which will have a clinical impact [101]. High specificity values lead to fewer false-positive results, and high sensitivity values lead to fewer false negatives [101]. This has an important impact on prognostic modeling and decision-making, namely, high specificity would trigger less often to prompt interventions with higher risk, and high sensitivity would trigger more often to prompt interventions with lower risk [101].

The first study to compare logistic regression models and ML algorithms was a retrospective study by Kate et al., who analyzed EMRs of 25,521 hospital stays of elderly patients and aimed to predict within the first 24 h of admission whether a patient would develop AKI during hospitalization. This study demonstrated only modest performance in all ML models (support vector machines, decision trees, and naïve Bayes), with an area under the receiver operating characteristic curve (AUROC) ranging from 0.621–0.664, and better performance of logistic regression with an AUROC of 0.743 [102].

A research group led by Bihorac performed a retrospective study of 50,318 adult surgical patients and compared four predictive ML modeling approaches for two major postoperative complications, using data from EMRs [103]. This study demonstrated that the choice of predictive modeling approach affected the risk prediction performance for postoperative AKI and sepsis; specifically, generalized additive models showed the best performance with an AUROC of 0.858 [103].

Davis et al. also compared several ML models (random forest, neural network, and naïve Bayes) and logistic regression methods to predict AKI in a retrospective study of 2003 patients [104]. Both methods had a good performance in detecting AKI, but importantly, over-time logistic regression methods required more updates than random forest or neural network methods to compensate overprediction [104].

Cheng et al. developed ML-based AKI prediction models using EMRs from 48,955 hospital admissions and concluded that the best model for predicting AKI within 24 h had an AUROC of 0.76 achieved by a random forest algorithm [105]. Indeed, this ML algorithm could predict AKI 2-days with AUC of 0.73 and 3-days prior with AUC of 0.700 [105].

Ibrahim et al. developed a clinical and proteomics AKI risk predictor with an ML approach (least absolute shrinkage and selection operator (LASSO) with logistic regression) in a prospective study of 889 patients undergoing coronary angiography [106]. The risk predictor included a history of diabetes, blood urea nitrogen/creatinine ratio, c-reactive protein, osteopontin, CD5 antigen-like, and Factor VII and had an AUROC of 0.790 for predicting procedural AKI [106].

Koola et al. analyzed a retrospective cohort of 504 cirrhotic patients and compared the ability of ML methods (logistic regression, naïve Bayes, support vector machines, random forest, and gradient boosting) to predict hepatorenal syndrome (HRS) [107]. This study demonstrated the ability to create a high-performance risk prediction algorithm to detect cases of HRS, with AUROC ranging between 0.730–0.930 [107].

Another mortality prediction model was constructed using the random forest algorithm in 19,044 AKI patients by Lin and colleagues [100]. Urine output, systolic blood pressure, age, serum bicarbonate, and heart rate were the most significant variables, predicting AKI-associated mortality [100]. This model had a great performance with an AUROC of 0.866 and could prove useful in avoiding delays of AKI treatment in high-mortality risk patients [100].

Koyner et al. developed a gradient boosting model, which could predict AKI in the emergency department, wards, and ICU [108]. Their model included data from 121,158 admissions, such as patient demographics, vital signs, laboratories, clinical interventions, and diagnostics, and demonstrated increasing accuracy across AKI severity, providing AUROC greater than 0.900 for renal replacement therapy requirement within 72 h [108].

Huang et al. performed a retrospective study of 947,091 patients submitted to percutaneous coronary intervention and compared logistic regression and gradient descent boosting to detect if ML algorithms could enhance AKI prediction [109]. Their algorithm had a good performance in detecting AKI with an AUROC 0.728 [109]. The risk prediction model included 12 variables, namely, age, heart failure, cardiogenic shock within 24 h, cardiac arrest within 24 h, diabetes, coronary artery disease, baseline renal function, admission source, body mass index, emergency status, and left ventricular ejection fraction [109].

In another retrospective study of 2,076,694 patients submitted to percutaneous coronary intervention, Huang et al. applied an ML method to predict AKI risk according to contrast volume [110]. The generalized additive model produced an AUROC of 0.777 (95% CI, 0.775–0.779) for predicting the risk of a creatinine level increase of at least 0.3 mg/dL [110]. The model was developed from a random 50% of the cohort, and performance was evaluated in the remaining 50% of the cohort. The association of contrast volume with AKI risk was nonlinear, and this model proved useful to quantify individual risk and adjust contrast volume to decrease AKI risk [110].

Tomasev et al. developed a recurrent neural network model, which predicted 55.8% of all inpatient episodes of AKI and 90.2% of all dialysis, requiring AKI up to 48 h in advance in 703,782 adult patients from inpatient and outpatient sites [111]. This ML model had a great performance with an AUROC of 0.921, and, at each time point, this model outputted the risk of AKI occurrence within the next 48 h, thus allowing for the prompt implementation of preventive and treatment strategies [111].

MySurgeryRisk is an ML algorithm recently developed and internally validated from a retrospective single-center cohort of 2911 adults who underwent surgery [112]. This random forest model combined preoperative and intraoperative variables and had an AUROC of 0.860 to predict the risk of developing postoperative AKI [112].

Flechet et al. conducted a prospective observational study of 252 critically ill patients and compared the AKI predictions by physicians and a random forest method, *AKIpredictor* [113]. There was no statistically significant difference in discrimination between physicians and *AKIpredictor;* however, physicians overestimated the risk, and *AKIpredictor* allowed for the selection of high-risk patients or reducing false positives, and *AKIpredictor* provided its prediction earlier than physicians [113].

Parreco et al. developed and compared different ML models (gradient boosted trees, logistic regression, and deep learning) to predict AKI from the laboratory values, vital signs, and slopes in

151,098 ICU admissions [114]. Gradient boosted trees method was the most accurate model with an AUROC of 0.834, for which the most important variable was the slope of the minimum creatinine [114].

Xu et al. investigated ML models (logistic regression, random forest. and gradient boosting decision tree) for predicting the mortality risk of 58,976 AKI patients admitted to an ICU, stratified according to AKI severity stages [115]. Gradient boosting decision tree presented a better performance than other models for mortality prediction [115].

Tran et al. developed an ML method (k-nearest neighbor) to predict AKI in 50 burn patients, which included measurements of neutrophil gelatinase-associated lipocalin (NGAL), UO, SCr, and N-terminal B-type natriuretic peptide (NT-proBNP) measured within the first 24 h of admission. This method performed greatly with an AUROC of 0.920 and achieved a 90%–100% accuracy for identifying AKI, with a mean time-to-AKI recognition within 18 h [116].

In 6682 critical care patients, Zhang et al. identified predictors of volume responsive AKI, such as age, urinary creatinine concentration, maximum blood urea nitrogen concentration, and albumin using ML methods [117]. Their model (gradient boosting) had an AUROC of 0.860 and could prove useful to stratify patients with oliguria responsive to fluids and prompt immediate therapeutic measures [117].

Zimmerman et al. conducted a retrospective cohort of 23,950 adult critical care patients and developed a predictive model by logistic regression for early prediction of AKI in the first 72 h. following ICU admission with an AUROC of 0.783 [118]. Their model included first-day measurements of physiologic variables but not medications and procedures, in order to detect which deterioration of patients' physiologic baselines are predictive of AKI [118]. This was cross-validated with ML algorithms, demonstrating an accurate and early prediction of AKI with their risk prediction score [118].

Rashidi and colleagues developed, internally validated, and compared ML models for early recognition of AKI in 50 burn and 51 trauma patients, including NGAL, NT-proBNP, SCr, and UO into the predictive model [119]. Their models were able to accurately predict AKI 62 h in advance [119].

Overall, ML algorithms have performed impressively, and sensitivity is favored over specificity in order to early detect as many cases of AKI, allowing for a higher number of false positives. The ML algorithms have also performed better than the currently used logistic regression in the majority of studies. These studies are summarized in Table 1.

Table 1. Machine learning studies on acute kidney injury (AKI) prediction.

Study	Design	Setting	N	AKI Definition	Timing of AKI	ML Algorithm	Predictive Ability	Sensitivity; Specificity; Confidence Interval	External Validation
Kate et al. (2016)	retrospective	medical and surgical	25,521	AKIN	during hospitalization	naïve Bayes; support vector machine; decision trees; logistic regression	AUROC 0.654 AUROC 0.621 AUROC 0.639 AUROC 0.660	75%; 61%; -	no
Thottakkara et al. (2016)	retrospective	surgical	50,318	KDIGO	post surgery	naïve Bayes; generalized additive model; logistic regression; support vector machine	AUROC 0.819 AUROC 0.858 AUROC 0.853 AUROC 0.857	77%; -; -	no
Davis et al. (2017)	retrospective	medical and surgical	2003	KDIGO	during hospitalization	random forest; neural network; naïve Bayes; logistic regression	AUROC 0.730 AUROC 0.720 AUROC 0.690 AUROC 0.780	-; -; 95% CI	no
Cheng et al. (2018)	retrospective	medical and surgical	60,534	KDIGO, AKIN, RIFLE	during hospitalization	random forest; AdaBoostM1; logistic regression	AUROC 0.765 AUROC 0.751 AUROC 0.763	69%; 71%; -	no
Ibrahim et al. (2018)	prospective	contrast	889	KDIGO	pre and post intervention	logistic regression	AUROC 0.790	77%; 75%: -	no

Table 1. *Cont.*

Study	Design	Setting	N	AKI Definition	Timing of AKI	ML Algorithm	Predictive Ability	Sensitivity; Specificity; Confidence Interval	External Validation
Koola et al. (2018)	retrospective	medical and surgical	504	KDIGO	during hospitalization	logistic regression; naïve Bayes; support vector machines; random forest; gradient boosting	AUROC 0.930 AUROC 0.730 AUROC 0.900 AUROC 0.910 AUROC 0.880	87%; 76%; -	no
Lin et al. (2018)	retrospective	ICU	19,044	KDIGO	during hospitalization	support vector machine	AUROC 0.860	-	no
Koyner et al. (2018)	retrospective	medical and surgical	121,158	KDIGO	24 h post admission	gradient boosting	AUROC 0.900	95% CI	no
Huang et al. (2018)	retrospective	PCI	947,091	AKIN	during hospitalization	gradient boost; logistic regression	AUROC 0.728 AUROC 0.717	-; -; 95% CI	no
Huang et al. (2019)	retrospective	PCI	2,076,694	AKIN	pre and post intervention	generalized additive model	AUROC 0.777	-; -; 95% CI	no
Tomašev et al. (2019)	retrospective	medical and surgical	703,782	KDIGO	during hospitalization	recurrent neural network	AUROC 0.921	95%; 70.3%; -	no
Adhikari et al. (2019)	retrospective	surgical	2901	KDIGO	post surgery	random forest	AUROC 0.860	68%; -; -	no
Flechet et al. (2019)	prospective	ICU	252	KDIGO	during hospitalization	random forest	AUROC 0.780	-; -; 95% CI	no

Table 1. *Cont.*

Study	Design	Setting	N	AKI Definition	Timing of AKI	ML Algorithm	Predictive Ability	Sensitivity; Specificity; Confidence Interval	External Validation
Parreco et al. (2019)	retrospective	medical and surgical	151,098	KDIGO	during hospitalization	gradient boosting; logistic regression; deep learning	AUROC 0.834 AUROC 0.827 AUROC 0.817	-; -; 95% CI	no
Xu et al. (2019)	retrospective	medical and surgical	58,976	KDIGO	during hospitalization	gradient boosting	AUROC 0.749	-	no
Tran et al. (2019)	prospective	burn	50	KDIGO	during hospitalization	k-nearest neighbor	AUROC 0.920	90%; -; -	no
Zhang et al. (2019)	retrospective	ICU	6682	KDIGO	24 h post admission	gradient boosting	AUROC 0.860	-; -; 95% CI	no
Zimmerman et al. (2019)	retrospective	ICU	46,000	KDIGO	72 h post admission	logistic regression; random forest; neural network	AUROC 0.783 AUROC 0.779 AUROC 0.796	68%; 34%; -	no
Rashidi et al. (2020)	retrospective and prospective	burn and trauma	50/51	KDIGO vs New Biomarkers	1st week post ICU admission	recurrent neural network	AUROC 0.920	-; -; 92% CI	no

AKI-acute kidney injury, AKIN-acute kidney injury network, AUROC-area under the receiver operating characteristic curve, ICU-intensive care unit, KDIGO-kidney disease improving global outcomes, ML-machine learning, PCI-percutaneous coronary intervention, RIFLE-risk, injury, failure, loss of kidney function, end-stage kidney disease.

These studies have demonstrated the efficacy of ML algorithms to detect clinical and laboratory characteristics associated with AKI risk and detection in big data studies. The future widespread use of ML algorithms could improve risk stratification of patients, early detection of AKI, and provide decision aid on treatment, ultimately improving patient care and increasing time and cost-efficiency. Furthermore, these algorithms could predict further adverse events and long-term prognosis, therefore, providing useful information to establish an individualized follow-up plan.

Despite the promising results, important limitations have to be considered [82]. Firstly, most ML approaches have performed positively in retrospective cohorts, and prospective implementation of these methods is still challenging [95,101]. None of these studies have external validation, and the variability in the availability of EMRs across centers limits the widespread use of these models [95,101]. The development of these risk prediction models requires a substantial amount of data from EMRs and computer-assisted risk prediction [82]. Furthermore, to guarantee detailed information on comorbidities, physiological and laboratory parameters and medication, and electronic connections between community and hospital data are necessary [82]. Logistic regression models are more familiar to clinicians than ML models, limiting data interpretation [103]. It is also important to note that neural networks are developed and tested in the same dataset, which limits generalizability [95,101]. Additionally, from a legal and ethical perspective, the inability to clarify what contributes to decision-making in neural networks is an important restriction in these models, which is conflicting to general data protection requirements [95,101].

7. Conclusions

AKI has a significant negative impact on short and long-term outcomes; thus, it is crucial to develop methods to identify patients at risk for AKI and to diagnose subclinical AKI. The increasing amount of evidence is encouraging the real-time implementation of these ML risk models as this does not require additional AKI biomarker testing. Combining these risk prediction models with early care bundles in the future is likely to improve patient outcomes.

Author Contributions: The authors participated as follows: J.G. drafted the article, T.B. participated in the acquisition of data, J.A.L. revised the article and approved the final version to be submitted for publication. All authors have read and agreed to the published version of the manuscript.

References

1. Kellum, J.A.; Prowle, J.R. Paradigms of acute kidney injury in the intensive care setting. *Nat. Rev. Nephrol.* **2018**, *14*, 217–230. [CrossRef] [PubMed]
2. Hoste, E.A.J.; Schurgers, M. Epidemiology of acute kidney injury: How big is the problem? *Crit. Care Med.* **2008**, *36* (Suppl. S36), S146–S151. [CrossRef] [PubMed]
3. Coca, S.G.; Yusuf, B.; Shlipak, M.G.; Garg, A.X.; Parikh, C.R. Long-term Risk of Mortality and Other Adverse Outcomes After Acute Kidney Injury: A Systematic Review and Meta-analysis. *Am. J. Kidney Dis.* **2009**, *53*, 961–973. [CrossRef] [PubMed]
4. Chertow, G.M.; Burdick, E.; Honour, M.; Bonventre, J.V.; Bates, D.W. Acute Kidney Injury, Mortality, Length of Stay, and Costs in Hospitalized Patients. *J. Am. Soc. Nephrol.* **2005**, *16*, 3365–3370. [CrossRef] [PubMed]
5. Chawla, L.S.; Bellomo, R.; Bihorac, A.; Goldstein, S.L.; Siew, E.D.; Bagshaw, S.M.; Bittleman, D.; Cruz, D.; Endre, Z.; Fitzgerald, R.L.; et al. Acute kidney disease and renal recovery: Consensus report of the Acute Disease Quality Initiative (ADQI) 16 Workgroup. *Nat. Rev. Nephrol.* **2017**, *13*, 241–257. [CrossRef] [PubMed]
6. Wald, R. Chronic Dialysis and Death Among Survivors of Acute Kidney Injury Requiring Dialysis. *JAMA* **2009**, *302*, 1179. [CrossRef] [PubMed]

7. De Corte, W.; Dhondt, A.; Vanholder, R.; De Waele, J.; Decruyenaere, J.; Sergoyne, V.; Vanhalst, J.; Claus, S.; Hoste, E.A. Long-term outcome in ICU patients with acute kidney injury treated with renal replacement therapy: A prospective cohort study. *Crit. Care* **2016**, *20*, 256. [CrossRef]
8. Susantitaphong, P.; Cruz, D.N.; Cerda, J.; Abulfaraj, M.; Alqahtani, F.; Koulouridis, I.; Jaber, B.L. Acute Kidney Injury Advisory Group of the American Society of Nephrology. World Incidence of AKI: A Meta-Analysis. *Clin. J. Am. Soc. Nephrol.* **2013**, *8*, 1482–1493. [CrossRef]
9. Uchino, S. Acute Renal Failure in Critically Ill PatientsA Multinational, Multicenter Study. *JAMA* **2005**, *294*, 813. [CrossRef]
10. Hoste, E.A.J.; Bagshaw, S.M.; Bellomo, R.; Cely, C.M.; Colman, R.; Cruz, D.N.; Edipidis, K.; Forni, L.G.; Gomersall, C.D.; Govil, D.; et al. Epidemiology of acute kidney injury in critically ill patients: The multinational AKI-EPI study. *Intensive Care Med.* **2015**, *41*, 1411–1423. [CrossRef]
11. Ympa, Y.P.; Sakr, Y.; Reinhart, K.; Vincent, J.-L. Has mortality from acute renal failure decreased? A systematic review of the literature. *Am. J. Med.* **2005**, *118*, 827–832. [CrossRef] [PubMed]
12. Waikar, S.S.; Curhan, G.C.; Wald, R.; McCarthy, E.P.; Chertow, G.M. Declining Mortality in Patients with Acute Renal Failure, 1988 to 2002. *J. Am. Soc. Nephrol.* **2006**, *17*, 1143–1150. [CrossRef] [PubMed]
13. Wald, R.; McArthur, E.; Adhikari, N.K.J.; Bagshaw, S.M.; Burns, K.E.; Garg, A.X.; Harel, Z.; Kitchlu, A.; Mazer, C.D.; Nash, D.M.; et al. Changing Incidence and Outcomes Following Dialysis-Requiring Acute Kidney Injury Among Critically Ill Adults: A Population-Based Cohort Study. *Am. J. Kidney Dis.* **2015**, *65*, 870–877. [CrossRef]
14. Hodgson, L.E.; Selby, N.; Huang, T.-M.; Forni, L.G. The Role of Risk Prediction Models in Prevention and Management of AKI. *Semin. Nephrol.* **2019**, *39*, 421–430. [CrossRef] [PubMed]
15. Khwaja, A. KDIGO Clinical Practice Guidelines for Acute Kidney Injury. *Nephron* **2012**, *120*, c179–c184. [CrossRef] [PubMed]
16. Thomas, M.E.; Blaine, C.; Dawnay, A.; Devonald, M.A.; Ftouh, S.; Laing, C.; Latchem, S.; Lewington, A.; Milford, D.V.; Ostermann, M. The definition of acute kidney injury and its use in practice. *Kidney Int.* **2015**, *87*, 62–73. [CrossRef] [PubMed]
17. Schinstock, C.A.; Semret, M.H.; Wagner, S.J.; Borland, T.M.; Bryant, S.C.; Kashani, K.B.; Larson, T.S.; Lieske, J.C. Urinalysis is more specific and urinary neutrophil gelatinase-associated lipocalin is more sensitive for early detection of acute kidney injury. *Nephrol. Dial. Transplant.* **2012**, *28*, 1175–1185. [CrossRef]
18. Han, W.K.; Bailly, V.; Abichandani, R.; Thadhani, R.; Bonventre, J.V. Kidney Injury Molecule-1 (KIM-1): A novel biomarker for human renal proximal tubule injury. *Kidney Int.* **2002**, *62*, 237–244. [CrossRef]
19. Ostermann, M.; Philips, B.J.; Forni, L.G. Clinical review: Biomarkers of acute kidney injury: Where are we now? *Crit. Care* **2012**, *16*, 233. [CrossRef]
20. Parikh, C.R.; Mishra, J.; Thiessen-Philbrook, H.; Dursun, B.; Ma, Q.; Kelly, C.; Dent, C.; Devarajan, P.; Edelstein, C.L. Urinary IL-18 is an early predictive biomarker of acute kidney injury after cardiac surgery. *Kidney Int.* **2006**, *70*, 199–203. [CrossRef]
21. Di Somma, S.; Magrini, L.; De Berardinis, B.; Marino, R.; Ferri, E.; Moscatelli, P.; Ballarino, P.; Carpinteri, G.; Noto, P.; Gliozzo, B.; et al. Additive value of blood neutrophil gelatinase-associated lipocalin to clinical judgement in acute kidney injury diagnosis and mortality prediction in patients hospitalized from the emergency department. *Crit. Care* **2013**, *17*, R29. [CrossRef] [PubMed]
22. Bennett, M.; Dent, C.L.; Ma, Q.; Dastrala, S.; Grenier, F.; Workman, R.; Syed, H.; Ali, S.; Barasch, J.; Devarajan, P. Urine NGAL Predicts Severity of Acute Kidney Injury After Cardiac Surgery: A Prospective Study. *Clin. J. Am. Soc. Nephrol.* **2008**, *3*, 665–673. [CrossRef] [PubMed]
23. Hall, I.E.; Yarlagadda, S.G.; Coca, S.G.; Wang, Z.; Doshi, M.; Devarajan, P.; Han, W.K.; Marcus, R.J.; Parikh, C.R. IL-18 and Urinary NGAL Predict Dialysis and Graft Recovery after Kidney Transplantation. *J. Am. Soc. Nephrol.* **2009**, *21*, 189–197. [CrossRef] [PubMed]
24. Jia, H.-M.; Huang, L.-F.; Zheng, Y.; Li, W.-X. Diagnostic value of urinary tissue inhibitor of metalloproteinase-2 and insulin-like growth factor binding protein 7 for acute kidney injury: A meta-analysis. *Crit. Care* **2017**, *21*. [CrossRef]
25. Bargnoux, A.-S.; Piéroni, L.; Cristol, J.-P. Analytical study of a new turbidimetric assay for urinary neutrophil gelatinase-associated lipocalin (NGAL) determination. *Clin. Chem. Lab. Med.* **2013**, *51*. [CrossRef]

26. Westhoff, J.H.; Tönshoff, B.; Waldherr, S.; Pöschl, J.; Teufel, U.; Westhoff, T.H.; Fichtner, A. Urinary Tissue Inhibitor of Metalloproteinase-2 (TIMP-2) • Insulin-Like Growth Factor-Binding Protein 7 (IGFBP7) Predicts Adverse Outcome in Pediatric Acute Kidney Injury. *PLoS ONE* **2015**, *10*, e0143628. [CrossRef]
27. Lima, C.; Macedo, E. Urinary Biochemistry in the Diagnosis of Acute Kidney Injury. *Dis. Markers* **2018**, *2018*, 1–7. [CrossRef]
28. Vanmassenhove, J.; Vanholder, R.; Nagler, E.; Van Biesen, W. Urinary and serum biomarkers for the diagnosis of acute kidney injury: An in-depth review of the literature. *Nephrol. Dial. Transplant.* **2012**, *28*, 254–273. [CrossRef]
29. Marx, D.; Metzger, J.; Pejchinovski, M.; Gil, R.B.; Frantzi, M.; Latosinska, A.; Belczacka, I.; Heinzmann, S.S.; Husi, H.; Zoidakis, J.; et al. Proteomics and Metabolomics for AKI Diagnosis. *Semin. Nephrol.* **2018**, *38*, 63–87. [CrossRef]
30. Kashani, K.; Cheungpasitporn, W.; Ronco, C. Biomarkers of acute kidney injury: The pathway from discovery to clinical adoption. *Clin. Chem. Lab. Med.* **2017**, *55*, 1074–1089. [CrossRef]
31. Cruz, D.N.; Ronco, C. Acute kidney injury in the intensive care unit: Current trends in incidence and outcome. *Crit. Care* **2007**, *11*, 149. [CrossRef] [PubMed]
32. Ali, T.; Khan, I.; Simpson, W.; Prescott, G.; Townend, J.; Smith, W.; Macleod, A. Incidence and Outcomes in Acute Kidney Injury: A Comprehensive Population-Based Study. *J. Am. Soc. Nephrol.* **2007**, *18*, 1292–1298. [CrossRef] [PubMed]
33. Lameire, N.H.; Bagga, A.; Cruz, D.; De Maeseneer, J.; Endre, Z.; Kellum, J.A.; Liu, K.D.; Mehta, R.L.; Pannu, N.; Van Biesen, W.; et al. Acute kidney injury: An increasing global concern. *Lancet* **2013**, *382*, 170–179. [CrossRef]
34. Grams, M.E.; Sang, Y.; Ballew, S.H.; Gansevoort, R.T.; Kimm, H.; Kovesdy, C.P.; Naimark, D.; Oien, C.; Smith, D.H.; Coresh, J.; et al. A Meta-analysis of the Association of Estimated GFR, Albuminuria, Age, Race, and Sex With Acute Kidney Injury. *Am. J. Kidney Dis.* **2015**, *66*, 591–601. [CrossRef] [PubMed]
35. De Zan, F.; Amigoni, A.; Pozzato, R.; Pettenazzo, A.; Murer, L.; Vidal, E. Acute Kidney Injury in Critically Ill Children: A Retrospective Analysis of Risk Factors. *Blood Purif.* **2019**, 1–7. [CrossRef] [PubMed]
36. Nie, S.; Tang, L.; Zhang, W.; Feng, Z.; Chen, X. Are There Modifiable Risk Factors to Improve AKI? *Biomed. Res. Int.* **2017**, *2017*, 1–9. [CrossRef]
37. Anderson, S.; Eldadah, B.; Halter, J.B.; Hazzard, W.R.; Himmelfarb, J.; Horne, F.M.; Kimmel, P.L.; Molitoris, B.A.; Murthy, M.; O'Hare, A.M.; et al. Acute Kidney Injury in Older Adults. *J. Am. Soc. Nephrol.* **2011**, *22*, 28–38. [CrossRef]
38. Chawla, L.S.; Eggers, P.W.; Star, R.A.; Kimmel, P.L. Acute Kidney Injury and Chronic Kidney Disease as Interconnected Syndromes. *N. Engl. J. Med.* **2014**, *371*, 58–66. [CrossRef]
39. Nie, S.; Feng, Z.; Xia, L.; Bai, J.; Xiao, F.; Liu, J.; Tang, L.; Chen, X. Risk factors of prognosis after acute kidney injury in hospitalized patients. *Front. Med.* **2017**, *11*, 393–402. [CrossRef]
40. Kane-Gill, S.L.; Sileanu, F.E.; Murugan, R.; Trietley, G.S.; Handler, S.M.; Kellum, J.A. Risk Factors for Acute Kidney Injury in Older Adults With Critical Illness: A Retrospective Cohort Study. *Am. J. Kidney Dis.* **2015**, *65*, 860–869. [CrossRef] [PubMed]
41. Gameiro, J.; Agapito Fonseca, J.; Jorge, S.; Lopes, J.A. Acute kidney injury in HIV-infected patients: A critical review. *HIV Med.* **2019**, *20*. [CrossRef] [PubMed]
42. Wyatt, C.M.; Arons, R.R.; Klotman, P.E.; Klotman, M.E. Acute renal failure in hospitalized patients with HIV: Risk factors and impact on in-hospital mortality. *AIDS* **2006**, *20*, 561–565. [CrossRef] [PubMed]
43. Singbartl, K.; Kellum, J.A. AKI in the ICU: Definition, epidemiology, risk stratification, and outcomes. *Kidney Int.* **2012**, *81*, 819–825. [CrossRef] [PubMed]
44. Lameire, N.; Van Biesen, W.; Vanholder, R. The changing epidemiology of acute renal failure. *Nat. Clin. Pract. Nephrol.* **2006**, *2*, 364–377. [CrossRef]
45. Liaño, F.; Junco, E.; Pascual, J.; Madero, R.; Verde, E. The spectrum of acute renal failure in the intensive care unit compared with that seen in other settings. The Madrid Acute Renal Failure Study Group. *Kidney Int. Suppl.* **1998**, *66*, S16–S24. [PubMed]
46. Ejaz, A.A.; Beaver, T.M.; Shimada, M.; Sood, P.; Lingegowda, V.; Schold, J.D.; Kim, T.; Johnson, R.J. Uric Acid: A Novel Risk Factor for Acute Kidney Injury in High-Risk Cardiac Surgery Patients? *Am. J. Nephrol.* **2009**, *30*, 425–429. [CrossRef] [PubMed]

47. Ejaz, A.A.; Kambhampati, G.; Ejaz, N.I.; Dass, B.; Lapsia, V.; Arif, A.A.; Asmar, A.; Shimada, M.; Alsabbagh, M.M.; Aiyer, R.; et al. Post-operative serum uric acid and acute kidney injury. *J. Nephrol.* **2012**, *25*, 497–505. [CrossRef]
48. Lapsia, V.; Johnson, R.J.; Dass, B.; Shimada, M.; Kambhampati, G.; Ejaz, N.I.; Arif, A.A.; Ejaz, A.A. Elevated Uric Acid Increases the Risk for Acute Kidney Injury. *Am. J. Med.* **2012**, *125*, 302.e9–302.e17. [CrossRef]
49. Guo, W.; Liu, Y.; Chen, J.-Y.; Chen, S.Q.; Li, H.L.; Duan, C.Y.; Liu, Y.H.; Tan, N. Hyperuricemia Is an Independent Predictor of Contrast-Induced Acute Kidney Injury and Mortality in Patients Undergoing Percutaneous Coronary Intervention. *Angiology* **2015**, *66*, 721–726. [CrossRef]
50. Kim, C.S.; Oak, C.Y.; Kim, H.Y.; Kang, Y.U.; Choi, J.S.; Bae, E.H.; Ma, S.K.; Kweon, S.S.; Kim, S.W. Incidence, Predictive Factors, and Clinical Outcomes of Acute Kidney Injury after Gastric Surgery for Gastric Cancer. *PLoS ONE* **2013**, *8*, e82289. [CrossRef]
51. Lee, E.-H.; Baek, S.-H.; Chin, J.-H.; Choi, D.K.; Son, H.J.; Kim, W.J.; Hahm, K.D.; Sim, J.Y.; Choi, I.C. Preoperative hypoalbuminemia is a major risk factor for acute kidney injury following off-pump coronary artery bypass surgery. *Intensive Care Med.* **2012**, *38*, 1478–1486. [CrossRef] [PubMed]
52. Wiedermann, C.J.; Wiedermann, W.; Joannidis, M. Hypoalbuminemia and acute kidney injury: A meta-analysis of observational clinical studies. *Intensive Care Med.* **2010**, *36*, 1657–1665. [CrossRef] [PubMed]
53. Delaney, A.P.; Dan, A.; McCaffrey, J.; Finfer, S. The role of albumin as a resuscitation fluid for patients with sepsis: A systematic review and meta-analysis. *Crit. Care Med.* **2011**, *39*, 386–391. [CrossRef] [PubMed]
54. Li, N.; Qiao, H.; Guo, J.-F.; Yang, H.Y.; Li, X.Y.; Li, S.L.; Wang, D.X.; Yang, L. Preoperative hypoalbuminemia was associated with acute kidney injury in high-risk patients following non-cardiac surgery: A retrospective cohort study. *BMC Anesthesiol.* **2019**, *19*, 171. [CrossRef] [PubMed]
55. Glance, L.G.; Wissler, R.; Mukamel, D.B.; Li, Y.; Diachun, C.A.; Salloum, R.; Fleming, F.J.; Dick, A.W. Perioperative Outcomes among Patients with the Modified Metabolic Syndrome Who Are Undergoing Noncardiac Surgery. *Anesthesiology* **2010**, *113*, 859–872. [CrossRef] [PubMed]
56. Kelz, R.R.; Reinke, C.E.; Zubizarreta, J.R.; Wang, M.; Saynisch, P.; Even-Shoshan, O.; Reese, P.P.; Fleisher, L.A.; Silber, J.H. Acute Kidney Injury, Renal Function, and the Elderly Obese Surgical Patient. *Ann. Surg.* **2013**, *258*, 359–363. [CrossRef]
57. Danziger, J.; Chen, K.P.; Lee, J.; Feng, M.; Mark, R.G.; Celi, L.A.; Mukamal, K.J. Obesity, Acute Kidney Injury, and Mortality in Critical Illness. *Crit. Care Med.* **2016**, *44*, 328–334. [CrossRef]
58. Billings, F.T.; Pretorius, M.; Schildcrout, J.S.; Mercaldo, N.D.; Byrne, J.G.; Ikizler, T.A.; Brown, N.J. Obesity and Oxidative Stress Predict AKI after Cardiac Surgery. *J. Am. Soc. Nephrol.* **2012**, *23*, 1221–1228. [CrossRef]
59. Karkouti, K.; Grocott, H.P.; Hall, R.; Jessen, M.E.; Kruger, C.; Lerner, A.B.; MacAdams, C.; Mazer, C.D.; de Medicis, É.; Myles, P.; et al. Interrelationship of preoperative anemia, intraoperative anemia, and red blood cell transfusion as potentially modifiable risk factors for acute kidney injury in cardiac surgery: A historical multicentre cohort study. *Can. J. Anesth. Can. d'anesthésie* **2014**, *62*, 377–384. [CrossRef]
60. Karkouti, K.; Wijeysundera, D.N.; Yau, T.M.; Callum, J.L.; Cheng, D.C.; Crowther, M.; Dupuis, J.Y.; Fremes, S.E.; Kent, B.; Laflamme, C.; et al. Acute Kidney Injury After Cardiac Surgery. *Circulation* **2009**, *119*, 495–502. [CrossRef]
61. Haase, M.; Bellomo, R.; Story, D.; Letis, A.; Klemz, K.; Matalanis, G.; Seevanayagam, S.; Dragun, D.; Seeliger, E.; Mertens, P.R.; et al. Effect of mean arterial pressure, haemoglobin and blood transfusion during cardiopulmonary bypass on post-operative acute kidney injury. *Nephrol. Dial. Transplant.* **2012**, *27*, 153–160. [CrossRef] [PubMed]
62. Lelubre, C.; Vincent, J.-L. Red blood cell transfusion in the critically ill patient. *Ann. Intensive Care* **2011**, *1*, 43. [CrossRef] [PubMed]
63. Koch, C.G.; Li, L.; Sessler, D.I.; Figueroa, P.; Hoeltge, G.A.; Mihaljevic, T.; Blackstone, E.H. Duration of Red-Cell Storage and Complications after Cardiac Surgery. *N. Engl. J. Med.* **2008**, *358*, 1229–1239. [CrossRef] [PubMed]
64. Tinmouth, A.; Fergusson, D.; Yee, I.C.; Hébert, P.C. Clinical consequences of red cell storage in the critically ill. *Transfusion* **2006**, *46*, 2014–2027. [CrossRef]
65. Moriyama, N.; Ishihara, M.; Noguchi, T.; Nakanishi, M.; Arakawa, T.; Asaumi, Y.; Kumasaka, L.; Kanaya, T.; Miyagi, T.; Nagai, T.; et al. Admission Hyperglycemia Is an Independent Predictor of Acute Kidney Injury in Patients With Acute Myocardial Infarction. *Circ. J.* **2014**, *78*, 1475–1480. [CrossRef]

66. Palomba, H.; de Castro, I.; Neto, A.L.C.; Lage, S.; Yu, L. Acute kidney injury prediction following elective cardiac surgery: AKICS Score. *Kidney Int.* **2007**, *72*, 624–631. [CrossRef]
67. Stolker, J.M.; McCullough, P.A.; Rao, S.; Inzucchi, S.E.; Spertus, J.A.; Maddox, T.M.; Masoudi, F.A.; Xiao, L.; Kosiborod, M. Pre-Procedural Glucose Levels and the Risk for Contrast-Induced Acute Kidney Injury in Patients Undergoing Coronary Angiography. *J. Am. Coll. Cardiol.* **2010**, *55*, 1433–1440. [CrossRef]
68. Giannini, F.; Latib, A.; Jabbour, R.J.; Ruparelia, N.; Aurelio, A.; Ancona, M.B.; Figini, F.; Mangieri, A.; Regazzoli, D.; Tanaka, A.; et al. Impact of post-procedural hyperglycemia on acute kidney injury after transcatheter aortic valve implantation. *Int. J. Cardiol.* **2016**, *221*, 892–897. [CrossRef]
69. Yoo, S.; Lee, H.-J.; Lee, H.; Ryu, H.-G. Association Between Perioperative Hyperglycemia or Glucose Variability and Postoperative Acute Kidney Injury After Liver Transplantation. *Anesth. Analg.* **2017**, *124*, 35–41. [CrossRef]
70. Shacham, Y.; Gal-Oz, A.; Leshem-Rubinow, E.; Arbel, Y.; Keren, G.; Roth, A.; Steinvil, A. Admission Glucose Levels and the Risk of Acute Kidney Injury in Nondiabetic ST Segment Elevation Myocardial Infarction Patients Undergoing Primary Percutaneous Coronary Intervention. *Cardiorenal Med.* **2015**, *5*, 191–198. [CrossRef]
71. Hoste, E.A.J.; Kellum, J.A.; Selby, N.M.; Arbel, Y.; Keren, G.; Roth, A.; Steinvil, A. Global epidemiology and outcomes of acute kidney injury. *Nat. Rev. Nephrol.* **2018**, *14*, 607–625. [CrossRef] [PubMed]
72. Kheterpal, S.; Tremper, K.K.; Englesbe, M.J.; O'Reilly, M.; Shanks, A.M.; Fetterman, D.M.; Rosenberg, A.L.; Swartz, R.D. Predictors of Postoperative Acute Renal Failure after Noncardiac Surgery in Patients with Previously Normal Renal Function. *Anesthesiology* **2007**, *107*, 892–902. [CrossRef] [PubMed]
73. Park, S.; Cho, H.; Park, S.; Lee, S.; Kim, K.; Yoon, H.J.; Park, J.; Choi, Y.; Lee, S.; Kim, J.H.; et al. Simple Postoperative AKI Risk (SPARK) Classification before Noncardiac Surgery: A Prediction Index Development Study with External Validation. *J. Am. Soc. Nephrol.* **2019**, *30*, 170–181. [CrossRef] [PubMed]
74. Silver, S.A.; Shah, P.M.; Chertow, G.M.; Harel, S.; Wald, R.; Harel, Z. Risk prediction models for contrast induced nephropathy: Systematic review. *BMJ* **2015**, h4395. [CrossRef]
75. Wilson, T.; Quan, S.; Cheema, K.; Zarnke., K.; Quinn, R.; de Koning, L.; Dixon, E.; Pannu, N.; James, M.T. Risk prediction models for acute kidney injury following major noncardiac surgery: Systematic review. *Nephrol. Dial. Transplant.* **2015**, gfv415. [CrossRef]
76. Hodgson, L.E.; Sarnowski, A.; Roderick, P.J.; Dimitrov, B.D.; Venn, R.M.; Forni, L.G. Systematic review of prognostic prediction models for acute kidney injury (AKI) in general hospital populations. *BMJ Open* **2017**, *7*, e016591. [CrossRef]
77. Malhotra, R.; Kashani, K.B.; Macedo, E.; Kim, J.; Bouchard, J.; Wynn, S.; Li, G.; Ohno-Machado, L.; Mehta, R. A risk prediction score for acute kidney injury in the intensive care unit. *Nephrol. Dial. Transplant.* **2017**, *32*, 814–822. [CrossRef]
78. Koyner, J.L.; Adhikari, R.; Edelson, D.P.; Churpek, M.M. Development of a Multicenter Ward–Based AKI Prediction Model. *Clin. J. Am. Soc. Nephrol.* **2016**, *11*, 1935–1943. [CrossRef]
79. Bedford, M.; Stevens, P.; Coulton, S.; Billings, J.; Farr, M.; Wheeler, T.; Kalli, M.; Mottishaw, T.; Farmer, C. Development of risk models for the prediction of new or worsening acute kidney injury on or during hospital admission: A cohort and nested study. *Health Serv. Deliv. Res.* **2016**, *4*, 1–160. [CrossRef]
80. Forni, L.G.; Dawes, T.; Sinclair, H.; Cheek, E.; Bewick, V.; Dennis, M.; Venn, R. Identifying the Patient at Risk of Acute Kidney Injury: A Predictive Scoring System for the Development of Acute Kidney Injury in Acute Medical Patients. *Nephron Clin. Pract.* **2013**, *123*, 143–150. [CrossRef]
81. Breidthardt, T.; Socrates, T.; Noveanu, M.; Klima, T.; Heinisch, C.; Reichlin, T.; Potocki, M.; Nowak, A.; Tschung, C.; Arenja, N.; et al. Effect and Clinical Prediction of Worsening Renal Function in Acute Decompensated Heart Failure. *Am. J. Cardiol.* **2011**, *107*, 730–735. [CrossRef] [PubMed]
82. Park, S.; Lee, H. Acute kidney injury prediction models. *Curr. Opin. Nephrol. Hypertens.* **2019**, *28*, 552–559. [CrossRef]
83. Flechet, M.; Güiza, F.; Schetz, M.; Wouters, P.; Vanhorebeek, I.; Derese, I.; Gunst, J.; Spriet, I.; Casaer, M.; Van den Berghe, G.; et al. AKIpredictor, an online prognostic calculator for acute kidney injury in adult critically ill patients: Development, validation and comparison to serum neutrophil gelatinase-associated lipocalin. *Intensive Care Med.* **2017**, *43*, 764–773. [CrossRef] [PubMed]
84. Thakar, C.V.; Arrigain, S.; Worley, S.; Yared, J.-P.; Paganini, E.P. A Clinical Score to Predict Acute Renal Failure after Cardiac Surgery. *J. Am. Soc. Nephrol.* **2005**, *16*, 162–168. [CrossRef] [PubMed]

85. Cheungpasitporn, W.; Kashani, K. Electronic Data Systems and Acute Kidney Injury. *Contrib. Nephrol.* **2016**, *187*, 73–83. [CrossRef] [PubMed]
86. James, M.T.; Hobson, C.E.; Darmon, M.; Mohan, S.; Hudson, D.; Goldstein, S.L.; Ronco, C.; Kellum, J.A.; Bagshaw, S.M. Acute Dialysis Quality Initiative (ADQI) Consensus Group. Applications for Detection of Acute Kidney Injury Using Electronic Medical Records and Clinical Information Systems: Workgroup Statements from the 15th ADQI Consensus Conference. *Can. J. Kidney Health Dis.* **2016**, *3*, 100. [CrossRef] [PubMed]
87. Selby, N.M.; Crowley, L.; Fluck, R.J.; McIntyre, C.W.; Monaghan, J.; Lawson, N.; Kolhe, N.V. Use of Electronic Results Reporting to Diagnose and Monitor AKI in Hospitalized Patients. *Clin. J. Am. Soc. Nephrol.* **2012**, *7*, 533–540. [CrossRef]
88. Lachance, P.; Villeneuve, P.-M.; Rewa, O.G.; Wilson, F.P.; Selby, N.M.; Featherstone, R.M.; Bagshaw, S.M. Association between e-alert implementation for detection of acute kidney injury and outcomes: A systematic review. *Nephrol. Dial. Transplant.* **2017**, gfw424. [CrossRef]
89. Kolhe, N.V.; Reilly, T.; Leung, J.; Fluck, R.J.; Swinscoe, K.E.; Selby, N.M.; Taal, M.W. A simple care bundle for use in acute kidney injury: A propensity score-matched cohort study. *Nephrol. Dial. Transplant.* **2016**, *31*, 1846–1854. [CrossRef]
90. Kolhe, N.V.; Staples, D.; Reilly, T.; Merrison, D.; Mcintyre, C.W.; Fluck, R.J.; Selby, N.M.; Taal, M.W. Impact of Compliance with a Care Bundle on Acute Kidney Injury Outcomes: A Prospective Observational Study. *PLoS ONE* **2015**, *10*, e0132279. [CrossRef]
91. Chandrasekar, T.; Sharma, A.; Tennent, L.; Wong, C.; Chamberlain, P.; Abraham, K.A. A whole system approach to improving mortality associated with acute kidney injury. *QJM Int. J. Med.* **2017**, *110*, 657–666. [CrossRef] [PubMed]
92. Hodgson, L.E.; Roderick, P.J.; Venn, R.M.; Yao, G.L.; Dimitrov, B.D.; Forni, L.G. The ICE-AKI study: Impact analysis of a Clinical prediction rule and Electronic AKI alert in general medical patients. *PLoS ONE* **2018**, *13*, e0200584. [CrossRef] [PubMed]
93. Sutherland, S.M.; Chawla, L.S.; Kane-Gill, S.L.; Hsu, R.K.; Kramer, A.A.; Goldstein, S.L.; Kellum, J.A.; Ronco, C.; Bagshaw, S.M. 15 ADQI Consensus Group. Utilizing Electronic Health Records to Predict Acute Kidney Injury Risk and Outcomes: Workgroup Statements from the 15 th ADQI Consensus Conference. *Can. J. Kidney Health Dis.* **2016**, *3*, 99. [CrossRef] [PubMed]
94. Sutherland, S.M.; Goldstein, S.L.; Bagshaw, S.M. Acute Kidney Injury and Big Data. *Contrib. Nephrol.* **2018**, *193*, 55–67. [CrossRef]
95. Hamet, P.; Tremblay, J. Artificial intelligence in medicine. *Metabolism* **2017**, *69*, S36–S40. [CrossRef] [PubMed]
96. Lee, J.-G.; Jun, S.; Cho, Y.-W.; Lee, H.; Kim, G.B.; Seo, J.B.; Kim, N. Deep Learning in Medical Imaging: General Overview. *Korean J. Radiol.* **2017**, *18*, 570. [CrossRef]
97. Kulikowski, C.A. Beginnings of Artificial Intelligence in Medicine (AIM): Computational Artifice Assisting Scientific Inquiry and Clinical Art—With Reflections on Present AIM Challenges. *Yearb. Med. Inform.* **2019**, *28*, 249–256. [CrossRef]
98. LeCun, Y.; Bengio, Y.; Hinton, G. Deep learning. *Nature* **2015**, *521*, 436–444. [CrossRef]
99. Collins, G.S.; Reitsma, J.B.; Altman, D.G.; Moons, K.G.M. Transparent Reporting of a multivariable prediction model for Individual Prognosis Or Diagnosis (TRIPOD): The TRIPOD Statement. *Ann. Intern. Med.* **2015**, *162*, 55. [CrossRef]
100. Lin, K.; Hu, Y.; Kong, G. Predicting in-hospital mortality of patients with acute kidney injury in the ICU using random forest model. *Int. J. Med. Inform.* **2019**, *125*, 55–61. [CrossRef]
101. Wilson, F.P. Machine Learning to Predict Acute Kidney Injury. *Am. J. Kidney Dis.* **2019**. [CrossRef]
102. Kate, R.J.; Perez, R.M.; Mazumdar, D.; Pasupathy, K.S.; Nilakantan, V. Prediction and detection models for acute kidney injury in hospitalized older adults. *BMC Med. Inform. Decis. Mak.* **2016**, *16*, 39. [CrossRef] [PubMed]
103. Thottakkara, P.; Ozrazgat-Baslanti, T.; Hupf, B.B.; Rashidi, P.; Pardalos, P.; Momcilovic, P.; Bihorac, A. Application of Machine Learning Techniques to High-Dimensional Clinical Data to Forecast Postoperative Complications. *PLoS ONE* **2016**, *11*, e0155705. [CrossRef] [PubMed]
104. Davis, S.E.; Lasko, T.A.; Chen, G.; Siew, E.D.; Matheny, M.E. Calibration drift in regression and machine learning models for acute kidney injury. *J. Am. Med. Inform. Assoc.* **2017**, *24*, 1052–1061. [CrossRef] [PubMed]

105. Cheng, P.; Waitman, L.R.; Hu, Y.; Liu, M. Predicting Inpatient Acute Kidney Injury over Different Time Horizons: How Early and Accurate? *AMIA Annu. Symp. Proc.* **2017**, *2017*, 565–574. Available online: http://www.ncbi.nlm.nih.gov/pubmed/29854121 (accessed on 20 January 2020).
106. Ibrahim, N.E.; McCarthy, C.P.; Shrestha, S.; Gaggin, H.K.; Mukai, R.; Magaret, C.A.; Rhyne, R.F.; Januzzi, J.L., Jr. A clinical, proteomics, and artificial intelligence-driven model to predict acute kidney injury in patients undergoing coronary angiography. *Clin. Cardiol.* **2019**, *42*, 292–298. [CrossRef]
107. Koola, J.D.; Davis, S.E.; Al-Nimri, O.; Parr, S.K.; Fabbri, D.; Malin, B.A.; Ho, S.B.; Matheny, M.E. Development of an automated phenotyping algorithm for hepatorenal syndrome. *J. Biomed. Inform.* **2018**, *80*, 87–95. [CrossRef]
108. Koyner, J.L.; Carey, K.A.; Edelson, D.P.; Churpek, M.M. The Development of a Machine Learning Inpatient Acute Kidney Injury Prediction Model. *Crit. Care Med.* **2018**, *46*, 1070–1077. [CrossRef]
109. Huang, C.; Murugiah, K.; Mahajan, S.; Li, S.X.; Dhruva, S.S.; Haimovich, J.S.; Wang, Y.; Schulz, W.L.; Testani, J.M.; Wilson, F.P.; et al. Enhancing the prediction of acute kidney injury risk after percutaneous coronary intervention using machine learning techniques: A retrospective cohort study. Rahimi K, ed. *PLoS Med.* **2018**, *15*, e1002703. [CrossRef]
110. Huang, C.; Li, S.-X.; Mahajan, S.; Testani, J.M.; Wilson, F.P.; Mena, C.I.; Masoudi, F.A.; Rumsfeld, J.S.; Spertus, J.A.; Mortazavi, B.J.; et al. Development and Validation of a Model for Predicting the Risk of Acute Kidney Injury Associated With Contrast Volume Levels During Percutaneous Coronary Intervention. *JAMA Netw. Open* **2019**, *2*, e1916021. [CrossRef]
111. Tomašev, N.; Glorot, X.; Rae, J.W.; Zielinski, M.; Askham, H.; Saraiva, A.; Mottram, A.; Meyer, C.; Ravuri, S.; Protsyuk, I.; et al. A clinically applicable approach to continuous prediction of future acute kidney injury. *Nature* **2019**, *572*, 116–119. [CrossRef]
112. Adhikari, L.; Ozrazgat-Baslanti, T.; Ruppert, M.; Madushani, R.W.M.A.; Paliwal, S.; Hashemighouchani, H.; Zheng, F.; Tao, M.; Lopes, J.M.; Li, X.; et al. Improved predictive models for acute kidney injury with IDEA: Intraoperative Data Embedded Analytics. *PLoS ONE* **2019**, *14*, e0214904. [CrossRef] [PubMed]
113. Flechet, M.; Falini, S.; Bonetti, C.; Güiza, F.; Schetz, M.; Van den Berghe, G.; Meyfroidt, G. Machine learning versus physicians' prediction of acute kidney injury in critically ill adults: A prospective evaluation of the AKIpredictor. *Crit. Care* **2019**, *23*, 282. [CrossRef] [PubMed]
114. Parreco, J.; Soe-Lin, H.; Parks, J.J.; Byerly, S.; Chatoor, M.; Buicko, J.L.; Namias, N.; Rattan, R. Comparing Machine Learning Algorithms for Predicting Acute Kidney Injury. *Am. Surg.* **2019**, *85*, 725–729. Available online: http://www.ncbi.nlm.nih.gov/pubmed/31405416 (accessed on 20 January 2020). [PubMed]
115. Xu, Z.; Luob, Y.; Adekkanattua, P.; Ancker, J.S.; Jiang, G.; Kiefer, R.C.; Pacheco, J.A.; Rasmussen, L.V.; Pathak, J.; Wang, F. Stratified Mortality Prediction of Patients with Acute Kidney Injury in Critical Care. *Stud. Health Technol. Inform.* **2019**, *264*, 462–466.
116. Tran, N.K.; Sen, S.; Palmieri, T.L.; Lima, K.; Falwell, S.; Wajda, J.; Rashidi, H.H. Artificial intelligence and machine learning for predicting acute kidney injury in severely burned patients: A proof of concept. *Burns* **2019**, *45*, 1350–1358. [CrossRef]
117. Zhang, Z.; Ho, K.M.; Hong, Y. Machine learning for the prediction of volume responsiveness in patients with oliguric acute kidney injury in critical care. *Crit. Care* **2019**, *23*, 112. [CrossRef]
118. Zimmerman, L.P.; Reyfman, P.A.; Smith, A.D.R.; Zeng, Z.; Kho, A.; Sanchez-Pinto, L.N.; Luo, Y. Early prediction of acute kidney injury following ICU admission using a multivariate panel of physiological measurements. *BMC Med. Inform. Decis. Mak.* **2019**, *19* (Suppl. S1), 16. [CrossRef]
119. Rashidi, H.H.; Sen, S.; Palmieri, T.L.; Blackmon, T.; Wajda, J.; Tran, N.K. Early Recognition of Burn- and Trauma-Related Acute Kidney Injury: A Pilot Comparison of Machine Learning Techniques. *Sci. Rep.* **2020**, *10*, 205. [CrossRef]

12

Physical Activity and the Development of Post-Transplant Diabetes Mellitus, and Cardiovascular- and All-Cause Mortality in Renal Transplant Recipients

Oyuntugs Byambasukh [1,2,*], Maryse C. J. Osté [3], António W. Gomes-Neto [3], Else van den Berg [3], Gerjan Navis [3], Stephan J. L. Bakker [3] and Eva Corpeleijn [1]

1 Department of Epidemiology, University Medical Center Groningen, University of Groningen, 9713 GZ Groningen, The Netherlands; e.corpeleijn@umcg.nl
2 Department of Internal Medicine, Mongolian National University of Medical Sciences, 976 Ulaanbaatar, Mongolia
3 Department of Nephrology, University Medical Center Groningen, University of Groningen, 9700 RB Groningen, The Netherlands; m.c.j.oste@umcg.nl (M.C.J.O.); a.w.gomes.neto@umcg.nl (A.W.G.-N.); e.van.den.berg@umcg.nl (E.v.d.B.); g.j.navis@umcg.nl (G.N.); s.j.l.bakker@umcg.nl (S.J.L.B.)
* Correspondence: o.byambasukh@umcg.nl or oyuntugs@mnums.edu.mn

Abstract: (1) Background: Little is currently known about the health impacts of daily-life moderate-to-vigorous physical activity (MVPA) in relation to the development of post-transplant diabetes mellitus (PTDM) and the long-term survival of renal transplant recipients (RTRs). (2) Methods: We analyzed self-reported data on MVPA within non-occupational and occupational domains, estimated with the SQUASH questionnaire, from a prospective cohort study of RTRs ($n = 650$) with a functioning graft exceeding 1 year. PTDM diagnoses were based on plasma glucose levels (≥126 mg/dL), HbA1c (≥6.5%), and the use of antidiabetic medication. Mortality data were retrieved from patient files up to the end of September 2015. (3) Results: During a median follow-up period of 5.3 years, 50 patients (10%) developed PTDM and 129 (19.8%) died. Of these deaths, 53 (8.9%) were caused by cardiovascular disease. Cox regression analyses showed that higher MVPA levels among patients were associated with a lower risk of PTDM (hazard ratio (HR); 95% confidence interval (95%CI) = 0.49; 0.25–0.96, $p = 0.04$), cardiovascular- (0.34; 0.15–0.77, $p = 0.01$), and all-cause mortality (0.37; 0.24–0.58, $p < 0.001$) compared with No-MVPA patients, independently of age, sex, and kidney function parameters. Associations of MVPA with cardiovascular and all-cause mortality remained significant and materially unchanged following further adjustments made for transplant characteristics, lifestyle factors, metabolic parameters, medication use, and creatinine excretion (muscle mass). However, the association between MVPA and PTDM was no longer significant after we adjusted for metabolic confounders and glucose levels. (4) Conclusion: Higher MVPA levels are associated with long-term health outcomes in RTRs.

Keywords: physical activity; renal transplant recipients; transplantation; post-transplant diabetes mellitus; cardiovascular mortality; mortality

1. Introduction

Renal transplantation is a more effective treatment strategy than chronic dialysis in patients with end-stage renal disease [1]. However, post-transplant patients are at an increased risk of developing cardiometabolic diseases that lead to high morbidity and mortality among renal transplant recipients (RTRs) [2,3]. The cardiovascular mortality rate is estimated to be 10 times higher for RTRs compared with the general population [2]. Moreover, approximately 20% of RTRs develop post-transplant diabetes mellitus (PTDM) [3]. This situation necessitates an investigation aimed at developing strategies for improving the management of long-term health outcomes in RTRs.

Studies have consistently found that physical activity (PA) is a modifiable factor that contributes to reducing the risk of cardiometabolic diseases and premature mortality within the general population [4,5]. However, there is limited data on the impacts of PA on RTRs [6–10]. Studies conducted on the benefits of PA have mostly focused on the intermediate outcomes of clinical trials entailing exercise training programmes [6–8]. A few studies found that a low PA is significantly associated with substantial weight gain and with risks of cardiovascular and all-cause mortality in RTRs [11–14]. Moreover, it remains unclear whether the benefits of increased PA in relation to patients' long-term outcomes are independent of their health and transplant characteristics (i.e., kidney function and duration of pre-transplant dialysis), lifestyle factors, and use of medication [11–13].

Clinical guidelines for the general population recommend the performance of at least 150 min of moderate-to-vigorous physical activity (MVPA) per week [15]. There are no specific clinical guidelines or recommendations for RTRs. A recent position statement on exercise for solid organ transplant recipients released in 2019 recommending that it is a key step toward raising awareness of the importance of exercise training in the patients among transplant professionals [16]. The available data show that the level of daily-life PA is lower for RTRs compared with individuals within the general population [17–19]. It is unclear whether individuals within the general population as well as RTRs can attain the recommended MVPA level by engaging in different domains of daily-life activities, such as non-occupational and occupational activities. Results showed that occupational MVPA should not be included within assessments of healthy daily-life PA and should not be deemed a substitute for leisure time MVPA. Specifically, it is not known whether both non-occupational and occupational PA can contribute to the improved health of RTRs [20–22].

Therefore, we aimed to investigate the association between daily-life MVPA and the risk of developing long-term health outcomes, such as PTDM as well as cardiovascular and all-cause mortality in RTRs sampled from a large prospective study. We also examined whether these associations were independent of several variables, including age, sex, kidney function, transplant characteristics, lifestyle factors, medication use, metabolic parameters, and anthropometric measures. Moreover, we assessed the benefits of non-occupational MVPA as well as total daily-life MVPA, including occupational PA.

2. Methods

2.1. Study Population

This study was conducted in a large single-center prospective cohort of stable outpatient RTR [23,24]. A total of 817 adult RTRs who met the study's eligibility criteria, namely having a functioning graft for at least 1 year and no history of alcohol and/or drug addiction, were invited to participate in the study. Further exclusions were apparent systemic diseases, such as malignancies or active infections. In total, 707 (86.5%) RTRs signed written informed consent. Baseline data were collected between November 2008 and May 2011. We excluded 57 RTRs, whose PA questionnaires were incomplete, from the analysis, leaving a total of 650 RTRs. Subsequently, 148 and 61 RTRs, respectively, with a history of diabetes and cardiovascular diseases (CVDs) prior to undergoing transplants, were excluded from the analyses of PA and the development of PTDM and cardiovascular mortality. The study was conducted according to the Helsinki Declaration and was approved by the UMCG's review board (METc 2008/186).

2.2. Measurements at Baseline

All baseline measurements have been previously described in greater detail elsewhere [25]. Body mass index (BMI) was calculated as weight (kg) divided by height squared (m^2). A semiautomatic device (Dinamap®1846; Critikon, Tampa, FL, USA) was used to measure blood pressure in a half-sitting position and the average of the final three readings of blood pressure was used. Information on medication was derived from patient records. Daily caloric intake and alcohol consumption were calculated from a validated Food Frequency questionnaire. Information on smoking was obtained by a questionnaire. The serum creatinine-based Chronic Kidney Disease Epidemiology Collaboration equation was used to calculate the estimated glomerular filtration rate (eGFR) [26]. Creatinine excretion—a marker of muscle mass—was calculated from the 24-h urine collection as described earlier [27].

2.3. *Assessment of Physical Activity*

The SQUASH is a validated questionnaire used to estimate habitual physical activities performed during a normal week [28]. The SQUASH is pre-structured into four domains: commuting, leisure time and sports, household, and occupational activities. Questions consisted of three main queries: days per week, average time per day, and intensity. In this study, we used activities at the moderate (4.0–6.5 MET) to vigorous (≥6.5 MET) level. Metabolic equivalent (MET) values were assigned to activities according to Ainsworth's Compendium of Physical Activities [29]. We used the combination of leisure-time and commuting (non-occupational) moderate-to-vigorous physical activity (MVPA) minutes per week (min/week) as a measure of PA in this study, since active commuting of high intensity and longer duration is often replacing sports activities, like cycling. We did not include occupational MVPA in the main analysis because of its health benefit is not clear in the general population [20–22,30]. In an additional analysis, we investigated the association between total MVPA, including occupational MVPA, with clinical endpoints. Participants were subdivided into three categories based on their levels of non-occupational MVPA. RTRs who did not engage in PA at a moderate-to-vigorous level were deemed 'inactive' (no-MVPA), and the remaining participants (MVPA > 0) were divided into two groups based on median values of non-occupational MVPA (less active, MVPA-1 and active, MVPA-2). The MVPA min/week (median, interquartile range (IQR)) was used to define the MVPA groups (MVPA-1 and MVPA-2): 5-197 (120, 60–150) and 200–1680 (360, 260–540).

2.4. *Endpoints of the Study*

Endpoints of interest in this study were post-transplant diabetes mellitus (PTDM), cardiovascular and all-cause mortality. PTDM was defined according to the presence of at least one of the following criteria: diabetes symptoms (e.g., polyuria, polydipsia, or unexplained weight loss) along with a non-fasting plasma glucose concentration of ≥200 mg/dL (11.1 mmol/L); fasting plasma glucose concentration (FPG) ≥ 126 mg/dL (7.0 mmol/L); start of antidiabetic medication; or HbA1c ≥ 6.5% (48 mmol/L). This definition matched the diagnostic criteria for diabetes applied by the American Diabetes Association, including HbA1c levels, as proposed by the expert panel constituted at the international consensus meeting on PTDM [31,32]. Cardiovascular mortality and all-cause mortality were monitored through continuous surveillance conducted within the outpatient program and retrieved from patients' files up to the end of September 2015. No participants were lost to follow-up.

2.5. *Statistical Analysis*

The patient characteristics are expressed as means with a standard deviation for normally distributed variables or as medians with interquartile range (25th to 75th percentile) for non-normally distributed variables and numbers with percentages in case of categorical data. The differences between groups were tested using 1-way analysis of variance tests or Kruskal–Wallis tests for normally and non-normally distributed continuous variables, respectively. The frequency distributions of categorical variables were analyzed using the Pearson Chi-Square test.

We adopted MVPA as a continuous and categorical variable in a Cox regression analysis. First, we tested associations of non-occupational MVPA, considered as a continuous variable, on clinical endpoints. In this analysis, MVPA (measured in min/week) was log-transformed to obtain a normal distribution. Thereafter, multivariate Cox regression analyses were performed to examine whether higher non-occupational MVPA is associated with lower risks of PTDM, cardiovascular mortality, and all-cause mortality independently of potential confounders which are clinically known confounders in the relating associations of physical activity with long-term outcomes [6,7,12–14,33]. In these analyses, we first adjusted for age and sex (model 1) as well as kidney function parameters, including eGFR, proteinuria, the time lapse between transplantation and the baseline measures, and primary renal disease (model 2). We further adjusted model 1 for transplant characteristics (acute rejection, preemptive transplantation, and living donor status) in model 3. Similarly, we adjusted model 1 for lifestyle factors, such as smoking, alcohol consumption, and daily caloric intake (model 4); calcineurin inhibitors and prednisolone used as immunosuppressive medication (model 5); systolic blood pressure, use of antihypertensive drugs, high-density lipoprotein cholesterol (HDL), and triglycerides (model 6), BMI and waist circumference (model 7), and 24-h creatinine excretion (model 8). With regard to potential collinearity (model 7), we tested the correlation between BMI and waist circumference ($r = 0.84$, $p < 0.001$ for men and $r = 0.81$, $p < 0.001$ for women). Then we performed Cox-regression analyses using separate models adjusted for BMI and waist circumference separately (Supplementary materials, Table S1. We found no differences relating to the confounding effects of total fat and fat distribution. Finally, we included those variables in the same model. In addition, we adjusted model 1 for baseline hemoglobin A1C and fasting plasma glucose (model 9) relating to the association between MVPA and PTDM. We also adjusted model 1 relating to the association between MVPA and PTDM for diet quality (Model 10). We furthermore investigated whether diet quality might modify the association of MVPA with development of PTDM by additional inclusion of a product-term of the continuous variables of diet quality and MVPA in the concerned model, to assess potential interaction between the two. Mediterranean diet score was used as diet quality and assessed with a 177-item validated food frequency questionnaire which is described in greater detail elsewhere [33]. All models (1-10) include up to 6 variables to fulfil the rule of thumb which allows 1 variable per 7–10 events. This is now fulfilled for all analyses [34,35]. Hazard ratios were reported with 95% confidence intervals. Proportional hazard assumptions were tested using the Schoenfield residuals method developed by Grambsch and Therneau [36]. Penalized splines were constructed to visualize the association of non-occupational MVPA with PTDM as well as cardiovascular and all-cause mortality independently of age and sex.

We performed additional analyses to explore the role of work within this population by investigating the associations between total MVPA, including occupational MVPA, and non-occupational MVPA with clinical endpoints for the RTRs who worked ($n = 322$, 49.5%). Occupational status was defined using the answers for the questions related to occupational PA. If responders answered as not applicable, we considered them as unemployed. Another subgroup analysis was performed to address changes in these associations across age categories. The population was categorized as being over or under 55 years of age, based on the WHO guideline on the prevention of CVD [37]. Finally, to rule out competing mortality risks associated with the occurrence of PTDM, we conducted competing risk analyses following the procedures outlined by Fine and Gray [38].

A two-sided statistical significance was set at $p < 0.05$ for all tests. All statistical analyses were performed using SPSS software V.22 (IBM Inc., Chicago, IL, USA,) R software V.3.2.2 (R Foundation for Statistical Computing, Vienna, Austria), STATA version 13.0 (StataCorp LP, College Station, TX, USA) and Graph Pad Prism 7 (Graph Pad Software Inc., La Jolla, CA, USA).

3. Results

3.1. Baseline Characteristics

A total of 650 RTRs (men: 56.3%, mean age: 51.8 ± 13.2 years old) were examined in this study. Baseline measurements were taken 5.7 years (median value; interquartile range (IQR): 1.9–12.1 years) post-transplantation. Of the total sample of RTRs, 37.8% ($n = 246$) did not perform daily MPVA at all within any domain. The other RTRs spent a median of 200 min (IQR = 120–360 min per week) engaged in non-occupational MVPA. Table 1 shows the baseline characteristics of RTRs according to their non-occupational MVPA levels. RTRs in the active groups (MVPA > 0) had lower values for BMI, waist circumference, and systolic blood pressure and higher creatinine excretion values compared with the values of the inactive group (no-MVPA). Moreover, higher alcohol consumption, lower concentrations of triglycerides and HDL-C, haemoglobin A1C, and less proteinuria and diabetes at the baseline level along with more 'living donors' were observed for the 'active' groups compared with the 'inactive' group. Table S2 presents the baseline characteristics of the RTRs according to the presence of clinical endpoints. Figure S1 further shows levels of daily MVPA according to the participants' ages and work status. As expected, total MVPA values, including those for occupational MVPA, were significantly higher in RTRs who were working (n = 322). However, when working status or age was considered, the levels of non-occupational MVPA did not differ significantly.

Table 1. Characteristics of the study population, according to MVPA level.

Variable	Total (n = 650)	No-MVPA (n = 246)	MVPA-1 (n = 201)	MVPA-2 (n = 203)	p-Value
Age (years)	52.6 ± 12.8	54.1 ± 11.8	51.9 ± 13.4	51.6 ± 13.3	0.08
Male gender (%, n)	56.3 (366)	56.1 (138)	55.7 (112)	57.1 (116)	0.96
Current smoking (%, n)	12.3 (80)	15.3 (36)	12.4 (25)	9.5 (19)	0.20
Occupational status: Employed * (%, n)	49.5 (322)	44.7 (110)	51.2 (103)	53.7 (109)	0.14
Alcohol use (g/day)	2.61 (0.1–11.1)	1.45 (0.1–9.7)	2.51 (0.1–9.7)	3.95 (0.1–14.1)	0.01
Total energy intake (kcal/d)	2174.9 ± 640.7	2114.7± 720.4	2247.5 ± 598.7	2173.2 ± 573.9	0.11
Non-occupational MVPA (min/week)	90 (0–240)	0	120 (60–150)	360 (260–540)	–
Anthropometric measures					
Body mass index (kg/m^2)	26.7 ± 4.84	27.9 ± 5.49	25.7 ± 4.26	26.1 ± 4.23	0.001
Waist circumference, men (cm)	101.1 ± 13.4	104.0 ± 13.7	98.9 ± 13.5	99.7 ± 12.4	0.01
Waist circumference, women (cm)	95.0 ± 15.8	99.7 ± 12.4	91.5 ± 14.6	93.1 ± 14.1	0.01
Creatinine excretion (mmol/24h)	11.7 ± 3.49	11.2 ± 3.80	11.8 ± 3.29	12.2 ± 3.23	0.01
Lipids and blood pressure					
Total cholesterol (mmol/L)	5.14 ± 1.11	5.18 ± 1.18	5.17 ± 1.10	5.07 ± 1.02	0.48
Triglyceride (mmol/L)	1.68 (1.2–2.33)	1.85 (1.3–2.6)	1.67 (1.2–2.4)	1.59 (1.2–2.05)	0.001
HDL-C in men (mmol/L)	1.27 ± 0.41	1.23 ± 0.41	1.27 ± 0.36	1.32 ± 0.45	0.21
HDL-C in women (mmol/L)	1.56 ± 0.51	1.39 ± 0.43	1.62 ± 0.54	1.70 ± 0.53	0.001
Systolic blood pressure (mm Hg)	136.2 ± 17.3	138.3 ± 18.5	135.6 ± 16.7	134.2 ± 16.3	0.04
Diastolic blood pressure (mm Hg)	82.8 ± 10.9	83.1 ± 11.2	82.5 ± 11.3	82.6 ± 10.3	0.77
Cardiovascular medication use					
Antihypertensive (%, n)	88 (572)	92.7 (228)	81.1 (163)	89.2 (181)	0.001
A2 antagonist (%, n)	14.8 (96)	15.4 (38)	12.9 (26)	15.8 (32)	0.68
ACE inhibitor (%, n)	32.2 (209)	32.1 (79)	30.3 (61)	34.0 (69)	0.74
RAAS blockers (%, n)	47.8 (311)	49.2 (121)	44.8 (90)	49.3 (100)	0.58
Beta-blockers (%, n)	63.2 (411)	63.4 (156)	62.2 (125)	64.0 (130)	0.93
Calcium channel blockers (%, n)	24.5 (159)	26.0 (64)	20.4 (41)	26.6 (54)	0.27
Diuretics (%, n)	40.0 (260)	52.0 (128)	27.4 (50)	37.9 (77)	0.001
Vitamin K antagonist (%, n)	11.4 (74)	13 (32)	10.4 (21)	10.3 (21)	0.60
mTOR inhibitor (%, n)	1.8 (12)	3.3 (8)	1 (2)	1 (2)	0.60
Anti-diabetic drugs (%, n)	14.8 (96)	18.7 (46)	14.4 (29)	10.3 (21)	0.045
Statin (%, n)	51.8 (337)	54.9 (135)	52.7 (106)	47.3 (96)	0.27
Glucose metabolism					
Fasting plasma glucose (mmol/L)	5.67 ± 1.82	5.78 ± 192	5.76 ± 2.13	5.46 ± 1.28	0.13
Heamoglobin A1C (%)	5.94 ± 0.78	6.03 ± 0.77	5.94 ± 0.90	5.83 ± 0.65	0.021
Kidney function					
eGFR (mL/min/1.73m^2)	52.0 ± 20.2	49.9 ± 22.1	53.8 ± 18.7	52.9 ± 18.8	0.09
Albumin excretion (mg/24h)	267.3 ± 734.6	307.2 ± 777.5	175.1 ± 378.5	308.7 ± 917.5	0.11
Proteinuria (%, n)	21.5 (140)	28.0 (69)	16.9 (34)	18.2 (37)	0.01

Table 1. *Cont.*

Variable	Total (n = 650)	No-MVPA (n = 246)	MVPA-1 (n = 201)	MVPA-2 (n = 203)	p-Value
Primary renal disease (%, n)					0.01
Glomerulosclerosis	28.8 (187)	30.1 (74)	28.4 (57)	27.6 (56)	
Glomerulonephritis	7.7 (50)	5.7 (14)	8.0 (16)	9.9 (20)	
Tubulointerstitial nephritis	11.8 (77)	9.8 (24)	12.9 (26)	13.3 (27)	
Polycystic kidney disease	20.9 (136)	20.7 (51)	19.9 (40)	22.2 (45)	
Renal hypodysplasia	3.5 (23)	4.1 (10)	3.0 (6)	3.4 (7)	
Renavascular diseases	5.7 (37)	7.7 (19)	4.0 (8)	4.9 (10)	
Diabetes mellitus	4.6 (30)	6.5 (16)	5.5 (11)	1.5 (3)	
Others	16.9 (110)	15.4 (38)	18.4 (37)	17.2 (35)	
Duration of dialysis before the transplantation (months)	25 (8–48)	29 (11–51)	19 (4–49)	25 (9–43)	0.51
Transplant characteristics					
Transplant vintage (months)	14.0 (2.0–39.5)	17.0 (2.0–41.0)	12.0 (2.0–44.8)	16.0 (0.5–41.0)	0.49
Cold ischemia time (h)	15.2 (2.8–21.1)	16.4 (3.6–22.0)	15.1 (2.6–21.3)	13.6 (2.5–20.5)	0.10
Living donor (%, n)	34.8 (226)	26.4 (65)	37.3 (75)	42.4 (86)	0.001
Pre-emptive transplant (%, n)	16.6 (108)	13.4 (33)	20.9 (42)	16.3 (33)	0.11
Acute rejection	27.2 (177)	27.2 (67)	27.9 (56)	26.6 (54)	0.96
Immunosuppressive medication					
Calcineurin inhibitor (%, n)	58.3 (379)	59.8 (147)	59.2 (119)	55.7 (113)	0.52
Proliferation inhibitor (%, n)	82.6 (537)	80.1 (197)	84.1 (169)	84.2 (171)	0.62
Prednisolone dose (mg)	10.0 (7.5–10.0)	10.0 (7.5–10.0)	10.0 (7.5–10.0)	10.0 (7.5–10.0)	0.48

Data are presented as mean ± SD or median (interquartile range) and percentage (%, number). MVPA = moderate-to-vigorous physical activity, HDL-C = high-density lipoprotein cholesterol, eGFR = estimated glomerular filtration rate, A2 = angiotensin 2, ACE = angiotensin-converting-enzyme, RAAS = renin–angiotensin–aldosterone system, mTOR = mammalian target of rapamycin. * the number of patients that do have employment.

3.2. Post-Transplant Diabetes Mellitus

A total of 50 RTRs (10%) had developed PTDM after a median follow-up period of 5.3 years (4.1–6.0 years). The multivariable Cox proportional hazard models showed that the group with the highest level of non-occupational MVPA was associated with a lower risk of PTDM (hazard ratio (HR); 95% CI = 0.49; 0.25–0.96, p = 0.04) compared with the no-MVPA group, independently of age, sex, and kidney function parameters (model 1, Table 2). This association remained significant after we made further adjustments for kidney function parameters, transplant characteristics, lifestyle factors, Mediterranean diet score and 24-h creatinine excretion quantities (considered as a marker of muscle mass) (models 2–4, 8, and 10). Following adjustments made for immunosuppressive medication (model 5), metabolic parameters (model 6), anthropometric measures (model 7), and baseline glucose levels (model 9), the highest level of MVPA was no longer associated with PTDM. However, when MVPA was applied as a continuous variable in the Cox regression analysis, as opposed to using groups of MVPA levels, a higher non-occupational MVPA was associated with a lower risk of PTDM independent of all of the above-mentioned confounders apart from the adjustment of metabolic parameters and glucose level.

Table 2. Association of non-occupational MVPA with long-term health outcomes.

Physical Activity	MVPA (cont.)		No-MVPA (Ref)	MVPA-1		MVPA-2	
	HR (95% CI)	*p*		HR (95% CI)	*p*	HR (95% CI)	*p*
			Post-transplant DM				
No. of events	50/502		23	14		13	
Model 1	0.88 (0.79–0.97)	0.01	1.00	0.57 (0.29–1.10)	0.09	0.49 (0.25–0.96)	0.04
Model 2	0.88 (0.79–0.98)	0.02	1.00	0.61 (0.31–1.20)	0.15	0.49 (0.25–0.96)	0.04
Model 3	0.88 (0.79–0.98)	0.02	1.00	0.55 (0.28–1.07)	0.08	0.48 (0.24–0.95)	0.04
Model 4	0.87 (0.79–0.97)	0.01	1.00	0.57 (0.29–1.12)	0.10	0.46 (0.22–0.94)	0.03
Model 5	0.89 (0.80–0.99)	0.03	1.00	0.59 (0.30–1.26)	0.11	0.52 (0.26–1.03)	0.06
Model 6	0.91 (0.82–1.01)	0.09	1.00	0.70 (0.36–1.40)	0.31	0.60 (0.29–1.22)	0.16
Model 7	0.88 (0.79–0.99)	0.03	1.00	0.63 (0.31–1.25)	0.19	0.50 (0.25–1.03)	0.06
Model 8	0.87 (0.79–0.97)	0.01	1.00	0.55 (0.29–1.08)	0.08	0.47 (0.24–0.93)	0.03
Model 9	0.91 (0.82–1.01)	0.12	1.00	0.72 (0.36–1.41)	0.34	0.59 (0.30–1.19)	0.14
Model 10	0.87 (0.78–0.97)	0.01	1.00	0.58 (0.32–1.25)	0.11	0.44 (0.21–0.92)	0.03
			Cardiovascular mortality				
No. of events	53/589		26	14		13	
Model 1	0.84 (0.74–0.94)	0.01	1.00	0.45 (0.22–0.94)	0.03	0.34 (0.15–0.77)	0.01
Model 2	0.84 (0.75–0.95)	0.01	1.00	0.49 (0.23–1.02)	0.06	0.35 (0.16–0.80)	0.01
Model 3	0.86 (0.76–0.96)	0.01	1.00	0.51 (0.25–1.05)	0.07	0.40 (0.18–0.91)	0.03
Model 4	0.87 (0.77–0.98)	0.02	1.00	0.56 (0.26–1.21)	0.14	0.43 (0.19–0.94)	0.046
Model 5	0.84 (0.74–0.94)	0.001	1.00	0.45 (0.21–0.93)	0.03	0.36 (0.16–0.81)	0.01
Model 6	0.85 (0.76–0.96)	0.001	1.00	0.49 (0.23–1.02)	0.06	0.38 (0.17–0.86)	0.02
Model 7	0.85 (0.75–0.96)	0.01	1.00	0.51 (0.23–1.11)	0.09	0.40 (0.17–0.92)	0.03
Model 8	0.87 (0.77–0.98)	0.02	1.00	0.55 (0.26–1.16)	0.12	0.44 (0.19–0.99)	0.051
			All-cause mortality				
No. of events	129/650		76	27		26	
Model 1	0.84 (0.78–0.89)	<0.001	1.00	0.39 (0.25–0.61)	<0.001	0.37 (0.24–0.58)	<0.001
Model 2	0.85 (0.79–0.91)	<0.001	1.00	0.43 (0.27–0.67)	<0.001	0.40 (0.26–0.63)	<0.001
Model 3	0.85 (0.79–0.91)	<0.001	1.00	0.41 (0.27–0.64)	<0.001	0.41 (0.26–0.64)	<0.001
Model 4	0.83 (0.77–0.89)	<0.001	1.00	0.41 (0.21–0.64)	<0.001	0.35 (0.22–0.58)	<0.001
Model 5	0.83 (0.78–0.89)	<0.001	1.00	0.39 (0.25–0.61)	<0.001	0.37 (0.23–0.58)	<0.001
Model 6	0.85 (0.79–0.91)	<0.001	1.00	0.42 (0.27–0.66)	<0.001	0.41 (0.26–0.65)	<0.001
Model 7	0.84 (0.78–0.89)	<0.001	1.00	0.40 (0.25–0.63)	<0.001	0.37 (0.23–0.59)	<0.001
Model 8	0.86 (0.80–0.92)	<0.001	1.00	0.45 (0.29–0.70)	<0.001	0.44 (0.28–0.69)	<0.001

DM = Diabetes mellitus, MVPA = moderate-to-vigorous physical activity. Model 1: adjusted for age and sex. Model 2: model 1 + adjustment for kidney function (eGFR, urinary protein excretion, time between transplantation and baseline, and primary renal disease). Model 3: model 1 + adjustment for transplant characteristics (acute rejection, pre-emptive transplantation, donor type). Model 4: model 1 + adjustment for lifestyle factors (smoking, alcohol consumption, daily caloric intake). Model 5: model 1 + adjustment for immunosuppressive medication (calcineurin inhibitors, prednisolonee). Model 6: model 1 + adjustment for lipids and blood pressure (systolic blood pressure, use of antihypertensive drugs, triglycerides, HDL-C). Model 7: model 1 + adjustment for BMI and waist circumference. Model 8: model 1 + adjustment for 24-h creatinine excretion. Model 9: model 1 + adjustment for fasting plasma glucose and HbA1c. Model 10: model 1 + adjustment for Mediterranean diet score.

3.3. Cardiovascular and All-Cause Mortality

During the follow-up period, 129 (19.8%) patients died. Of these deaths, 53 (8.9%) were caused by cardiovascular disease (CVD). In the multivariable Cox proportional hazard models, the highest level of non-occupational MVPA was associated with a lower risk of cardiovascular mortality (HR; 95% CI = 0.34; 0.15–0.77, $p = 0.01$) compared with the no-MVPA group, independently of age, sex, and kidney function parameters (model 1–2, Table 2). This association remained significant after further adjustments were made for transplant characteristics, immunosuppressive medication, metabolic parameters, and anthropometric measures (models 3, 5–7). However, the association was no longer significant after adjusting for lifestyle factors (model 4) and creatinine excretion (model 8). Moreover, the association of MVPA with cardiovascular mortality was sustained independently of all of the potential confounders when non-occupational MVPA was applied as a continuous variable in the Cox regression (models 1–9, Table 2).

With regard to all-cause mortality, the group with the highest level of non-occupational MVPA was associated with a lower risk of all-cause mortality (HR; 95% CI = 0.37; 0.24–0.58, $p < 0.001$) compared with the no-MVPA group (model 1, Table 2). This association remained significant after we adjusted for potential confounders (models 2–8). However, the association weakened after we adjusted for transplant characteristics (model 3), metabolic parameters (model 6), and creatinine excretion (model 8). When log-transformed non-occupational MVPA was applied as a continuous variable in the Cox regression analysis, the association was independent of all of the above-mentioned confounders, apart from creatinine excretion (model 8), remaining materially unchanged.

To illustrate these associations further, age-and sex-adjusted penalized splines and the Kaplan-Meier survival curves are shown in Figures 1 and 2.

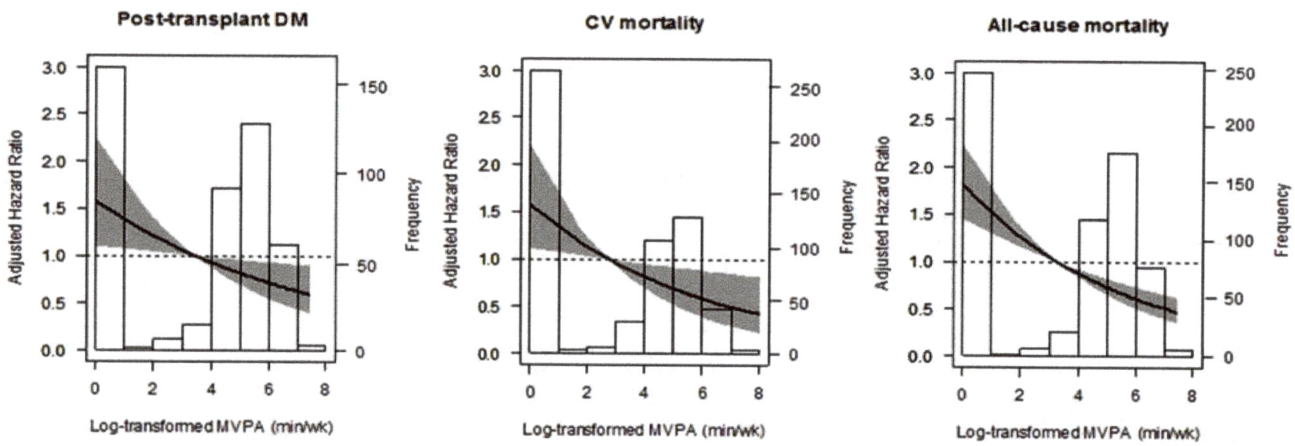

Figure 1. Association between non-occupational MVPA and post-transplant diabetes mellitus (PTDM), Cardiovascular (CV)mortality, and all-cause mortality in renal transplant recipients (RTRs).

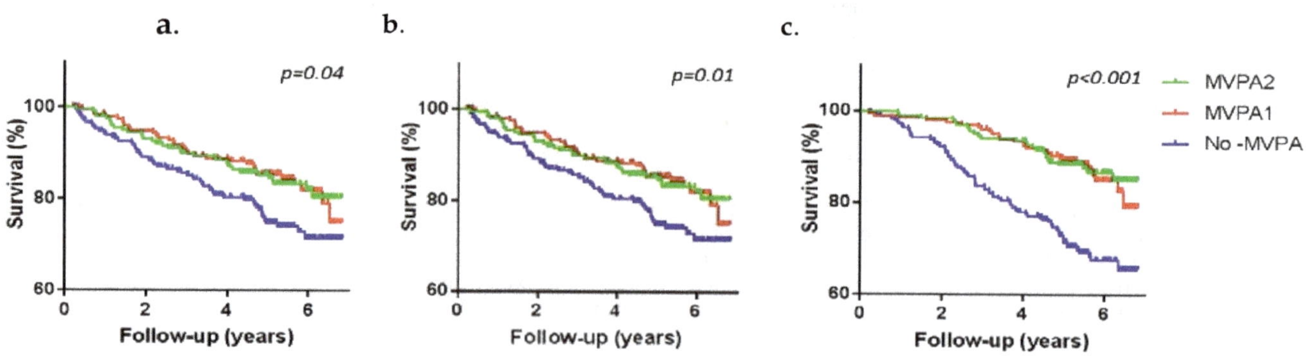

Figure 2. Probability of survival for PTDM (**a**), cardiovascular mortality (**b**), and all-cause mortality (**c**) according to non-occupational MVPA level.

3.4. Additional Analyses

Additional analyses of the subgroup of working RTRs revealed that the inclusion of occupational PA in the estimate of MVPA resulted in the attenuation of the HRs of all of the significant and non-significant associations (Table 3). The association of non-occupational MVPA with cardiovascular and all-cause mortality was stronger compared with that of total MVPA, which includes occupational MVPA.

Table 3. Additional analysis on the associations of MVPA with long-term health outcomes in RTRs who are working (n = 322).

Physical Activity	MVPA (cont.)		No-MVPA		MVPA > 0		
	HR^ (95% CI)	*p*-value	N *	Reference	N *	HR^^ (95% CI)	*p*-Value
Post-transplant DM							
Non-occupational PA	0.87 (0.74–1.03)	0.113	10	1.00	10	0.46 (0.18–1.13)	0.076
Total PA	0.91 (0.78–1.06)	0.212	8	1.00	12	0.48 (0.20–1.20)	0.056
Cardiovascular mortality							
Non-occupational PA	0.63 (0.48–0.83)	0.001	12	1.00	3	0.11 (0.11–0.42)	0.001
Total PA	0.75 (0.63–0.91)	0.003	9	1.00	6	0.23 (0.10–0.58)	0.051
All-cause mortality							
Non-occupational PA	0.76 (0.66–0.87)	<0.01	25	1.00	11	0.21 (0.14–0.51)	<0.01
Total PA	0.82 (0.74–0.92)	0.001	19	1.00	17	0.30 (0.18–0.58)	<0.01

Total PA was the sum of non-occupational and occupational MVPA in min/week. DM = diabetes mellitus, MVPA = moderate-to-vigorous physical activity, HR=hazard ratio, CVD = cardiovascular disease, N * = number of events. ^ Analyses were adjusted for age, gender, and kidney function parameters. ^^ Analyses were adjusted for age and gender (kidney function parameters excluded in this analysis due to fulfill the rule of thumb).

Age-stratified analyses revealed that associations of MVPA with long-term health outcomes were stronger in older adults (Figure 3).

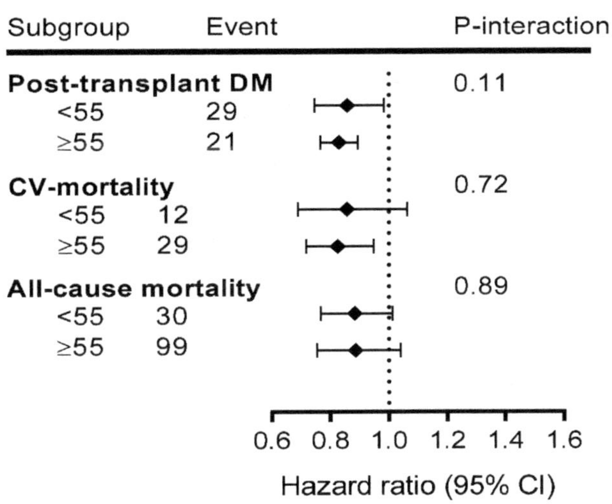

Figure 3. Subgroup analysis for the associations of MVPA with long-term health outcomes over age categories.

The results of the competing risk analyses showed that there was no strong influence of a competing risk of all-cause mortality on the association of MVPA with PTDM. For instance, the competing HR was 0.51 (0.30–0.92, p = 0.04) for the highest MVPA with PTDM after adjusting for age and sex. By comparison, the HR was 0.49 (0.25–0.96, p = 0.04, model 1, Table 2) when competing risks were discounted.

4. Discussion

We found that increased daily-life MVPA is associated with a reduced risk of PTDM, cardiovascular mortality, and all-cause mortality in RTRs independently of age, sex, baseline kidney function parameters, transplant characteristics, and other lifestyle habits. The association of MVPA with PTDM was affected by the adjustments we made for baseline glucose levels and metabolic parameters, but it did not seem to be affected by other potential confounders, notably anthropometric and immunosuppressive medication. The associations of MVPA with cardiovascular and all-cause mortality were not substantially affected by adjustments made for the above-mentioned confounders. These results confirm the importance of PA in the long-term healthcare management of RTRs.

Previous studies have found that PTDM is highly prevalent in RTRs [3,39]. However, data on lifestyle interventions for improving glucose tolerance or observational data on the association of increased PA with incidences of PTDM are lacking [13,40]. An intervention study showed that lifestyle modifications, including the incorporation of exercise training, improved 2-h postprandial glucose levels in RTRs who were glucose intolerant [40]. One observational study found that higher levels of PA are associated with a lower risk of glucose intolerance in RTRs [13]. However, this study entailed a cross-sectional design and did not test whether this association of PA is independent of other potential confounders. In our longitudinal study, the association of MVPA with PTDM was found to be independent of age, sex, baseline kidney function parameters, transplant characteristics, and other lifestyle factors, such as smoking, alcohol use, and diet (daily caloric intake and Mediterranean diet score). However, the association was affected by adjustments made for immunosuppressive medication, anthropometric measures (BMI and waist circumference), baseline glucose levels, and metabolic parameters. It is widely accepted that obesity is associated with the development of diabetes within the general population [41]. The use of immunosuppressive medications play a role in the development of PTDM through a pathway of stimulation of gluconeogenesis affecting increased blood glucose which can leads to insulin resistance in combination with other mechanisms [39]. However, when we applied log-transformed continuous MVPA, significant associations were observed after we adjusted for immunosuppressive medication and anthropometric measures, indicating that statistical power issues may also play a role. Thus, further large-scale studies of a longer duration should be conducted to explore whether or not MVPA is associated with PTDM independently of immunosuppressive medication and obesity. Furthermore, diet is an important factor in the development of diabetes. A previous analysis by Osté et al. for our study population showed that Mediterranean style diet predicts the development of PTDM [33]. We found that the association between MVPA and PTDM became slightly stronger when adjusted for Mediterranean diet score indicating the importance of diet, but there was no effect modification by diet quality (P-interaction = 0.147).

A previous study, investigating another sample of RTRs, found that a lower PA is strongly associated with an increased risk of cardiovascular and all-cause mortality [14]. In their Cox regression analyses, these authors found that the association was independent of potential confounders, including the history of CVD, muscle mass, and Framingham CVD risk score factors. However, they did not adjust for some clinical variables, such as kidney function and transplant characteristics (e.g., transplant vintage and donor type). Our study supports an independent association of PA with the risk of cardiovascular and all-cause mortality. Many studies have pointed to the benefit of PA within the general population in preventing premature mortality [4,5]. One of the mechanisms proposed to explain the effects of increased PA entails the improvement of all organ systems, especially the cardiovascular system. Specifically in RTRs, improved cardiovascular function is associated with improvements in kidney function. Increased physical activity can support perfusion and oxygen delivery in the kidneys. Studies have shown that higher levels of daily-life PA are associated with a lower risk of renal function decline within the general population and in patients with chronic kidney disease [42–44]. Consequently, increased PA, by improving kidney function, may be of benefit for long-term graft survival. This effect may also be due to improvements in metabolic dysfunctions, such as insulin resistance, impaired glucose tolerance, dyslipidemia, and hypertension, all of which are related to (central) adiposity [45–47]. Furthermore, a number of studies on diet analysed in-depth the effect of dietary factors on the same outcomes such as PTDM, renal function decline and mortality [23–25,33,48]. They suggest that lifestyle is very important for RTR, however, it should be noted that MVPA in daily life has not gotten that much attention. Taken together, these findings suggest that the improvement of daily-life MVPA needs to be evaluated as a therapy for improving patients' long-term survival.

Within this RTR population, MVPA levels were lower than those within the general population. In our study, 38% of RTRs were inactive (no-MVPA), whereas in the Lifelines cohort, a population-based study for which the same questionnaire (SQUASH) and comparable data processing methods were used, the prevalence of inactivity (no-MVPA) was 10% (n = 125,402, 40.5% males, median age of 45) [30,49]. Even in different age groups and gender, it was lower, ranging between 7.5% (n = 42,661, 40% of males, median age of 40) and 12.5% (n = 34,506, 45.6% of males, median age of 56) in the Lifelines. Lower PA levels among RTRs may be attributed to lower muscle mass (a structural abnormality) and muscle weakness (a functional abnormality) [6]. Our descriptive analysis indicated that inactive RTRs had a lower 24-h creatinine excretion value (a marker of muscle mass) compared with that of active RTRs. We also found that the duration of pre-transplantation dialysis was longer in inactive RTRs, although not significantly so. Studies concluded that low muscle mass can be caused by low PA levels [6,7,9]. This conclusion is in line with our findings, indicating that the association was slightly attenuated after we adjusted for renal factors and muscle mass but that the effect of PA remained evident. Actually a shorter time on dialysis would thus also help post-transplant health because studies showed that the level of PA declines in patients with end-stage kidney diseases and it increases after transplantation [7]. Finally, both recovery of activity after transplantation, as well as prevention of inactivity and loss of muscle mass in people with longstanding kidney disease is important for long-term health after transplantation.

A growing body of evidence is showing that occupational MVPA may have no clear benefit on health in the general population [20–22,30,49]. This was tested in our study including a specific patient population, the RTR. Even in the case of RTR, where being at work may be indicative of relatively good health, individuals who were much more active in terms of their occupational MVPA may not obtain any additional benefits for health. A clear mechanism that prevents occupational PA from generating health benefits is missing. There is always the possibility of residual confounding by factors such as sex, socioeconomic status, work-related stress, and body weight in the association between occupational PA and health outcomes [20,22,30,49]. Studies attempted to explore the possibility of residual confounding, but also found no clear association of occupational MVPA and health outcomes. Thus, we suggest that it is important to be aware that occupational MVPA should not be considered as a substitute for leisure time MVPA in RTR.

The potential benefit of PA seems to be more pronounced in older adults, a phenomenon that was described before in the general population [50]. In the general population, studies concluded that the benefit of PA can be gained more easily when there is more room for improvement, like as in older people. However, it might also be that its effects will be potentially outweighed by other, more important clinical factors (e.g., comorbidities and medication use). Therefore, we attempted to test the effect of physical activity in specific groups such as in RTR in two age groups. We found that a higher MVPA is strongly associated with the development of long-term outcomes such as PTDM and cardiovascular mortality in younger and older adults, but is especially stronger in older adults. Thus, older RTR who are able to remain active despite their longstanding condition are likely to remain relatively healthy.

The strengths of this study include its prospective design, long duration, and complete follow-up. Another strength is we included stable RTRs after transplantation and studied relevant clinical outcomes. Nevertheless, there are some limitations to our study. The observational nature of the study precludes us from drawing conclusions regarding causality. A limitation of this study was its use of self-reporting, which is subject to recall bias, for the PA assessment. However, the SQUASH questionnaire has been validated within general as well as specific populations, such as patients who have undergone total hip arthroplasty and those with ankylosing spondylitis [28,51,52]. Furthermore, PA was assessed at a single point in time. However, in RTR, after 1-year of transplantation, PA is increased by 30% and remained materially unchanged the next 5-years [18]. In this study, we included RTR > 1 year graft functioning with a median of 5.7 years post-transplantation. Another limitation is that we could not fully control for the history of all cardiometabolic diseases in the association of MVPA with all-cause mortality. Patients with a history of diabetes or CVD before the transplantation were excluded from the analyses on the association between MVPA and PTDM or CV mortality. However, cardiometabolic diseases might be more prevalent in 'No-MVPA' group after transplantation as well. A limitation is that we could not have data on functional evaluations, like e.g., a 6 min walking test, which could have provided important information on cardiovascular efficiency. Finally, single-center nature of study, which mainly consisted of white people is unclear whether our findings can be extrapolated to other populations. It would be relevant to repeat our study in other patient populations.

5. Conclusions

Higher daily-life MVPA is associated with a reduced risk of PTDM as well as cardiovascular and all-cause mortality in RTRs, suggesting that PA has a positive influence on the long-term health management of RTRs. The associations of MVPA with cardiovascular and all-cause mortality were not substantially affected by adjustments made for potential confounders, such as age, sex, baseline kidney function parameters, transplant characteristics, lifestyle habits, metabolic parameters, anthropometric measures, and immunosuppressive medication. The association of MVPA with PTDM was affected by adjustments of metabolic parameters and glucose levels. The potentially beneficial effects of daily-life PA apply to non-occupational activities at the moderate-to-vigorous level (e.g., commuting, leisure activities, or sport). By contrast, a higher level of occupational MVPA is not directly associated with the development of long-term outcomes. The associations of non-occupational MVPA and the risk of PTDM and cardiovascular mortality were also stronger in older adults. Finally, we suggest that because of the long-term importance of PA, it should be embedded in the healthcare management of RTRs. Furthermore, large scale interventional studies are needed to test the ab initio effect of physical activity after transplantation on the development of post-transplant diabetes mellitus.

Author Contributions: Conceptualization, O.B., S.J.L.B., E.C., G.N., and E.v.d.B.; methodology, O.B., M.C.J.O., A.W.G.-N., E.v.d.B., G.N., S.J.L.B., and E.C.; validation, O.B. and E.C.; formal analysis, O.B. and M.C.J.O.; writing—original draft preparation, O.B. and E.C.; writing—review and editing, M.C.J.O., A.W.G.-N., E.v.d.B., G.N., S.J.L.B., and E.C.; supervision, S.J.L.B. and E.C.; All authors have read and agreed to the published version of the manuscript.

References

1. Ponton, P.; Rupolo, G.P. Quality-of-life change after kidney transplantation. *Transplant. Proc.* **2001**, *33*, 1887–1889. [CrossRef]
2. Neale, J. Cardiovascular risk factors following renal transplant. *World J. Transplant.* **2015**, *5*, 183–195. [CrossRef] [PubMed]
3. Chadban, S. New-onset diabetes after transplantation—Should it be a factor in choosing an immunosuppressant regimen for kidney transplant recipients. *Nephrol. Dial. Transplant.* **2008**, *23*, 1816–1818. [CrossRef] [PubMed]
4. Irons, B.K.; Mazzolini, T.A.; Greene, R.S. Delaying the Onset of Type 2 Diabetes Mellitus in Patients with Prediabetes. *Pharmacotherapy* **2004**, *24*, 362–371. [CrossRef] [PubMed]
5. Lee, I.-M.; Patrick, J. Skerrett. Physical activity and all-cause mortality: What is the dose-response relation? *Med. Sci. Sports Exerc.* **2001**, *33*, S459–S474. [CrossRef] [PubMed]
6. Calella, P.; Hernández-Sánchez, S.; Garofalo, C.; Ruiz, J.R.; Carrero, J.J.; Bellizzi, V. Exercise training in kidney transplant recipients: A systematic review. *J. Nephrol.* **2019**, *32*, 567–579. [CrossRef]
7. Zelle, D.M.; Klaassen, G.; Van Adrichem, E.; Bakker, S.J.L.; Corpeleijn, E.; Navis, G. Physical inactivity: A risk factor and target for intervention in renal care. *Nat. Rev. Nephrol.* **2017**, *13*, 152. [CrossRef]

8. Macdonald, J.H.; Kirkman, D.; Jibani, M. Kidney Transplantation: A Systematic Review of Interventional and Observational Studies of Physical Activity on Intermediate Outcomes. *Adv. Chronic Kidney Dis.* **2009**, *16*, 482–500. [CrossRef]
9. Bellizzi, V.; Cupisti, A.; Capitanini, A.; Calella, P.; D'Alessandro, C. Physical activity and renal transplantation. *Kidney Blood Press. Res.* **2014**, *39*, 212–219. [CrossRef]
10. Takahashi, A.; Hu, S.L.; Bostom, A. Physical Activity in Kidney Transplant Recipients: A Review. *Am. J. Kidney Dis.* **2018**, *72*, 433–443. [CrossRef]
11. Kang, A.W.; Garber, C.E.; Eaton, C.B.; Risica, P.M. Physical Activity and Cardiovascular Risk among Kidney Transplant Patients. *Med. Sci. Sport. Exerc.* **2019**, *51*, 1154–1161. [CrossRef] [PubMed]
12. Zelle, D.M.; Kok, T.; Dontje, M.L.; Danchell, E.I.; Navis, G.; Van Son, W.J.; Bakker, S.J.L.; Corpeleijn, E. The role of diet and physical activity in post-transplant weight gain after renal transplantation. *Clin. Transplant.* **2013**, *27*, E484–E490. [CrossRef] [PubMed]
13. Orazio, L.; Hickman, I.; Armstrong, K.; Johnson, D.; Banks, M.; Isbel, N. Higher Levels of Physical Activity Are Associated With a Lower Risk of Abnormal Glucose Tolerance in Renal Transplant Recipients. *J. Ren. Nutr.* **2009**, *19*, 304–313. [CrossRef] [PubMed]
14. Zelle, D.M.; Corpeleijn, E.; Stolk, R.P.; de Greef, M.H.G.; Gans, R.O.B.; van der Heide, J.J.H.; Navis, G.; Bakker, S.J.L. Low physical activity and risk of cardiovascular and all-cause mortality in renal transplant recipients. *Clin. J. Am. Soc. Nephrol.* **2011**, *6*, 898–905. [CrossRef] [PubMed]
15. World Health Organization. *Global Recommendations on Physical Activity for Health*; World Health Organization: Geneva, Switzerland, 2010.
16. Janaudis-Ferreira, T.; Mathur, S.; Deliva, R.; Howes, N.; Patterson, C.; Räkel, A.; So, S.; Wickerson, L.; White, M.; Avitzur, Y.; et al. Exercise for Solid Organ Transplant Candidates and Recipients: A Joint Position Statement of the Canadian Society of Transplantation and CAN-RESTORE. *Transplantation* **2019**, *103*, e220–e238. [CrossRef]
17. Dontje, M.L.; de Greef, M.H.G.; Krijnen, W.P.; Corpeleijn, E.; Kok, T.; Bakker, S.J.L.; Stolk, R.P.; van der Schans, C.P. Longitudinal measurement of physical activity following kidney transplantation. *Clin. Transplant.* **2014**, *28*, 394–402. [CrossRef]
18. Nielens, H.; Lejeune, T.M.; Lalaoui, A.; Squifflet, J.P.; Pirson, Y.; Goffin, E. Increase of physical activity level after successful renal transplantation: A 5 year follow-up study. *Nephrol. Dial. Transplant.* **2001**, *16*, 134–140. [CrossRef]
19. Gordon, E.J.; Prohaska, T.R.; Gallant, M.P.; Sehgal, A.R.; Strogatz, D.; Conti, D.; Siminoff, L.A. Prevalence and determinants of physical activity and fluid intake in kidney transplant recipients. *Clin. Transplant.* **2010**, *24*, E69–E81. [CrossRef]
20. Lund, T.; Labriola, M.; Christensen, K.B.; Bültmann, U.; Villadsen, E. Physical work environment risk factors for long term sickness absence: Prospective findings among a cohort of 5357 employees in Denmark. *Br. Med. J.* **2006**, *332*, 449–451. [CrossRef]
21. Huai, P.; Xun, H.; Reilly, K.H.; Wang, Y.; Ma, W.; Xi, B. Physical activity and risk of hypertension a meta-analysis of prospective cohort studies. *Hypertension* **2013**, *62*, 1021–1026. [CrossRef]
22. Larsson, C.A.; Krøll, L.; Bennet, L.; Gullberg, B.; Råstam, L.; Lindblad, U. Leisure time and occupational physical activity in relation to obesity and insulin resistance: A population-based study from the Skaraborg Project in Sweden. *Metabolism.* **2012**, *61*, 590–598. [CrossRef] [PubMed]
23. Van den Berg, E.; Engberink, M.F.; Brink, E.J.; Van den Berg, E.; Engberink, M.F.; Brink, E.J.; van Baak, M.A.; Joosten, M.M.; Gans, R.O.B.; Navis, G.; et al. Dietary acid load and metabolic acidosis in renal transplant recipients. *Clin. J. Am. Soc. Nephrol.* **2012**, *7*, 1811–1818. [CrossRef] [PubMed]
24. Van Den Berg, E.; Engberink, M.F.; Brink, E.J.; Van Baak, M.A.; Gans, R.O.B.; Navis, G.; Bakker, S.J.L. Dietary protein, blood pressure and renal function in renal transplant recipients. *Br. J. Nutr.* **2013**, *109*, 1463–1470. [CrossRef] [PubMed]
25. Van den Berg, E.; Johanna, M.; Geleijnse, E.; Brink, J.; van Baak, M.A.; van der Heide, J.J.H.; Gans, R.O.B.; Navis, G.; Bakker, S.J.L. Sodium intake and blood pressure in renal transplant recipients. *Nephrol. Dial. Transplant.* **2012**, *27*, 3352–3359. [CrossRef] [PubMed]
26. Levey, A.S.; Kramer, H.J.; Griffin, K.A.; Vellanki, K.; Leehey, D.J.; Bansal, V.K.; Markossian, T.W.; Levey, A.; Stevens, L.; Schmid, C.; et al. A New Equation to Estimate Glomerular Filtration Rate. *Ann. Intern. Med.* **2009**, *150*, 604–612. [CrossRef] [PubMed]

27. Oterdoom, L.H.; Gansevoort, R.T.; Schouten, J.P.; de Jong, P.E.; Gans, R.O.B.; Bakker, S.J.L. Urinary creatinine excretion, an indirect measure of muscle mass, is an independent predictor of cardiovascular disease and mortality in the general population. *Atherosclerosis* **2009**, *207*, 534–540. [CrossRef] [PubMed]
28. Wendel-Vos, G.C.W.; Schuit, A.J.; Saris, W.H.M.; Kromhout, D. Reproducibility and relative validity of the short questionnaire to assess health-enhancing physical activity. *J. Clin. Epidemiol.* **2003**, *56*, 1163–1169. [CrossRef]
29. Ainsworth, B.E.; Haskell, W.L.; Herrmann, S.D.; Meckes, N.; Bassett, D.R.; Tudor-Locke, C.; Greer, J.L.; Vezina, J.; Whitt-Glover, M.C.; Leon, A.S. 2011 compendium of physical activities: A second update of codes and MET values. *Med. Sci. Sports Exerc.* **2011**, *43*, 1575–1581. [CrossRef]
30. Byambasukh, O.; Snieder, H.; Corpeleijn, E. The relation between leisure time, commuting and occupational physical activity with blood pressure in 125,402 adults: The Lifelines cohort. *J. Am. Heart Assoc.* **2019**, *8*, e0814313.
31. Davidson, J.; Wilkinson, A.; Dantal, J.; Dotta, F.; Haller, H.; Hernandez, D.; Kasiske, B.L.; Kiberd, B.; Krentz, A.; Legendre, C.; et al. New-onser diabetes after transplantation: 2003 International Consensus Guidelines. *Transplantation* **2003**, *75*, SS3–SS24. [CrossRef]
32. Sharif, A.; Hecking, M.; De Vries, A.P.J.; Porrini, E.; Hornum, M.; Rasoul-Rockenschaub, S.; Berlakovich, G.; Krebs, M.; Kautzky-Willer, A.; Schernthaner, G.; et al. Proceedings from an international consensus meeting on posttransplantation diabetes mellitus: Recommendations and future directions. *Am. J. Transplant.* **2014**, *14*, 1992–2000. [CrossRef] [PubMed]
33. Osté, M.C.J.; Corpeleijn, E.; Navis, G.J.; Keyzer, C.A.; Soedamah-Muthu, S.S.; Van Den Berg, E.; Postmus, D.; De Borst, M.H.; Kromhout, D.; Bakker, S.J.L. Mediterranean style diet is associated with low risk of new-onset diabetes after renal transplantation. *BMJ Open Diabetes Res. Care* **2017**, *5*, e000283. [CrossRef] [PubMed]
34. Vittinghoff, E.; McCulloch, C.E. Relaxing the rule of ten events per variable in logistic and cox regression. *Am. J. Epidemiol.* **2007**, *165*, 710–718. [CrossRef] [PubMed]
35. Spaderna, H.; Zahn, D.; Pretsch, J.; Connor, S.L.; Zittermann, A.; Schulze Schleithoff, S.; Bramstedt, K.A.; Smits, J.M.A.; Weidner, G. Dietary habits are related to outcomes in patients with advanced heart failure awaiting heart transplantation. *J. Card. Fail.* **2013**, *19*, 240–250. [CrossRef]
36. Grambsch, P.M.; Therneau, T.M. Proportional hazards tests and diagnostics based on weighted residuals. *Biometrika* **1994**, *81*, 515–526. [CrossRef]
37. Shah, S. *Prevention of Cardiovascular Disease: Guideline for Assessment and Management of Cardiovascular Risk*; World Health Organization: Geneva, Switzerland, 2007.
38. Fine, J.P.; Gray, R.J. A Proportional Hazards Model for the Subdistribution of a Competing Risk. *J. Am. Stat. Assoc.* **1999**, *94*, 496–509. [CrossRef]
39. Weir, M.R.; Fink, J.C. Risk for posttransplant diabetes mellitus with current immunosuppressive medications. *Am. J. Kidney Dis.* **1999**, *34*, 1–13. [CrossRef]
40. Sharif, A.; Moore, R.; Baboolal, K. Influence of lifestyle modification in renal transplant recipients with postprandial hyperglycemia. *Transplantation* **2008**, *85*, 353–358. [CrossRef]
41. Sullivan, P.W.; Morrato, E.H.; Ghushchyan, V.; Wyatt, H.R.; Hill, J.O. Obesity, inactivity, and the prevalence of diabetes and diabetes-related cardiovascular comorbidities in the U.S., 2000–2002. *Diabetes Care* **2005**, *28*, 1599. [CrossRef]
42. Robinson-Cohen, C.; Katz, R.; Mozaffarian, D.; Dalrymple, L.S.; De Boer, I.; Sarnak, M.; Shlipak, M.; Siscovick, D.; Kestenbaum, B. Physical activity and rapid decline in kidney function among older adults. *Arch. Intern. Med.* **2009**, *169*, 2116–2123. [CrossRef]
43. Robinson-Cohen, C.; Littman, A.J.; Duncan, G.E.; Weiss, N.S.; Sachs, M.C.; Ruzinski, J.; Kundzins, J.; Rock, D.; de Boer, I.H.; Ikizler, T.A.; et al. Physical Activity and Change in Estimated GFR among Persons with CKD. *J. Am. Soc. Nephrol.* **2014**, *25*, 399–406. [CrossRef] [PubMed]
44. Gordon, E.J.; Prohaska, T.R.; Gallant, M.P.; Sehgal, A.R.; Strogatz, D.; Yucel, R.; Conti, D.; Siminoff, L.A. Longitudinal analysis of physical activity, fluid intake, and graft function among kidney transplant recipients. *Transpl. Int.* **2009**, *22*, 990–998. [CrossRef]
45. Koivisto, V.A.; Yki-Järvinen, H.; DeFronzo, R.A. Physical training and insulin sensitivity. *Diabetes. Metab. Rev.* **1986**, *1*, 445–481. [CrossRef] [PubMed]
46. Whelton, S.P.; Chin, A.; Xin, X.; He, J. Effect of aerobic exercise on blood pressure: A meta-analysis of randomized, controlled trials. *Ann. Intern. Med.* **2002**, *136*, 493–503. [CrossRef] [PubMed]

47. Wood, P.D.; Stefanick, M.L.; Williams, P.T.; Haskell, W.L. The Effects on Plasma Lipoproteins of a Prudent Weight-Reducing Diet, With or Without Exercise, in Overweight Men and Women. *N. Engl. J. Med.* **1991**, *325*, 461–466. [CrossRef] [PubMed]
48. Osté, M.C.J.; Gomes-Neto, A.W.; Corpeleijn, E.; Gans, R.O.B.; de Borst, M.H.; van den Berg, E.; Soedamah-Muthu, S.S.; Kromhout, D.; Navis, G.J.; Bakker, S.J.L. Dietary Approach to Stop Hypertension (DASH) diet and risk of renal function decline and all-cause mortality in renal transplant recipients. *Am. J. Transplant.* **2018**, *10*, 2523–2533. [CrossRef] [PubMed]
49. Byambasukh, O.; Zelle, D.; Corpeleijn, E. Physical Activity, Fatty Liver, and Glucose Metabolism Over the Life Course. *Am. J. Gastroenterol.* **2019**, *114*, 907–915. [CrossRef]
50. Crandall, J.; Schade, D.; Ma, Y.; Fujimoto, W.Y.; Barrett-Connor, E.; Fowler, S.; Dagogo-Jack, S.; Andres, R. The influence of age on the effects of lifestyle modification and metformin in prevention of diabetes. *J. Gerontol. A Biol. Sci. Med. Sci.* **2006**, *61*, 1075–1081.
51. Wagenmakers, R.; Van Den Akker-Scheek, I.; Groothoff, J.W.; Zijlstra, W.; Bulstra, S.K.; Kootstra, J.W.J.; Wendel-Vos, G.C.W.; Van Raaij, J.J.A.M.; Stevens, M. Reliability and validity of the short questionnaire to assess health-enhancing physical activity (SQUASH) in patients after total hip arthroplasty. *BMC Musculoskelet. Disord.* **2008**, *9*, 141. [CrossRef]
52. Arends, S.; Hofman, M.; Kamsma, Y.P.T.; van der Veer, E.; Houtman, P.M.; Kallenberg, C.G.M.; Spoorenberg, A.; Brouwer, E. Daily physical activity in ankylosing spondylitis: Validity and reliability of the IPAQ and SQUASH and the relation with clinical assessments. *Arthritis Res. Ther.* **2013**, *15*, R99. [CrossRef]

13

Weekend Effect and in-Hospital Mortality in Elderly Patients with Acute Kidney Injury: A Retrospective Analysis of a National Hospital Database in Italy

Fabio Fabbian [1,2,*], Alfredo De Giorgi [1], Emanuele Di Simone [1], Rosaria Cappadona [2], Nicola Lamberti [3], Fabio Manfredini [3,4], Benedetta Boari [1], Alda Storari [5] and Roberto Manfredini [1,2]

1 Clinica Medica Unit, Azienda Ospedaliero-Universitaria, I-44121 Ferrara, Italy; degiorgialfredo@libero.it (A.D.G.); emanuele.disimone@uniroma1.it (E.D.S.); benedetta.boari@unife.it (B.B.); roberto.manfredini@unife.it (R.M.)
2 Department of Medical Sciences, University of Ferrara, I-44121 Ferrara, Italy; rosaria.cappadona@unife.it
3 Department of Biomedical and Specialty Surgical Sciences, University of Ferrara, I-44121 Ferrara, Italy; nicola.lamberti@unife.it (N.L.); fabio.manfredini@unife.it (F.M.)
4 Neuroscience and Rehabilitation Department, Azienda Ospedaliero-Universitaria, I-44121 Ferrara, Italy
5 Nephrology and Dialysis Unit, Azienda Ospedaliero-Universitaria, I-44121 Ferrara, Italy; a.storari@ospfe.it
* Correspondence: f.fabbian@ospfe.it

Abstract: Background: The aim of this study was to relate the weekend (WE) effect and acute kidney injury (AKI) in elderly patients by using the Italian National Hospital Database (NHD). Methods: Hospitalizations with AKI of subjects aged ≥ 65 years from 2000–2015 who were identified by the ICD-9-CM were included. Admissions from Friday to Sunday were considered as WE, while all the other days were weekdays (WD). In-hospital mortality (IHM) was our outcome, and the comorbidity burden was calculated by the modified Elixhauser Index (mEI), based on ICD-9-CM codes. Results: 760,664 hospitalizations were analyzed. Mean age was 80.5 ± 7.8 years and 52.2% were males. Of the studied patients, 9% underwent dialysis treatment, 24.3% were admitted during WE, and IHM was 27.7%. Deceased patients were more frequently comorbid males, with higher age, treated with dialysis more frequently, and had higher admission during WE. WE hospitalizations were more frequent in males, and in older patients with higher mEI. IHM was independently associated with dialysis-dependent AKI (OR 2.711; 95%CI 2.667–2.755, $p < 0.001$), WE admission (OR 1.113; 95%CI 1.100–1.126, $p < 0.001$), and mEI (OR 1.056; 95% CI 1.055–1.057, $p < 0.001$). Discussion: Italian elderly patients admitted during WE with AKI are exposed to a higher risk of IHM, especially if they need dialysis treatment and have high comorbidity burden.

Keywords: acute kidney injury; weekend effect; in-hospital mortality; comorbidity; dialysis; elderly

---

1. Introduction

The negative clinical impact of the so-called weekend (WE) effect has been a matter of debate since the past two decades. Different research groups have reported poorer outcomes for patients admitted on WE compared to weekdays (WD). A milestone study published in 2001, conducted on almost 4 million acute care admissions from emergency departments in Ontario, Canada, found that patients with some serious medical conditions had higher in-hospital mortality (IHM) if they were admitted on a WE than on a WD [1]. A few years later, Cram et al. confirmed a modest increase in mortality after WE admission for all admissions, either unscheduled or emergency department admissions [2]. Our group also documented a higher IHM for some cardiovascular events, such as acute heart failure (OR 1.33) [3], and acute pulmonary embolism (OR 1.18) [4]. A systematic review evaluated 97 studies enrolling more than 51 million subjects, and patients admitted on WE had a significantly higher overall mortality, independent of factors including the levels of staffing, procedure rates and delays, and illness severity [5]. Another systematic review and meta-analysis focused on United Kingdom (UK) hospitals confirmed that WE admissions had higher odds of mortality than those admitted during WD, as well as when measures of case mix severity were included in the models. On the other hand, the WE effect was not significant when clinical registry data was used [6]. Finally, Chen et al. performed a large meta-analysis (68 studies, 640 million admissions), and found that risk of mortality during all WE admissions was 1.16, although it was greater for elective admissions than emergency ones [7]. A first consideration is that differences in hospital care associated with the day of the week (measured by indicators including short term mortality) can vary depending on the place, time, and reason for hospital admission [8]. On one hand, medical and nursing understaffing, shortage of diagnostic or procedural services, and the presence of inexperienced residents have been suggested as possible causes [9]. On the other, temporal aspects of onset of acute vascular diseases may also play a role, and it is possible that these diseases do not present with equal severity relative to time, that is, day of the week or hour of the day [10,11]. A single-center study on acute coronary syndromes (ACSs) showed that although there were fewer ACS admissions than expected on nights and WE, the proportion of patients with ACS presenting with ST-elevation myocardial infarctions was 64% higher on WE [12]. Again, in their large study on pulmonary embolism admissions, Nanchal et al. reported a 19% increase in patients admitted on WE [13], but WE admissions showed significantly worse parameters of severity, such as the need for mechanical ventilation, thrombolytic therapy use, and the use of vasopressors. A further confirmation to this hypothesis comes from the results of a study conducted on more than 500,000 unselected emergency admissions in the UK, evaluating and adjusting for multiple confounders including demographics, comorbidities, and admission characteristics, and common hematology and biochemistry test results. Hospital workload was not associated with mortality, suggesting that the WE effect could be associated with patient-level differences at admission rather than reduced hospital staffing or services [14]. Therefore, the debate about clinical impact of the WE effect is still open. Acute kidney injury (AKI) is a frequent finding in hospitalized subjects, especially in people who are 65 years old or older [15–17]. However, available data about admissions due to renal diseases are scarce; therefore, we wanted to explore the possible relationship between the WE effect and AK by using the National Hospital Database (NHD).

2. Experimental Section

2.1. Patient Selection and Eligibility

This retrospective study was conducted in agreement with the Declaration of Helsinki of 1975, revised in 2013. Subject identifiers were deleted before data analysis with the aim of maintaining data anonymity and confidentiality; therefore, none of the patients could be identified, either in this paper or in the database. The study was conducted in agreement with the existent Italian disposition-by-law (G.U. n.76, 31 March 2008), and due to the study design, ethics committee approval was not necessary.

We accessed the National Hospital Database (NHD), provided by the Italian Ministry of Health (SDO Database, Ministry of Health, General Directorate for Health Planning), selecting all hospitalizations complicated by AKI between 1 January 2000, and 31 December 2015. This database stores data of all hospitalizations both in public and private Italian hospitals. Based on the International Classification of Diseases, 9th Revision, Clinical Modification (ICD-9-CM), the hospital discharge record files contain information such as gender, age, date and department of admission and discharge, vital status at discharge (in-hospital death vs. discharged alive), main diagnosis, up to five co-morbidities, and up to six procedures/interventions. For this analysis, patients' names and all other potential identifiers were removed by the Ministry of Health from the database, following the national disposition-by-law in terms of privacy. A consecutive number for each patient was the only identifier. Although in clinical settings the term AKI has replaced the term acute renal failure, in administrative database codes the latter term is usually the reference term. We selected patients aged ≥65 years in whom the ICD-9-CM code 584.xx identified AKI when used as a first or second discharge diagnosis. As for a temporal definition, midnight Friday to midnight Sunday was considered as WE, while all the other days were assumed as WD. The nine main national festive days in Italy (1 January, 25 April, 1 May, 2 June, 15 August, 2 November, 8 December, 25 December, and 26 December), when occurring on WD, were considered as WE.

2.2. Data Analysis

In-hospital mortality (IHM) was the hard clinical outcome indicator. In order to evaluate the comorbidity burden, a novel score from our group, a modified Elixhauser Index (mEI) [18], was calculated based on the guidelines set by Quan et al [19]. To calculate the score, the following conditions were considered: age, gender, presence of chronic kidney disease (CKD), neurological disorders, lymphoma, solid tumor with metastasis, ischemic heart disease, congestive heart disease, coagulopathy, fluid and electrolyte disorders, liver disease, weight loss, and metastatic cancer. The original score was corrected, removing the diagnosis of previous AKI; therefore, the points assigned to renal diseases were considered only if CKD was recorded. The points for each condition ranged from 0 to 16, and the total score calculated could vary between 0 and 89. When the score was >40, the risk of IHM was >60%. The score, based on administrative data, was calculated automatically. Table 1 reports single items and relative score. Finally, dialysis treatment was also taken into consideration (code ICD-9-CM 39.95).

Table 1. Items and relative assigned score to calculate in-hospital mortality (IHM).

Items	Score
Age 0–60 (years)	0
Age 61–70 (years)	3
Age 71–80 (years)	7
Age 81–90 (years)	11
Age 91+ (years)	16
Chronic kidney disease	1
Male gender	2
Neurological disorders	3
Lymphoma	4
Solid tumor without metastasis	4
Ischemic heart disease	5
Congestive heart failure	5
Coagulopathy	8
Fluid and electrolyte disorders	8
Liver disease	10
Cachexia	11
Metastatic cancer	12

2.3. Statistical Analysis

A descriptive analysis of the whole population, i.e., absolute numbers, percentages, and means ± SD, was performed. Univariate analysis was carried out by using the Chi-Squared test, Student *t*-tests, Mann–Whitney U-test, and ANOVA as appropriate, comparing survivors and deceased subjects, and AKI patients admitted during the WE or WD. Moreover, in order to evaluate the relationship between the WE effect and IHM, the latter was considered as the dependent variable in a logistic regression analysis, while demography, comorbidity score, and dialysis-dependent AKI were considered as independent variables. Odds ratios (ORs) with their 95% confidence intervals (95% CI) were reported. All p-values were 2-tailed, and p-value <0.5 was considered significant. SPSS 13.0 for Windows (SPSS IN., Chicago, IL, USA, 2004) was used for statistical analysis.

3. Results

The total sample consisted of 760,664 hospitalizations due to AKI, 52.2% were men, with a mean age of 80.5 ± 7.8 years, and 9% underwent dialysis treatment. Of these patients, 24.3% were admitted during WE and 27.7% died during hospitalization (Table 2).

Table 2. Demographic features of the considered sample (AKI: acute kidney injury, WE: weekend effect).

Total Number of Records	760,664
Men (*n* (%))	397,174 (52.2)
Women (*n* (%))	361,490 (47.8)
Age (years)	80.5 ± 7.8
Comorbidity score	14.57 ± 6.21
Dialysis dependent AKI (*n* (%))	68,563 (9)
Patients admitted during WE (*n* (%))	184,727 (24.3)
Deceased subjects (*n* (%))	210,661 (27.7)

IHM was significantly higher in men (51.8% vs. 48.2%, $p < 0.001$). Deceased subjects were more likely to be older (81.9 ± 7.9 vs. 80 ± 7.7 years, $p < 0.001$), to have higher comorbidity score (15.96 ± 6.48 vs. 14.04 ± 6.02, $p < 0.001$), to be treated with dialysis (17.7% vs. 6.8%, $p < 0.001$), and to show higher admission during WE (25.8% vs. 23.7%, $p < 0.001$), compared to survivors (Table 3).

Table 3. Comparison between survivors and deceased subjects.

	Survivors *n* = 550,003	Deceased *n* = 210,661	*p*
Men (*n* (%))	288,120 (52.4)	109,054 (51.8)	<0.001
Women (*n* (%))	261,883 (47.6)	101,607 (48.2)	
Age (years)	80 ± 7.7	81.9 ± 7.9	<0.001
Comorbidity score	14.04 ± 6.02	15.96 ± 6.48	<0.001
Dialysis dependent AKI (*n* (%))	37,598 (6.8)	31,055 (17.7)	<0.001
Patients admitted during WE (*n* (%))	130,318 (23.7)	54,409 (25.8)	<0.001

Patients admitted during WE were more likely to be male (51.5% vs. 48.5%, $p < 0.001$), older (mean age 81 ± 7.8 vs. 80.4 ± 7.8 years, $p < 0.001$), and had a higher comorbidity score (14.75 ± 6.2 vs. 14.52 ± 6.22, $p < 0.001$). No difference was found for prevalence of dialysis dependent AKI (Table 4).

Table 4. Comparison between subjects admitted during weekdays (WD) or weekends (WE).

	WD Admissions *n* = 575,937	WE Admissions *n* = 184,727	*p*
Men (*n* (%))	302,010 (52.4)	95,164 (51.5)	<0.001
Women (*n* (%))	273,927 (47.6)	89,563 (48.5)	
Age (years)	80.4 ± 7.8	81 ± 7.8	<0.001
Dialysis dependent AKI (*n* (%))	52,075 (9)	16,578 (9)	NS
Comorbidity score	14.52 ± 6.22	14.75 ± 6.2	<0.001

NS: non-significant.

At the logistic regression analysis, IHM was independently associated, in decreasing order, with dialysis-dependent AKI, WE admission, and comorbidity score (Table 5). As for the comorbidity score, the risk of death raised of 5.6% for every 1-point increase.

Table 5. Logistic regression analysis showing factors independently associated with in-hospital mortality. OR: Odds Ratio; 95%CI: 95% confidence intervals; WE: weekend.

	OR	95% Confidence Intervals	*p*
Dialysis dependent AKI	2.711	2.667–2.755	<0.001
WE admission	1.113	1.100–1.126	<0.001
Comorbidity score	1.056	1.055–1.057	<0.001

4. Discussion

In this study, based on a large national database of hospitalizations, the day of admission had a significant clinical impact on elderly subjects with AKI. The WE effect was independently associated with IHM, along with dialysis treatment and comorbidity burden. The OR for IHM was 1.113, and this finding confirmed previous results from our group, also drawn by analysis of the NHD records, regarding pulmonary embolism (OR 1.15) [20], and acute aortic dissection or rupture (OR 1.34) [21]. The importance of a diverse level of emergency has been underlined by previous studies. Concha et al. studied the 7-day post-admission time patterns of excess mortality following WE admission to investigate whether the phenomenon could be due to poorer quality of care or a case selection. After evaluation of mortality risk for WE and WD, adjusting for age, sex, Charlson Comorbidity Index (CCI), and diagnostic group, they found that WE mortality was diverse for different diagnostic groups, and concluded that the WE effect is probably not a uniform phenomenon, but rather a complex cluster of different causal pathways, even associated with quite different risk profiles [22]. Similar results were reported by Roberts et al., who evaluated 30-day mortality for WE admissions in England and Wales. The WE effect was more evident for disorders with high mortality during the acute phase, and negligible for less acute ones [23].

Moreover, the presence of comorbidities plays a primary role in determining IHM. In the present study, in fact, the OR of comorbidity score is lower than that of presence of dialysis and age, but the risk of death raised of 4.2% for every 1-point increase. In a previous study conducted by our group, we showed that CCI was significantly higher in subjects admitted during WE, and significantly contributed to clinical outcome, along with gender and age. In logistic regression analysis, in fact, admission on WE, CCI, male sex, and age were significantly associated with IHM [24].

To the best of our knowledge, this is the first study considering the relationship between the WE effect and IHM in elderly patients hospitalized because of AKI. The question of whether the WE effect also exists in renal diseases is still matter of debate, because the number of available studies is limited, and results are not univocal. We are aware of only three studies considered the relationship between WE admission and AKI, conducted in the United States (USA), United Kingdom (UK), and Wales, respectively. James et al. analyzed data from the U.S. Nationwide Inpatient Sample and selected more than 200,000 admissions reporting AKI as the primary diagnosis. The prevalence of WE admission was 21% and WE hospitalizations were independently associated with IHM [25]. Kolhe et al. conducted a study on more than 53,000 dialysis-dependent AKI patients. The prevalence of WE admission was 23%, and WE admissions were significantly associated with higher mortality in the unadjusted model, but not in the multivariable analysis [26]. Finally, Holmes et al. did not find any WE effect for mortality associated with hospital-acquired AKI [27]. None of these studies, however, included comorbidity analysis.

A higher interest in the WE effect has been shown to investigate possible negative outcomes in renal transplantation, but results have not demonstrated any negative outcome thus far. In the U.S., Baid-Agrawal et al. did not confirm the hypothesis that kidney transplants performed during WE could have worse outcomes than those performed during WD. In fact, the day of surgery did not affect death, length of hospitalization after transplantation, delayed allograft function, acute rejection within the first year of transplant, and patient and allograft survival at 1 month and at 1 year after transplantation [28]. In Germany, Schütte-Nütgen et al. found no differences between subjects transplanted on WD or WE in terms of 3-year patient and graft survival, frequencies of delayed graft function, acute rejections, 1-year estimated glomerular filtration rate, and length of hospital stay [29]. Again, in England, Anderson et al. did not confirm the relationship between WE and mortality, rehospitalization, and kidney allograft failure/rejection [30]. Moreover, a study of the Australia and New Zealand Dialysis and Transplant registry concluded that timing of transplantation did not impact on allograft outcome [31]. Also, our group tested this hypothesis on all cases of the Emilia-Romagna region, but did not find any risk of adverse outcome related to the WE effect, observing only that WE admissions were characterized by longer duration of hospitalization [32].

On the other hand, WE admission seems to negatively influence outcomes in dialysis patients, although the available evidence is strictly limited to a couple of studies. In the U.S., Sakhuja et al. reported that WE admissions were more likely to have higher IHM, higher mortality during the first 3 days of admission, longer hospital stays, and less likely to be discharged to home. Moreover, time to death was shorter compared with WD admissions [33]. Finally, data from the Australia and New Zealand Dialysis and Transplant Registry reported higher rates of hospitalization secondary to peritonitis on WE compared to WD [34].

In our present study, dialysis-dependent AKI and the WE effect were independently associated with IHM; it could be that the two factors negatively impact patients' survival and complications.

Limitations

We are aware that a major limitation is introduced by the study design: retrospective, based on administrative data, and with no possibility to assess whether AKI was cause or complication of hospitalization. We observed that day-of-week of hospital admission has a significant impact on outcome, but we cannot extrapolate from the administrative database some important items, such as cause of admission and death, intensive care level or hospitals' facilities, device use, type of treatment, and impact of clinical or biochemical parameters. It is known that administrative databases, born to be used for other reasons (i.e., reimbursement), lack specific clinical information and may cause possible misclassification of outcomes, thereby generating confounding factors [35]. Moreover, we did not identify AKI on the basis of international Kidney Disease Improving Global Outcomes (KDIGO) guidelines [36], nor differentiate patients on the basis of the cause of AKI and the treatment setting, with the exception of dialysis treatment.

We previously stated that medical and nursing understaffing, shortage of diagnostic or procedural services, and the presence of inexperienced residents could be related to WE effect [9]. Unfortunately, administrative databases do not allow us investigate these aspects, being conceived for financial reasons.

Some years ago, concerns about WE effect were raised due to three main potential limitations of administrative databases: (1) coding mistakes, (2) insufficient consideration of comorbidity, and (3) failure to consider the severity or acuity of patients [37]. According to several authors, the performance of ICD-9-CM for diagnosis of acute renal failure showed poor sensitivity, and high specificity, while positive and negative predictive value could differ [38–41]. However, Grams et al. underlined that sensitivity was significantly higher when the selected individuals were aged ≥ 65 years; moreover, AKI diagnosed by administrative data detected more severe disease and higher IHM mortality [41]. Due to this reason, we decided to focus on patients aged > 65 years. Finally, we also have to underline some strengths of our study: (1) a high number of records derived from a national database, (2) the long period of time analyzed, and (3) the utilization of a hard outcome indicator, such as IHM.

5. Conclusions

The global population is ageing, and the prevalence of elderly subjects is increasing. Older adults are projected to increase enormously by 2050, rising to more than 400 million [42]. Chronic illnesses and disability causing hospitalization are frequent in the last decades of life and AKI is a frequent cause of morbidity and mortality as shown by the U.S. Renal Data Services (USRDS) 2018 [43]. The latter data demonstrated an increasing incidence rate of AKI over the past several years, in the elderly population.

Patients over the age of 65 who required dialysis continued to have substantially higher mortality compared to general population [43]. Last year, our group demonstrated that in-hospital mortality was a frequent complication in elderly subjects with AKI discharge codes, involving more than a quarter of admissions. The increasing burden of comorbidity, dialysis-dependent AKI, and sepsis were the major risk factors for mortality [16]. Comorbidity is a well-known risk factor affecting survival in dialysis patients [44]; however, predictors of short-term survival in renal patients are still a matter of debate.

Multi-morbidity is crucial for defining the prognosis of the aged population [45], and our findings suggest that pre-existing diseases diagnosed prior to admission may be associated with the outcome of an acute condition such as AKI (especially if AKI needs dialysis treatment). In elderly hospitalized subjects with AKI, WE effect seems to be a risk factor for IHM, even adjusting for comorbidity and advanced AKI stage. Thus, elderly patients admitted on Saturday or Sunday should deserve careful attention and evaluation, and consideration should be taken of their higher risk of IHM.

Author Contributions: Conceptualization, A.D.G., F.F., and R.M..; methodology, F.F, A.D.G., E.D.S., N.L. and F.M.; software, A.D.G., and E.D.S.; validation, E.D.S., N.L., F.M, and A.S.; formal analysis, F.F., A.D.G., N.L., and F.M.; investigation, E.D.S., B.B.; and A.S.; resources, R.C., A.S., and R.M.; data curation, A.D.G., E.D.S., R.C., N.L., and F.M.; writing—original draft preparation, F.F., and B.B.; writing—review and editing, F.F., and R.M.; visualization, A.D.G., R.C., and B.B.; supervision, F.F., B.B., A.S., and R.M.; project administration, R.C., B.B., and R.M; funding acquisition, F.F., and R.M. All authors have read and agreed to the published version of the manuscript.

Acknowledgments: We thank Massimo Gallerani, head of Medical Department, Azienda Ospedaliero-Universitaria "S.Anna", Ferrara, Italy, for precious help in obtaining data from the Italian Ministry of Health.

References

1. Bell, C.M.; Redelmeier, D.A. Mortality among Patients Admitted to Hospitals on Weekends as Compared with Weekdays. *N. Engl. J. Med.* **2001**, *345*, 663–668. [CrossRef] [PubMed]
2. Cram, P.; Hillis, S.L.; Barnett, M.; E Rosenthal, G. Effects of weekend admission and hospital teaching status on in-hospital mortality. *Am. J. Med.* **2004**, *117*, 151–157. [CrossRef] [PubMed]
3. Gallerani, M.; Boari, B.; Manfredini, F.; Mari, E.; Maraldi, C.; Manfredini, R. Weekend versus weekday hospital admissions for acute heart failure. *Int. J. Cardiol.* **2011**, *146*, 444–447. [CrossRef] [PubMed]
4. Imberti, D.; Ageno, W.; Dentali, F.; Manfredini, R.; Gallerani, M. Higher mortality rate in patients hospitalised for acute pulmonary embolism during weekends. *Thromb. Haemost.* **2011**, *106*, 83–89. [CrossRef] [PubMed]
5. Pauls, L.; Johnson-Paben, R.; Mcgready, J.; Murphy, J.; Pronovost, P.J.; Wu, C. The Weekend Effect in Hospitalized Patients: A Meta-Analysis. *J. Hosp. Med.* **2017**, *12*, 760–766. [CrossRef] [PubMed]
6. Honeyford, K.; Cecil, E.; Lo, M.; Bottle, A.; Aylin, P. The weekend effect: Does hospital mortality differ by day of the week? A systematic review and meta-analysis. *BMC Heal. Serv. Res.* **2018**, *18*, 870. [CrossRef]
7. Chen, Y.-F.; Armoiry, X.; Higenbottam, C.; Cowley, N.; Basra, R.; Watson, S.I.; Tarrant, C.; Boyal, A.; Sutton, E.; Wu, C.-W.; et al. Magnitude and modifiers of the weekend effect in hospital admissions: A systematic review and meta-analysis. *BMJ Open* **2019**, *9*, e025764. [CrossRef] [PubMed]
8. Fedeli, U.; Gallerani, M.; Manfredini, R. Factors Contributing to the Weekend Effect. *JAMA* **2017**, *317*, 1582. [CrossRef] [PubMed]
9. Kostis, W.J.; Demissie, K.; Marcella, S.W.; Shao, Y.-H.; Wilson, A.C.; E Moreyra, A. Weekend versus Weekday Admission and Mortality from Myocardial Infarction. *N. Engl. J. Med.* **2007**, *356*, 1099–1109. [CrossRef] [PubMed]
10. Manfredini, R.; Salmi, R.; Gallerani, M. Weekend effect for pulmonary embolism and other acute cardiovascular diseases. *Chest* **2013**, *143*, 275–276. [CrossRef]
11. Manfredini, R.; Manfredini, F.; Salmi, R.; Gallerani, M. Weekend admissions and increased risk for mortality: Less urgent treatments only? *JAMA Neurol.* **2013**, *70*, 131–132. [CrossRef] [PubMed]

12. LaBounty, T.; Eagle, K.A.; Manfredini, R.; Fang, J.; Tsai, T.; Smith, D.; Rubenfire, M. The impact of time and day on the presentation of acute coronary syndromes. *Clin. Cardiol.* **2006**, *29*, 542–546. [CrossRef] [PubMed]
13. Nanchal, R.; Kumar, G.; Taneja, A.; Patel, J.; Deshmukh, A.; Tarima, S.; Jacobs, E.R.; Whittle, J. From the Milwaukee Initiative in Critical Care Outcomes Research (MICCOR) Group of Investigators Pulmonary embolism: The weekend effect. *Chest* **2012**, *142*, 690–696. [CrossRef] [PubMed]
14. Walker, A.S.; Mason, A.M.; Quan, T.P.; Fawcett, N.J.; Watkinson, P.; Llewelyn, M.J.; Stoesser, N.; Finney, J.; Davies, J.; Wyllie, D.H.; et al. Mortality risks associated with emergency admissions during weekends and public holidays: An analysis of electronic health records. *Lancet* **2017**, *390*, 62–72. [CrossRef]
15. Gameiro, J.; Fonseca, J.A.; Jorge, S.; Lopes, J.A. Acute Kidney Injury Definition and Diagnosis: A Narrative Review. *J. Clin. Med.* **2018**, *7*, 307. [CrossRef]
16. Fabbian, F.; Savriè, C.; De Giorgi, A.; Cappadona, R.; Simone, D.; Boari, B.; Storari, A.; Gallerani, M.; Manfredini, R.; De Giorgi, A.; et al. Acute Kidney Injury and In-Hospital Mortality: A Retrospective Analysis of a Nationwide Administrative Database of Elderly Subjects in Italy. *J. Clin. Med.* **2019**, *8*, 1371. [CrossRef]
17. Thongprayoon, C.; Hansrivijit, P.; Kovvuru, K.; Kanduri, S.R.; Torres-Ortiz, A.; Acharya, P.; Gonzalez-Suarez, M.L.; Kaewput, W.; Bathini, T.; Cheungpasitporn, W. Diagnostics, Risk Factors, Treatment and Outcomes of Acute Kidney Injury in a New Paradigm. *J. Clin. Med.* **2020**, *9*, 1104. [CrossRef]
18. Fabbian, F.; De Giorgi, A.; Maietti, E.; Gallerani, M.; Pala, M.; Cappadona, R.; Manfredini, R.; Fedeli, U. A modified Elixhauser score for predicting in-hospital mortality in internal medicine admissions. *Eur. J. Intern. Med.* **2017**, *40*, 37–42. [CrossRef]
19. Quan, H.; Sundararajan, V.; Halfon, P.; Fong, A.; Burnand, B.; Luthi, J.-C.; Saunders, L.D.; Beck, C.A.; Feasby, T.E.; Ghali, W.A. Coding Algorithms for Defining Comorbidities in ICD-9-CM and ICD-10 Administrative Data. *Med Care* **2005**, *43*, 1130–1139. [CrossRef]
20. Gallerani, M.; Fedeli, U.; Pala, M.; De Giorgi, A.; Fabbian, F.; Manfredini, R. Weekend Versus Weekday Admission and In-Hospital Mortality for Pulmonary Embolism: A 14-Year Retrospective Study on the National Hospital Database of Italy. *Angiology* **2017**, *69*, 236–241. [CrossRef]
21. Gallerani, M.; Volpato, S.; Boari, B.; Pala, M.; De Giorgi, A.; Fabbian, F.; Gasbarro, V.; Bossone, E.; Eagle, K.; Carle, F.; et al. Outcomes of weekend versus weekday admission for acute aortic dissection or rupture: A retrospective study on the Italian National Hospital Database. *Int. J. Cardiol.* **2013**, *168*, 3117–3119. [CrossRef] [PubMed]
22. Concha, O.P.; Gallego, B.; Hillman, K.; Delaney, G.P.; Coiera, E. Do variations in hospital mortality patterns after weekend admission reflect reduced quality of care or different patient cohorts? A population-based study. *BMJ Qual. Saf.* **2013**, *23*, 215–222. [CrossRef] [PubMed]
23. Roberts, E.S.; Thorne, K.; Akbari, A.; Samuel, D.G.; Williams, J.G. Weekend emergency admissions and mortality in England and Wales. *Lancet* **2015**, *385*, 1829. [CrossRef]
24. De Giorgi, A.; Fabbian, F.; Tiseo, R.; Misurati, E.; Boari, B.; Zucchi, B.; Signani, F.; Salmi, R.; Gallerani, M.; Manfredini, R. Weekend hospitalization and inhospital mortality: A gender effect? *Am. J. Emerg. Med.* **2015**, *33*, 1701–1703. [CrossRef] [PubMed]
25. James, M.T.; Wald, R.; Bell, C.M.; Tonelli, M.; Hemmelgarn, B.R.; Waikar, S.S.; Chertow, G.M. Weekend hospital admission, acute kidney injury, and mortality. *J. Am. Soc. Nephrol.* **2010**, *21*, 845–851. [CrossRef]
26. Kolhe, N.V.; Fluck, R.J.; Taal, M.W. Effect of weekend admission on mortality associated with severe acute kidney injury in England: A propensity score matched, population-based study. *PLoS ONE* **2017**, *12*, e0186048. [CrossRef]
27. Holmes, J.; Rainer, T.; Geen, J.; Williams, J.D.; Phillips, A.O. Welsh AKI Steering Group Adding a new dimension to the weekend effect: An analysis of a national data set of electronic AKI alerts. *Qjm Int. J. Med.* **2018**, *111*, 249–255. [CrossRef]
28. Baid-Agrawal, S.; Martus, P.; Feldman, H.; Kramer, H. Weekend versus weekday transplant surgery and outcomes after kidney transplantation in the USA: A retrospective national database analysis. *BMJ Open* **2016**, *6*, e010482. [CrossRef]
29. Schütte-Nütgen, K.; Thölking, G.; Dahmen, M.; Becker, F.; Kebschull, L.; Schmidt, R.; Pavenstädt, H.; Suwelack, B.; Reuteret, S. Is there a "weekend effect" in kidney transplantation? *PLoS ONE* **2017**, *12*, e0190227. [CrossRef]
30. Anderson, B.M.; Mytton, J.L.; Evison, F.; Ferro, C.J.; Sharif, A. Outcomes After Weekend Admission for Deceased Donor Kidney Transplantation. *Transplantation* **2017**, *101*, 2244–2252. [CrossRef]

31. Lim, W.H.; Coates, P.T.; Russ, G.R.; Russell, C.; He, B.; Jaques, B.; Pleass, H.; Chapman, J.R.; Wong, G. Weekend effect on early allograft outcome after kidney transplantation- a multi-centre cohort study. *Transpl. Int.* **2018**, *32*, 387–398. [CrossRef] [PubMed]
32. Manfredini, R.; Gallerani, M.; De Giorgi, A.; Boari, B.; Lamberti, N.; Manfredini, F.; Storari, A.; La Manna, G.; Fabbian, F. Lack of a "Weekend Effect" for Renal Transplant Recipients: The Hospital Database of the Emilia-Romagna Region of Italy. *Angiology* **2017**, *68*, 366–373. [CrossRef] [PubMed]
33. Sakhuja, A.; Schold, J.D.; Kumar, G.; Dall, A.; Sood, P.; Navaneethan, S.D. Outcomes of Patients Receiving Maintenance Dialysis Admitted Over Weekends. *Am. J. Kidney Dis.* **2013**, *62*, 763–770. [CrossRef] [PubMed]
34. Johnson, D.W.; Clayton, P.; Cho, Y.; Badve, S.V.; Hawley, C.; McDonald, S.; Boudville, N.; Wiggins, K.J.; Bannister, K.; Brown, F. Weekend Compared with Weekday Presentations of Peritoneal Dialysis–Associated Peritonitis. *Perit. Dial. Int.* **2012**, *32*, 516–524. [CrossRef] [PubMed]
35. Mazzali, C.; Duca, P. Use of administrative data in health care research. *Intern. Emerg. Med.* **2015**, *10*, 517–524. [CrossRef] [PubMed]
36. Clinical Practice Guideline for Acute Kidney Injury. Available online: https://kdigo.org/wp-content/uploads/2016/10/KDIGO-2012-AKI-Guideline-English.pdf (accessed on 8 June 2020).
37. Black, N. Higher Mortality in Weekend Admissions to the Hospital. *JAMA* **2016**, *316*, 2593–2594. [CrossRef]
38. Waikar, S.S.; Wald, R.; Chertow, G.M.; Curhan, G.C.; Winkelmayer, W.C.; Liangos, O.; Sosa, M.A.; Jaber, B.L. Validity of International Classification of Diseases, Ninth Revision, Clinical Modification Codes for Acute Renal Failure. *J. Am. Soc. Nephrol.* **2006**, *17*, 1688–1694. [CrossRef]
39. Vlasschaert, M.E.; Bejaimal, S.A.; Hackam, D.G.; Quinn, R.; Cuerden, M.S.; Oliver, M.J.; Iansavichus, A.; Sultan, N.; Mills, A.; Garg, A.X. Validity of Administrative Database Coding for Kidney Disease: A Systematic Review. *Am. J. Kidney Dis.* **2011**, *57*, 29–43. [CrossRef]
40. Tomlinson, L.A.; Riding, A.M.; Payne, R.A.; Abel, G.A.; Tomson, C.R.; Wilkinson, I.B.; Roland, M.O.; Chaudhry, A.N. The accuracy of diagnostic coding for acute kidney injury in England—A single centre study. *BMC Nephrol.* **2013**, *14*, 58. [CrossRef]
41. Grams, M.E.; Waikar, S.S.; MacMahon, B.; Whelton, S.; Ballew, S.; Coresh, J. Performance and Limitations of Administrative Data in the Identification of AKI. *Clin. J. Am. Soc. Nephrol.* **2014**, *9*, 682–689. [CrossRef]
42. Available online: www.who.int/ageing/population/global_health.pdf (accessed on 8 June 2020).
43. Saran, R.; Robinson, B.; Abbott, K.C.; Bragg-Gresham, J.; Chen, X.; Gipson, D.; Gu, H.; Hirth, R.A.; Hutton, D.; Jin, Y.; et al. US Renal Data System 2019 Annual Data Report: Epidemiology of Kidney Disease in the United States. *Am. J. Kidney Dis.* **2019**, *75*, A6–A7. [CrossRef] [PubMed]
44. Floege, J.; Gillespie, I.; Kronenberg, F.; Anker, S.D.; Gioni, I.; Richards, S.; Pisoni, R.L.; Robinson, B.M.; Marcelli, D.; Froissart, M.; et al. Development and validation of a predictive mortality risk score from a European hemodialysis cohort. *Kidney Int.* **2015**, *87*, 996–1008. [CrossRef] [PubMed]
45. Barnett, K.; Mercer, S.; Norbury, M.; Watt, G.; Wyke, S.; Guthrie, B. Epidemiology of multimorbidity and implications for health care, research, and medical education: A cross-sectional study. *Lancet* **2012**, *380*, 37–43. [CrossRef]

14

The *Macrophage Migration Inhibitory Factor* (*MIF*) Promoter Polymorphisms (rs3063368, rs755622) Predict Acute Kidney Injury and Death after Cardiac Surgery

Luisa Averdunk [1,2], Jürgen Bernhagen [3,4,5], Karl Fehnle [6], Harald Surowy [2], Hermann-Josef Lüdecke [2], Sören Mucha [7,8], Patrick Meybohm [9], Dagmar Wieczorek [2], Lin Leng [10], Gernot Marx [1], David E. Leaf [11,12], Alexander Zarbock [13], Kai Zacharowski [9], on behalf of the RIPHeart Study Collaborators [†], Richard Bucala [10,*,‡] and Christian Stoppe [1,14,*,‡]

1 Department of Intensive Care Medicine, University Hospital Aachen, Rheinisch Westphälische Technische Hochschule Aachen, 52074 Aachen, Germany; luisa.aver@gmail.com (L.A.); gmarx@ukaachen.de (G.M.)

2 Institute of Human Genetics and Department of Pediatrics, Medical Faculty, Heinrich Heine University, 40225 Düsseldorf, Germany; harald.surowy@uni-duesseldorf.de (H.S.); Hermann-Josef.Luedecke@uni-duesseldorf.de (H.-J.L.); dagmar.wieczorek@hhu.de (D.W.)

3 Department of Vascular Biology, Institute for Stroke and Dementia Research, Klinikum der Universität München, Ludwig-Maximilians-University Munich, 80333 Munich, Germany; Juergen.Bernhagen@med.uni-muenchen.de

4 German Center for Cardiovascular Research (DZHK), Partner Site Munich Heart Alliance, 10785 Berlin, Germany

5 Munich Cluster for Systems Neurology (EXC 2145 SyNergy), 81377 Munich, Germany

6 Algora: Statistics and Clinical Research GmbH, 85540 Haar, Germany; karl.fehnle@algora.de

7 Institute of Clinical Molecular Biology, Christian Albrechts University of Kiel, 24118 Kiel, Germany; s.mucha@ikmb.uni-kiel.de

8 Institute for Cardiogenetics, University of Lübeck, Ratzeburger Allee 160, 23562 Lübeck, Germany

9 Department of Anesthesiology, Intensive Care Medicine & Pain Therapy, University Hospital Frankfurt, Goethe University, 60323 Frankfurt, Germany; meybohm_p@ukw.de (P.M.); kai.zacharowski@kgu.de (K.Z.)

10 Department of Internal Medicine, Yale University School of Medicine, New Haven, CT 06510, USA; lin.leng@yale.edu

11 Division of Renal Medicine, Brigham and Women's Hospital, Boston, MA 02115, USA; deleaf@bwh.harvard.edu

12 Harvard Medical School, Boston, MA 02115, USA

13 Intensive Care and Pain Medicine, Department of Anesthesiology, University of Münster, 48149 Münster, Germany; zarbock@uni-muenster.de

14 Department of Anesthesiology, Intensive Care Medicine and Pain Therapy, University Hospital Würzburg, 97080 Würzburg, Germany

* Correspondence: richard.bucala@yale.edu (R.B.); christian.stoppe@gmail.com (C.S.);

† RIPHeart Study Collaborators are listed at the end of the manuscript. See Supplemental Acknowledgments for consortium details.

‡ Contributed equally as last authors.

Abstract: Background: Macrophage Migration Inhibitory Factor (MIF) is highly elevated after cardiac surgery and impacts the postoperative inflammation. The aim of this study was to analyze whether the polymorphisms $CATT_{5–7}$ (rs5844572/rs3063368,"-794") and G>C single-nucleotide polymorphism (rs755622,-173) in the *MIF* gene promoter are related to postoperative outcome. Methods: In 1116 patients undergoing cardiac surgery, the *MIF* gene polymorphisms were analyzed and serum MIF was measured by ELISA in 100 patients. Results: Patients with at least one extended repeat allele ($CATT_7$) had a significantly higher risk of acute kidney injury (AKI) compared to others (23% vs. 13%; OR 2.01 (1.40–2.88), p = 0.0001). Carriers of $CATT_7$ were also at higher risk of death (1.8% vs. 0.4%; OR 5.12 (0.99–33.14), p = 0.026). The GC genotype was associated with

AKI (20% vs. GG/CC:13%, OR 1.71 (1.20–2.43), $p = 0.003$). Multivariate analyses identified $CATT_7$ predictive for AKI (OR 2.13 (1.46–3.09), $p < 0.001$) and death (OR 5.58 (1.29–24.04), $p = 0.021$). $CATT_7$ was associated with higher serum MIF before surgery (79.2 vs. 50.4 ng/mL, $p = 0.008$). Conclusion: The $CATT_7$ allele associates with a higher risk of AKI and death after cardiac surgery, which might be related to chronically elevated serum MIF. Polymorphisms in the *MIF* gene may constitute a predisposition for postoperative complications and the assessment may improve risk stratification and therapeutic guidance.

Keywords: acute kidney injury; genetic polymorphisms; risk prediction; (cardiac) surgery; inflammatory cytokines; clinical studies

1. Introduction

Conventional open-heart surgery is performed annually in more than one million patients worldwide, and the incidence of postoperative sequelae including acute organ dysfunction remains high [1,2]. A more precise identification of patients' risk for postoperative complications is desirable both for prognostic guidance and for the application of earlier and more effective interventions. While clinical scoring systems such as the well-established EuroSCORE were primarily developed for the preoperative risk stratification of mortality in cardiac surgery patients, only limited evidence exists about its value for postoperative organ dysfunction and other complications [3]. The identification of genomic risk alleles could be especially helpful to more accurately predict outcomes and to enable personalized medicine approaches.

Oxidative stress and a systemic inflammatory response contribution to the pathogenesis of postoperative organ dysfunctions following cardiac surgery [4]. Macrophage migration inhibitory factor (MIF) is a stress-regulating cytokine that increases in the circulation after cardiac surgery [5]. Within the *MIF* gene promoter, two polymorphisms, a G>C single nucleotide polymorphism 270 bases before *MIF* transcription start (−270) (originally described as −173; HGVS nomenclature: NM_002415.2 c.−270G>C, rs755622) and a CATT tetranucleotide repeat $CATT_{5\text{-}7}$ (rs3063368), have been associated with disease severity of multiple chronic inflammatory diseases, including osteoporosis, ankylosing spondylitis, and multiple sclerosis [6–8]. A higher number of CATT repeats has been reported to increase *MIF* promotor activity and to be associated with higher circulating MIF concentrations in different autoimmune and chronic inflammatory conditions [9–12]. The clinical significance of functional polymorphisms in *MIF* for postoperative outcome after cardiac surgery is unknown. In this study, we analyzed 1116 patients who underwent elective cardiac surgery with a cardiopulmonary bypass. We analyzed whether *MIF* promoter polymorphisms impact the risk of postoperative organ dysfunction and mortality in patients undergoing cardiac surgery. In a subset of patients, we also examined the correlation between *MIF* genotypes and circulating MIF levels.

2. Materials and Methods

2.1. Study Design and Patients

The present study is a predefined sub-study performed in cardiac surgery patients of the Remote Ischemic Preconditioning Heart (RIPHeart) study (January 2011–May 2014), which investigated whether upper limb remote ischemic conditioning reduced mortality and the incidence of myocardial infarction, stroke, and acute kidney injury (AKI) in adults scheduled for elective cardiac surgery requiring a cardiopulmonary bypass [13]. As the initial intervention study did not show group differences, this *MIF* polymorphism study includes all patients irrespective of the initial group assignment [13]. The trial was undertaken in compliance with International Conference on Harmonisation Good Clinical Practice guidelines, the Declaration of Helsinki (2008), and European Directive 2001/20/CE regarding the conduct of clinical trials (4 April 2001). The study was registered at ClinicalTrials.gov (NCT01067703). The study protocol was approved by the ethics committees of the University of Kiel, Aachen, and all participating centers of this prospective multicenter study.

Patients scheduled for elective cardiac surgery with use of cardiopulmonary bypass (e.g., coronary artery bypass graft (CABG), valve surgery, ascending aorta replacement) were eligible for this study. Of the 1403 patients screened for the study, blood samples were available from 1196 patients. Seven patients were excluded due to missing outcome data and 70 patients were excluded due to missing genotype information (Supplemental Figure S1). Thus, data from 1119 patients were included in the current study. The $CATT_8$ genotype was excluded from analysis because of its low frequency ($N = 3$), which is in accord with prior reports [14].

Blood samples were collected before surgery, at 45 min after cardiopulmonary bypass (CPB) initiation, at 2 min after opening of the cross-clamp (reperfusion), at 15 min after weaning from CPB, and at 1, 6, and 24 h after admission to ICU. Blood samples were processed no later than 2 h after collection and were stored at −70 °C or −20 °C until further transfer. The final study visit took place either before hospital discharge, or at the latest 30 days after ICU admission.

2.2. Outcome Measures

The primary exposure was the *MIF* genotype, which we analyzed according to the following groups: alleles (e.g., carriers of at least one C allele), genotypes (e.g., GC), and individual genotype combinations (e.g., $CATT_{5,7}$-GC). The endpoints were the association between the *MIF* genotype and the incidence of postoperative organ dysfunctions, including AKI, myocardial infarction, new onset of atrial fibrillation, stroke, delirium, and death. Each of these outcome parameters were analyzed as single events, and in the composite outcome "multiple organ dysfunction", when patients suffered from more than one organ dysfunction.

According to the KDIGO Clinical Practice Guideline 2012, AKI was defined as a ≥ 5-fold increase of serum creatinine from baseline, and a urine output of ≤0.5 mL/kg/h for more than 6 h, or the use of renal replacement therapy within 72 h [15]. However, a total creatinine increase of ≥ 0.3 mg/dL was not considered a diagnostic criterion for AKI, as this criterion had not yet been established in 2011 when the data collection started. Non-fatal myocardial infarction was defined by biomarker values more than five times higher than the 99th percentile of the normal reference range combined with new pathological Q-waves or new left bundle branch block within the first 72 h, standard clinical criteria for myocardial infarction from 72 h on, new ischemic finding by echocardiography or angiography, or myocardial infarction diagnosed at autopsy [16]. New onset of atrial fibrillation was defined as a new onset within the first four days after surgery [13]. The occurrence of postoperative delirium was assessed with the CAM-ICU score (preoperative, 24, 48, 72, and 96 h after surgery) [17]. Stroke was defined by any new, temporary or permanent, focal or global neurological deficit, or evidence of stroke on autopsy, and was evaluated according to the National Institutes of Health Stroke Scale (≥4 points) [18].

Myocardial infarction, atrial fibrillation, and stroke were analyzed until hospital discharge with a maximum of 14 days after surgery.

2.3. ELISA

Serum was available from 100 patients in the RIPheart Study. Serum MIF levels were quantified by ELISA in duplicates as previously described and according to the manufacturer's instructions (R&D Systems, Minneapolis, MN, USA) ([5]). Samples were diluted 1:10 before analysis to obtain measures in the valid assay range.

2.4. Nomenclature and Genotyping of the Tetranucleotide Repeat Polymorphism $CATT_n$ (rs3063368)

In adherence to the U.S. National Library of Medicine dbSNP database (ncbi.nlm.nih.gov/snp/), the tetranucleotide repeat polymorphism formerly described as rs5844572, referring to the $CATT_6$

allele, will be referred to with the reference SNP number rs3063368, which comprises the multiallelic repeat polymorphism $CATT_n$ present at this site. The tetranucleotide repeat polymorphism is located at position chr22:23893566-23893569: (GRCh38.p12) (ncbi.nlm.nih.gov/snp/rs3063368), and based on older transcript annotations (NM_002415.2) -794 nucleotides, or based on more accurate transcript annotations (NM_002415.2) -909 nucleotides upstream of the start codon. The repeat polymorphism is a deletion, or respectively a duplication, of TTCA tetranucleotide repeats. In parallel with former publications, in this study this SNP will be referred to as a tetranucleotide 5-, 6-, 7-, or 8- fold repeat of CATT. The DNA sequence of this SNP is illustrated in Supplemental Figure S2 (UCSC Genome Browser, genome.ucsc.edu).

EDTA-anticoagulated whole blood was used for genotyping. DNA was extracted with the Autopure LS automated system according to the manufacturer's recommendations (Qiagen, Hilden, Germany).

For the analysis of the tetranucleotide repeat (rs3063368), as formerly described, a fragment length polymorphism PCR with fluorescently labeled primers and fragment length analysis via capillary electrophoresis was applied [10]. Of note, with this technique a phase analysis with the rs755622 single nucleotide polymorphism (SNP) is not possible. DNA was amplified in a Mastercycler gradient (Eppendorf AG, Germany). The PCR reaction mix contained 2.5 μL 10× PCR buffer, 3 μL (25 mM) MgCl2, 2 μL dNTP Mix, 0.8 μL of each primer, 0.15 μL (1 U) Taq polymerase, and 13.75 μL of purified DNA, in a total end volume of 25 μL. The PCR consisted of the following steps: an initial denaturation step (95 °C, 12 min), 35 amplification cycle (95 °C, 30 s; X (primer annealing temperature see Supplemental Table S1, 30 s; 72 °C, 30 s) and a final elongation step (72 °C, 10 min). The reverse primer was labeled with 6-Carboxyfluorescein (6-FAM) [19]. The PCR was performed in a SimpliAmp Thermal Cycler (Life Technologies, Carlsbad, CA, USA). The PCR products were subjected to capillary electrophoresis on an ABI 3730XL Genetic Analyzer (Applied Biosystems, Foster City, CA, USA). Data collection was performed with Data Collection v3.0 software (Applied Biosystems, Foster City, CA, USA) and the results were analyzed by GeneMapper ID v5 software (Applied Biosystems, Foster City, CA, USA).

2.5. Nomenclature and Genotyping of the SNP G>C Substitution (rs755622)

The SNP rs755622 is a substitution of G>C in the non-coding region at position chr22:23,894,205 (GRCh38.p12). Based on the older transcript annotations (NM_002415.1), this SNP has been formerly described with the position NM_002415.1:m.-173. According to the more accurate transcript annotation (NM_002415.2), the G>C substitution is located at position NM_002415.2:m.-178 and NM_002415.2:c.-270 G>C. (The start codon is located at position chr22:23,894,475.)

DNA was extracted from EDTA-anticoagulated whole blood with Autopure (Qiagen, Hilden, Germany). Genotyping of the SNP rs755622 G>C was performed using an Assays-on-Demand® allelic discrimination on a TaqMan platform according to the manufacturer's instructions (ThermoFisher Scientific, Waltham, MA, USA). The polymerase chain reaction (PCR) contained 10 ng of genomic DNA, 10 μL TaqMan master mix, and 0.125 μL of 40× assay mix. PCR was performed using 96-well plates on an ABI 9700 thermal cycler (Applied Biosystems, Foster City, CA, USA) (reaction conditions 50 °C for 2 min, 95 °C for 10 min, followed by 40 cycles of 95 °C for 15 s and 60 °C for 1 min). The TaqMan 7700 platform was used to perform an end-plate reading using the allelic discrimination option.

Sample and marker quality control (QC) was performed with PLINK (v1.9; https://www.cog-genomics.org/plink/1.9)(PMID:25722852).

2.6. Statistics

Baseline characteristics were analyzed using of Wilcoxon Rank Sum test for continuous variables and Fisher's exact test for binary variables. Associations between *MIF* polymorphisms and outcome parameters were analyzed using univariate logistic regression and results are presented together with odds ratios and 95% confidence intervals.

Multivariable logistic regression analysis was performed to analyze the influence of relevant baseline variables. Model selection was based on the postoperative complication (dependent variable) and the genotype (independent variable). Further variables were selected on the basis of univariate analyses and significant differences. Model selection was accomplished by a backward elimination or a stepwise procedure.

Serum MIF levels at individual time points were compared using Wilcoxon Rank Sum test according to the *MIF* genotype. Analyses were calculated with SAS 9.4 (SAS Institute Inc., Cary, NC, USA) and SPSS (IBM SPSS, version 21.0, Armonk, NY, USA). All p-Values refer to two-sided tests, and $p < 0.05$ was considered statistically significant.

2.7. Study Approval

Each patient provided written informed consent prior to inclusion in the study.

3. Results

3.1. Patients, Baseline Characteristics, and Postoperative Complications

The median age was 68 years and 25.1% were females (Table 1). Postoperative AKI was associated with older age ($p < 0.001$), female gender ($p = 0.007$), the intake of aspirin ($p = 0.01$), lower baseline hemoglobin (<14 g/dL) ($p < 0.001$), peripheral artery disease ($p = 0.02$), hypertension ($p = 0.01$), insulin-dependent diabetes mellitus (IDDM) ($p = 0.01$), and a higher EuroSCORE ($p < 0.001$) (Table 1). Death was associated with older age ($p = 0.03$) and IDDM ($p = 0.03$) (Table 1).

Table 1. Baseline and operative characteristics by AKI and death.

	AKI					Death				
	Yes (N = 170)		No (N = 946)		p-Value	Yes (N = 8)		No (N = 1108)		p-Value
Demographics										
Age, years	72	(66–77)	67	(58–73)	**<0.001**	73	(70–80)	68	(59–73)	**0.03**
Sex (female)	57	(33.5)	223	(23.6)	**0.007**	3	(37.5)	277	(25.0)	0.42
Active smokers	32	(18.8)	198	(20.9)	0.61	1	(12.5)	229	(20.7)	1.00
Medication										
Beta blockers	109	(64.1)	587	(62.1)	0.67	6	(75.0)	690	(62.3)	0.72
ACE inhibitors	91	(53.5)	478	(50.5)	0.51	3	(37.5)	566	(51.1)	0.50
Cholesterol-lowering drug	110	(64.7)	624	(66.0)	0.79	6	(75.0)	728	(65.7)	0.72
Insulin	21	(12.4)	77	(8.1)	0.08	3	(37.5)	95	(8.6)	**0.03**
Aspirin	128	(75.3)	619	(65.4)	**0.01**	4	(50.0)	743	(67.1)	0.45
Clopidogrel	17	(10)	76	(8.0)	0.37	2	(25.0)	91	(8.2)	0.14
Comorbidities										
Hypertension	153	(90.0)	772	(81.6)	**0.01**	6	(75.0)	919	(82.9)	0.63
Ischemic heart disease	132	(77.6)	706	(74.6)	0.39	5	(62.5)	833	(75.2)	0.42
Previous MI						1	(12.5)	315	(28.4)	0.45
Congestive heart disease	43	(25.3)	193	(20.4)	0.15	2	(25.0)	234	(21.1)	0.68
PAD	20	(11.8)	62	(6.6)	**0.02**	2	(25.0)	80	(7.2)	0.68
COPD	15	(8.8)	80	(8.5)	0.88	0	0	95	(8.6)	1.00
Chronic kidney disease	24	(14.1)	107	(11.3)	0.30	1	(12.5)	130	(11.7)	1.00
IDDM	56	(32.9)	219	(23.2)	**0.01**	4	(50.0)	271	(24.5)	0.11
Laboratory, at baseline										
Serum creatinine mg/dL	0.92	(0.8–1.1)	0.91	(0.8–1.1)	0.66	0.99	(0.73–1.14)	0.91	(0.80–1.07)	0.82
Hemoglobin, g/dL	13.6	(12.5–14.6)	14.2	(13.4–14.9)	**<0.001**	13.6	(12.1–14.4)	14.1	(13.2–14.9)	0.31
EuroSCORE										
	5	(3–7)	4	(2–6)	**<0.001**	6	(5–8)	4	(2–6)	**0.03**
Type of surgery										
CABG (alone)	64	(37.6)	434	(45.9)		3	(37.5)	495	(44.7)	
Aortic valve *	37	(12.8)	190	(20.1)		2	(12.5)	225	(20.3)	
Mitral valve *	6	(3.5)	32	(3.4)	0.26	0	(37.5)	38	(3.4)	0.25
Aorta ascendens *	3	(1.8)	30	(3.2)		0	(25.0)	33	(3.0)	
Combined procedures	57	(33.5)	245	(25.9)		2	25.0	300	(27.1)	
Other type of surgery	3	(1.8)	15	(1.6)		1	12.5	17	(1.5)	

Data are expressed as the median and interquartile range (Q1–Q3) or absolute numbers and (percentage). The association of baseline characteristics with AKI and death was analyzed by Wilcoxon rank sum or Fisher's exact test. ACE, angiotensin converting enzyme; CABG, coronary artery bypass graft; COPD, chronic obstructive pulmonary disease; IDDM, insulin-dependent diabetes mellitus; MI, myocardial infarction; PAD, peripheral artery disease, *, replacement or reconstruction (alone). Bold fonts indicate p-values < 0.05.

3.2. Genotype Frequencies

The most common genotypes were $CATT_{6,6}$-GG (32.3%) and $CATT_{5,6}$-GG (30.9%) (Table 2); 24.8% of patients carried at least one $CATT_7$ allele; 29.6% of patients were heterozygous and 2.3% of patients were homozygous carriers of the G>C substitution. The allele frequencies in our study cohort were comparable to the frequencies published in the reference database gnomAD (Table 1) [20]. The frequency of the GC genotype and the $CATT_7$-repeat allele was higher than in patients with AKI compared to patients without AKI (X^2 test for trend, $p = 0.001$) (Figure 1).

Table 2. Frequencies of the *MIF* $CATT_{5-7}$ repeat allele (rs3063368) and the G>C single-nucleotide polymorphism (rs755622) in 1116 patients undergoing cardiac surgery.

$CATT_{5-7}$ Repeat Allele Carrier Frequencies (rs3063368)			
	N Carriers	%	**Allele Frequency (Europe) %** [1]
$CATT_5$	488	43.7	- *
$CATT_6$	957	85.8	84.3
$CATT_7$	277	24.8	24.9
G>C SNP Genotype Frequencies (rs755622)			
	***N* Genotypes**	%	**Allele Frequency (Europe) %** [1]
GG (homozygous)	762	68.3	65.2
GC (heterozygous)	328	29.4	31.7
CC (homozygous)	26	2.3	3.1
Individual Genotype Combination Frequencies (rs3063368 & rs755622)			
	N	%	
$CATT_{5,5}$-GG	68	6.1	
CATT $_{5,6}$-GG	329	29.5	
CATT $_{6,6}$-GG	360	32.3	
CATT $_{5,7}$-GG	2	0.2	
CATT $_{6,7}$-GG	3	0.3	
CATT $_{5,5}$-CG	3	0.3	
CATT $_{5,6}$-CG	16	1.4	
CATT $_{6,6}$-CG	63	5.6	
CATT $_{5,7}$-CG	69	6.2	
CATT $_{6,7}$-CG	176	15.8	
CATT $_{7,7}$-CG	1	0.1	
CATT $_{5,7}$-CC	1	0.1	
CATT $_{6,7}$-CC	10	0.9	
CATT $_{7,7}$-CC	15	1.3	
All	1116	100.00	

The most frequent genotypes observed were CATT $_{5,6}$-GG (29.5%), CATT $_{6,6}$-GG (32.3%), and CATT $_{6,7}$-CG (15.8%). The frequency of the polymorphisms was comparable to the frequency in the general reference population (Europe) [1]; SNP, Single nucleotide polymorphism; $CATT_7$, patients carrying at least one $CATT_7$ allele. Data presented as absolute numbers and percentage. [1] calculated from reference gnomAD Database (including >7500 genomes from unrelated non-Finnish European individuals sequenced as part of various population genetic studies) [20]. * As $CATT_5$ is the wildtype allele, there is no information regarding $CATT_5$ in the gnomAD Database.

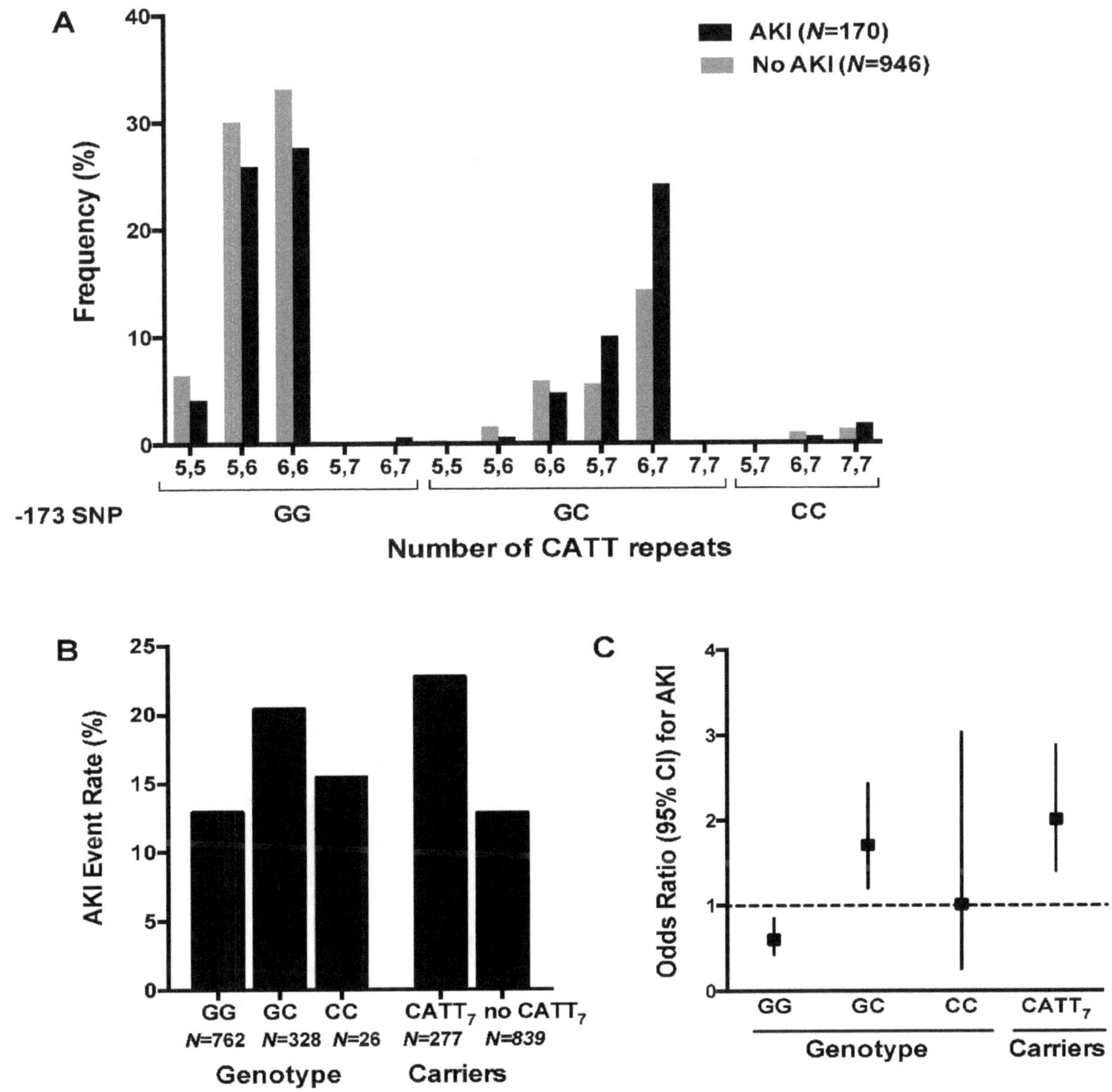

Figure 1. Frequency distribution of the CATT microsatellite repeat (rs3063368) and the G>C SNP (rs755622) in patients with AKI versus patients not affected by AKI after cardiac surgery. (**A**) In patients with AKI, the frequency of the GC genotype and the $CATT_7$ allele is higher than in patients without AKI (X^2 test for trend, $p = 0.001$). (**B**) The AKI event rate was higher in patients with the GC genotype (20%) versus patients with the CC or the GG genotype (13%), and higher in $CATT_7$ carriers (23%) compared to non-carriers. (**C**) Patients carrying the GC genotype or the $CATT_7$ allele had a significantly increased relative risk of AKI compared to all other patients.

3.3. Association of the Tetranucleotide Repeat $CATT_{5-7}$ (rs3063368) and the G>C Single-Nucleotide Polymorphism (rs755622) with Postoperative Outcome

All patients ($N = 1116$) were examined for the association between the two polymorphisms in the *MIF* promoter and risk of postoperative complications. The overall incidence of AKI after cardiac surgery was 15.2% ($N = 170$) (Table 3). Patients who were either homozygous or heterozygous carriers of the *MIF* $CATT_7$ allele had a significantly increased risk of AKI after cardiac surgery when compared to all other patients (22.7% vs. 12.8%, OR 2.01, 95% CI 1.40–2.88, $p = 0.0001$) (Table 4).

Table 3. Absolute and relative frequency of postoperative complications. * Patients affected by at least two of the predefined organ dysfunctions.

	Patients (N = 1116)	
	N	%
Death	8	0.7
Myocardial infarction (MI)	93	8.3
Stroke	24	2.2
Delirium	144	12.9
Acute kidney injury (AKI)	170	15.2
Stage 1	108	9.7
Stage 2	38	3.4
Stage 3	24	2.1
Atrial Fibrillation	245	21.9
Multiple Complications (≥) *	139	12.4

Table 4. Association of the *MIF* promoter polymorphisms with AKI.

MIF Polymorphism	AKI (N = 170) Patients Carrying This Allele/Genotype		Patients NOT Carrying this Allele/Genotype				p-Value
	N	Incidence, %	N	Incidence, %	OR	(95% CI)	
CATT Repeat Allele Carriers (rs3063368)							
$CATT_5$	69	14.1	101	16.1	0.86	(0.61–1.21)	0.401
$CATT_6$	143	14.9	27	17.0	0.86	(0.54–1.40)	0.551
$CATT_7$	**63**	**22.7**	**107**	**12.8**	**2.01**	**(1.40–2.88)**	**0.0001**
Genotypes							
G>C (rs755622)							
GG	**99**	**12.9**	**71**	**20.1**	**0.60**	**(0.42–0.85)**	**0.0031**
GC	**67**	**20.4**	**103**	**13.1**	**1.71**	**(1.20–2.43)**	**0.0025**
CC	4	15.4	166	15.2	1.01	(0.25–3.03)	1.000
CATT repeat (rs3063368)							
$CATT_{5,5}$	7	9.9	163	15.6	0.59	(0.22–1.32)	0.233
$CATT_{5,6}$	45	13.0	125	16.2	0.78	(0.52–1.13)	0.178
$CATT_{5,7}$	17	23.6	153	14.7	1.80	(0.95–3.25)	0.060
$CATT_{6,6}$	55	13.0	115	16.6	0.75	(0.52–1.07)	0.122
$CATT_{6,7}$	**43**	**22.8**	**127**	**13.7**	**1.86**	**(1.23–2.77)**	**0.003**
$CATT_{7,7}$	3	18.8	167	15.2	1.29	(0.23–4.76)	0.723
Individual genotype combinations *							
$CATT_{5,5}$-GG (6.1%)	7	10.3	163	15.6	0.62	(0.24–1.40)	0.297
$CATT_{5,6}$-GG (29.5%)	44	13.4	126	16.0	0.81	(0.55–1.19)	0.275
$CATT_{6,6}$-GG (32.3%)	47	13.1	123	16,3	0.77	(0.53–1.12)	0.182
$CATT_{6,6}$-CG (5.6%)	8	12.7	162	15.4	0.80	(0.32–1.73)	0.718
$CATT_{5,7}$-CG (6.2%)	**17**	**24.6**	**153**	**14.6**	**1.91**	**(1.01–3.46)**	**0.036**
$CATT_{6,7}$-CG (15.8%)	**41**	**23.3**	**129**	**13.7**	**1.91**	**(1.25–2.87)**	**0.002**

The incidence of AKI was higher among patients carrying the $CATT_7$ allele, in patients with the GC or $CATT_{6,7}$ genotype, and in patients with the genotype combinations $CATT_{5,7}$-CG and $CATT_{6,7}$-CG. AKI, acute kidney injury; CI, confidence interval; OR, odds ratio; SNP, Single nucleotide polymorphism; $CATT_7$, patients carrying at least one $CATT_7$ allele. * genotype combinations with a frequency of >5%. Data presented as absolute numbers and percentage. p-value calculated by Fisher exact test; bold fonts indicate p-values < 0.05.

Patients carrying the G>C SNP were also at increased risk of AKI (20.4% vs. 13.1%, OR 1.71, 95% CI 1.20–2.43, p = 0.0025) (Table 4). The 26 homozygote carriers of the CC genotype did not show an increased risk of AKI when compared to others (p = 1.000).

Multiple complications, defined as at least two of the predefined organ dysfunctions, were observed in 12.4% of patients (N = 139) (Table 3). The $CATT_7$ repeat and the G>C SNP were significantly associated with the occurrence of multiple postoperative complications when compared to all other genotypes ($CATT_7$: 17.7% vs. 10.7%, OR 1.79, 95% CI 1.20–2.65, $p = 0.003$; GC: 16.8% vs. 10.7%, OR 1.69, 95% CI 1.15–2.47, $p = 0.007$) (Table 5).

Table 5. Association of the *MIF* promoter polymorphisms with multiple complications *.

MIF Polymorphism	Multiple Complications * (N = 139) Patients Carrying this Allele/Genotype		Patients NOT Carrying this Allele/Genotype				*p*-Value
	N	Incidence, %	*N*	Incidence, %	OR	(95% CI)	
-CATT repeat allele carriers (rs3063368)							
CATT $_5$	50	10.3	89	14.2	0.69	(0.47–1.01)	0.055
CATT $_6$	120	12.5	19	12.0	1.06	(0.62–1.88)	0.898
CATT $_7$	**49**	**17.7**	**90**	**10.7**	**1.79**	**(1.20–2.65)**	**0.003**
Genotypes							
G>C (rs755622)							
GG	**80**	**10.1**	**59**	**16.7**	**0.59**	**(0.40–0.86)**	**0.005**
GC	**55**	**16.8**	**84**	**10.7**	**1.69**	**(1.15–2.47)**	**0.007**
CC	4	15.4	135	12.4	1.29	(0.32–3.87)	0.554
CATT repeat (rs3063368)							
CATT $_{5,5}$	4	5.6	135	12.9	0.40	(0.10–1.11)	0.092
CATT $_{5,6}$	33	9.6	106	13.8	0.66	(0.42–1.02)	0.050
CATT $_{5,7}$	13	18.1	126	12.1	1.61	(0.78–3.06)	0.140
CATT $_{6,6}$	53	12.5	86	12.4	1.01	(0.69–1.48)	1.000
CATT $_{6,7}$	**34**	**18.0**	**105**	**11.3**	**1.72**	**(1.09–2.66)**	**0.015**
CATT $_{7,7}$	2	12.5	137	12.5	1.00	(0.11–4.45)	1.000
Individual genotype combinations †							
CATT $_{5,5}$-GG (6.1%)	4	5.9	135	12.9	0.42	(0.11–1.16)	0.126
CATT $_{5,6}$-GG (29.5%)	32	9.7	107	13.6	0.68	(0.44–1.05)	0.091
CATT $_{6,6}$-GG (32.3%)	44	12.2	95	12.6	0.97	(0.65–1.44)	0.923
CATT $_{6,6}$-CG (5.6%)	9	14.3	130	12.4	1.18	(0.50–2.49)	0.693
CATT $_{5,7}$-CG (6.2%)	13	18.4	126	12.0	1.70	(0.83–3.25)	0.127
CATT $_{6,7}$-CG (15.8%)	**32**	**18.2**	**107**	**11.4**	**1.73**	**(1.08–2.70)**	**0.018**

The incidence of multiple complications was higher among patients carrying the $CATT_7$ allele, in patients with the GC or CATT $_{6,7}$ genotype, and in patients with the genotype combinations CATT $_{5,7}$-CG and CATT $_{6,7}$-CG. CI, confidence interval; OR, odds ratio; SNP, Single nucleotide polymorphism; $CATT_{7x}$, patients carrying at least one $CATT_7$ allele. † genotype combinations with a frequency of > 5%. * Patients affected by at least two of the predefined organ dysfunctions. † defined as at least two of the predefined organ dysfunctions. Data presented as absolute numbers and percentage. *p*-value calculated by Fisher's exact test; bold fonts indicate *p*-values < 0.05.

The incidence of death during the first 30 days after surgery was 0.7% ($N = 8$) (Table 3). The mortality of carriers of the *MIF* $CATT_7$ allele was significantly higher compared to patients not carrying the $CATT_7$ repeat (1.81% vs. 0.36%, $p = 0.026$, OR 5.12, 95% CI 0.99–33.14) (Table 6). Likewise, patients with the *MIF* $CATT_{6,7}$ repeat genotype also had an increased risk of death when compared to all other patients (2.1% vs. 0.4%, OR 4.99, 95% CI 0.92–26.98, $p = 0.032$). Mortality rates in carriers of the GC genotype were increased with borderline significance (1.5% vs. 0.4%, OR 4.05, 95% CI 0.78–26.20, $p = 0.053$).

There was no significant difference in the incidence of AKI or death in heterozygous or homozygous carriers of the C allele or the CATT7 repeat allele (AKI-C-allele: 20.4% vs. 15.4%, OR 1.41 (0.47–4.24), $p = 0.537$; AKI-CATT7: 21.7% vs. 18.8%, OR 1.11 (0.30–4.05), $p = 0.879$; death-C allele: 0% vs. 1.5%, OR 0.90 (0.05–16.75), $p = 0.526$; death-CATT7: 0% vs. 1.9%; OR 0.66 (0.03–12.54), $p = 0.589$). While *MIF* promoter polymorphisms were significantly associated with AKI, multiple complications, and death, no significant association was found with regards to the incidence of postoperative myocardial infarction, atrial fibrillation, stroke, or delirium (Supplemental Tables S2–S5).

Table 6. Association of the *MIF* promoter polymorphisms with death.

MIF Polymorphism	Death ($N = 8$) Patients Carrying This Allele/Genotype		Patients NOT Carrying This Allele/Genotype				*p*-Value
	N	Incidence, %	*N*	Incidence, %	OR	(95% CI)	
CATT repeat allele carriers (rs3063368)							
CATT 5	2	0.4	6	1.0	0.43	(0.04–2.40)	0.478
CATT 6	7	0.7	1	0.6	1.16	(0.15–52.80)	1.000
CATT 7	**5**	**1.8**	**3**	**0.4**	**5.12**	**(0.99–33.14)**	**0.026**
Genotypes							
G>C (rs755622)							
GG	3	0.4	5	1.4	0.28	(0.04–1.43)	0.118
GC	5	1.5	3	0.4	4.05	(0.78–26.20)	0.053
CC	0	0	8	0.7	0.00	(0.00–19.77)	1.000
CATT repeat (rs3063368)							
CATT 5,5	0	0	8	0.8	0.00	(0.00–6.75)	1.000
CATT 5,6	1	0.3	7	0.9	0.32	(0.01–2.49)	0.447
CATT 5,7	1	1.4	7	0.7	2.09	(0.05–16.59)	0.415
CATT 6,6	2	0.5	6	0.9	0.54	(0.05–3.06)	0.717
CATT 6,7	**4**	**2.1**	**4**	**0.4**	**4.99**	**(0.92–26.98)**	**0.032**
CATT 7,7	0	0	8	0.7	0.00	(0.00–33.33)	1.000
Individual genotype combinations *							
CATT 5,5-GG (6.1%)	0	0	8	0.8	0.00	(0.00–7.07)	1.000
CATT 5,6-GG (29.5%)	1	0.3	7	0.9	0.34	(0.01–2.66)	0.449
CATT 6,6-GG (32.3%)	2	0.6	6	0.8	0.70	(0.07–3.93)	1.000
CATT 6,6-CG (5.6%)	0	0	8	0.8	0.00	(0.00–7.68)	1.000
CATT 5,7-CG (6.2%)	1	1.5	7	0.7	2.18	(0.05–17.39)	0.401
CATT 6,7-CG (15.8%)	**4**	**2.3**	**4**	**0.4**	**5.44**	**(1.00–29.44)**	**0.025**

The incidence of death was higher among patients carrying the $CATT_7$ allele, in patients with the CATT $_{6,7}$ genotype, and in patients with the genotype combination CATT $_{6,7}$-CG.; OR, odds ratio; SNP, Single nucleotide polymorphism; $CATT_7$, patients carrying at least one $CATT_7$ allele. * genotypes with a frequency of > 5%. Data presented as absolute numbers and percentage. *p*-value calculated by Fisher's exact test; bold fonts indicate *p*-values < 0.05.

3.4. MIF Genotypes as a Predictor of AKI in Multivariable Analyses

To assess if the *MIF* genotype improves preoperative risk prediction, a multivariable logistic regression was performed for AKI and death. For risk modeling, all baseline patients' characteristics (Table 1), including the well-established EuroSCORE, a preoperative risk stratification tool, were considered, and a logistic regression parameter selection procedure was performed. For the prediction of AKI, the variables EuroSCORE, hemoglobin, hypertension, and the presence of the *MIF* $CATT_7$ allele were selected. When adjusted for these variables, the *MIF* $CATT_7$ allele remained a significant predictor of AKI (OR 2.13, 95% CI, 1.46–3.1) (Table 7). The resulting model had an AUC of 0.71 (95% CI, 0.67–0.76).

For prediction of death, the statistical variable selection procedure resulted in a model containing the variables EuroSCORE, insulin-dependent diabetes, and the *MIF* $CATT_7$ allele. The presence of a *MIF* $CATT_7$ repeat allele significantly improved the prediction of postoperative mortality in this model (OR 5.58, 95% CI 1.29–24.04, $p = 0.021$). The resulting model had an AUC (receiver operating statistics—area under the curve) of 0.874 (95% CI, 0.786–0.962) (Table 7, Figure 2). In summary, the *MIF* $CATT_7$ allele is a significant predisposing risk factor for AKI and death after cardiac surgery.

The multivariable logistic regression model for AKI includes the variables *MIF* $CATT_7$ allele carriers and arterial hypertension as binary variables, and EuroSCORE and hemoglobin levels as continuous variables (according to Table 7). The model for death includes the variables *MIF* $CATT_7$ carrier status and insulin-dependent diabetes as binary variables and EuroSCORE as a continuous variable. AUC, area under the curve; CI, confidence interval.

Table 7. Predictors of Acute Kidney Injury (AKI) and death using multivariable logistic regression.

Variable	ß	OR	(95% CI)	*p*-Value
AKI (*N* = 170) *	−1.066			
CATT7 carrier	0.755	2.13	(1.46–3.09)	**<0.001**
EuroSCORE	0.202	1.22	(1.38–1.32)	**<0.001**
Hemoglobin	−0.183	0.83	(0.74–0.94)	**0.004**
Hypertension	0.701	2.03	(1.11–3.72)	**0.022**
Death (*N* = 8) †	−6.709			
CATT7 carrier	1.719	5.58	(1.29–24.04)	**0.021**
EuroSCORE	0.342	1.41	(1.05–1.88)	**0.021**
IDDM	1.923	6.84	(1.55–30.26)	**0.011**

In addition to the well-established EuroSCORE and other baseline characteristics, the *MIF* CATT7 was identified as a significant predictor of AKI and death. AKI, acute kidney injury; OR, odds ratio; CI, confidence interval. IDDM, insulin-dependent diabetes mellitus. Bold fonts indicate p-values < 0.05. * Area under the curve (AUC), 0.71; 95% CI, 0.67 - 0.76; Hosmer und Lemeshow Goodness-of-Fit Test, 0.8432. † Area under the curve (AUC), 0.87; 95% CI, 0.79–0.96; Hosmer und Lemeshow Goodness-of-Fit Test, 0.9702.

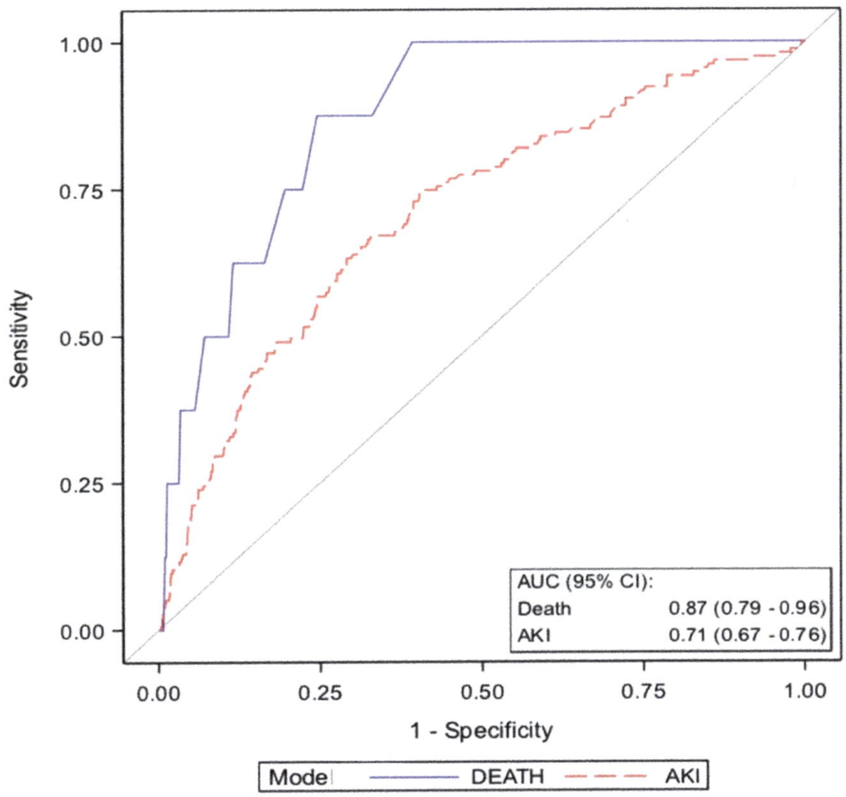

Figure 2. Receiver operating characteristics (ROC) curves for the prediction of AKI (red) and death (blue) after elective cardiac surgery. The grey line indicates the reference values of a diagnostic test that is no better than chance level.

3.5. MIF Serum Levels Before Surgery Are Increased in Patients Carrying the CATT7 Allele

To assess the association of the *MIF* promoter polymorphisms and the circulating MIF levels in cardiac surgery patients, perioperative kinetics of serum MIF were analyzed in 100 patients in relation to the underlying *MIF* polymorphisms. In patients carrying at least one CATT7 allele (CATT7), serum MIF was significantly elevated before surgery (79.2 vs. 50.4 ng/mL, $p = 0.008$) and one hour after surgery (154.8 vs. 79.5 ng/mL, $p = 0.02$) (Figure 3). The comparison of all other alleles, genotypes, and individual genotype combinations did not show significant differences between groups.

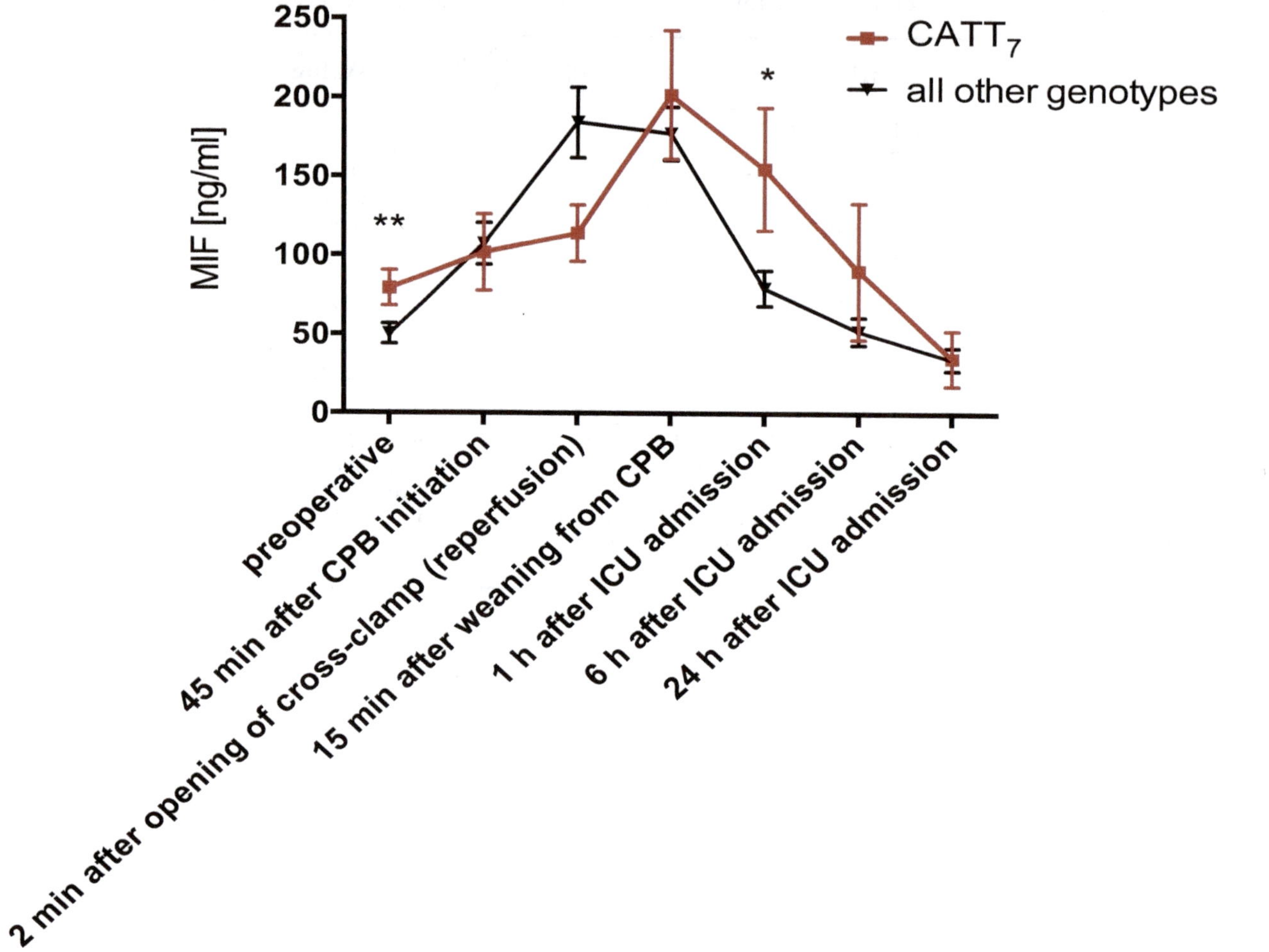

Figure 3. Perioperative kinetics of serum MIF in patients undergoing cardiac surgery. * $P < 0.05$, ** $P < 0.01$.

Serum MIF was quantified with ELISA in 100 patients. Patients heterozygous or homozygous for the *MIF* CATT$_7$ allele had significantly increased serum MIF before surgery (preoperative) and significantly lower serum MIF 1 h after surgery. Data are means ± SEM. ** $p < 0.01$, * $p < 0.05$ versus other groups at the corresponding time point (difference between groups) analyzed by Wilcoxon Rank Sum test.

4. Discussion

MIF is an inflammatory cytokine that is rapidly released from preformed intracellular pools in response to diverse cellular and systemic stressors, including ischemia-reperfusion, endotoxemia and surgery [21]. Previous studies demonstrated a significant peak of circulating MIF during cardiac surgery, as well as an association between circulating MIF and adverse postoperative outcomes [5,22–24]. Two polymorphisms in the *MIF* gene regulatory region, a CATT$_{5\text{-}7}$ microsatellite repeat (rs3063368) and a -270 (formerly described as -173) G>C single-nucleotide polymorphism (rs755622), which is in linkage disequilibrium with CATT$_7$, have been studied regarding their association with different pathologic conditions (e.g., pulmonary tuberculosis, acute coronary syndrome, carotid artery atherosclerosis, systemic lupus erythematosis, multiple sclerosis) [8,14,25–28]. However, the impact of the *MIF* gene polymorphisms on postoperative outcomes after cardiac surgery has not been analyzed.

The cardiac surgery patients in the present study displayed similar allele frequencies of the *MIF* CATT$_{5\text{-}7}$ microsatellite repeat (rs3063368) and G>C single nucleotide variant (rs755622) as in the general population [20]. Approximately 25% of patients carried at least one longer CATT repeat (CATT$_7$) (rs3063368) and 30% carried at least one C allele (rs755622). Demographic characteristics and procedural data revealed no significant differences between genotypes. Heterozygous or homozygous carriers of the $CATT_7$ allele had an almost 5-fold increased risk of death after cardiac surgery. Patients carrying either the $CATT_7$ or the C allele had an approximately 2-fold increased risk of suffering from AKI or multiple organ dysfunctions. While the risk for AKI was 12.8% in patients not carrying a $CATT_7$ allele, it was 22.7% for carriers of the $CATT_7$ allele. In addition to the well-established EuroSCORE, the *MIF* $CATT_7$ was identified as a significant predictor of death and development of AKI in a multivariable logistic regression model. The reason why we observed no significant association between homozygosity of the CC genotype might be attributed to the very low number of patients ($N = 26$, frequency 2.3%), but should be reevaluated in larger cohorts.

The *MIF* promoter microsatellite was suggested to influence MIF mRNA expression, as assessed by luciferase reporter assays in normal and patient cells [11,14]. The longer $CATT_7$ repeat further has been associated with higher serum MIF levels in various patient cohorts, including those with coronary artery disease [10,29,30]. In this study, we found that patients carrying the $CATT_7$ allele had higher serum MIF preoperatively and one hour after surgery, but serum MIF did not differ at the other intra- and postoperative timepoints.

In recent literature, MIF has already been associated with AKI in divergent clinical settings of septic shock, liver transplantation, glomerulonephritis, and renal allograft rejection [31–34].

However, there are indications that MIF can have a protective role against renal tubular injury in experimental models of ischemic AKI [23,35]. In one study, high MIF serum levels during cardiac surgery were associated with a reduced risk of postoperative AKI [23]. This contrasts with our observation of the $CATT_7$ and G>C, that are the proposed high expression alleles, being associated with AKI. An important risk factor for postoperative AKI is pre-existing chronic kidney disease (CKD), genetic studies support an association between the presence of at least one *MIF* G>C allele (rs755622) with chronic kidney and cardiovascular disease [36,37]. In a cross-sectional study MIF serum levels were significantly increased in patients with CKD [38]. It is well established that chronic kidney disease (CKD) predisposes to AKI [39]. Therefore, it can be speculated that the association between proposed high expression *MIF* genotypes with AKI is related to CKD that may inflate the risk for postoperative AKI. We suggest that preoperatively, chronically elevated MIF serum levels are associated with detrimental effects and may need to be discriminated from high intraoperative MIF serum levels, which might in fact mediate organ-protective effects during ischemia-reperfusion. This is in line with the notion that acute elevations of MIF serum levels may ameliorate ischemia-reperfusion injury after cardiac surgery, whereas long-term elevations in MIF may aggravate inflammatory pathways in atherosclerosis [40,41]. The observation of MIF correlating with markers of oxidative stress (8-hydroxy-2-deoxyguanosine) and endothelial activation (ICAM-1) in a cohort of CKD patients, supports the thesis that chronically elevated MIF levels might contribute to cardiovascular and associated CKD [38].

Mechanistically, MIF induces intracellular signal cascades via binding to its receptors including the cardioprotective CD74/AMPK kinase axis and the MIF CXC motif chemokine receptors, CXCR2, CXCR4, or CXCR7. Serum MIF may influence the expression of MIF receptors, and there are indications from mouse models that genetic *MIF* deficiency downregulates the expression of the MIF-signalling co-receptor CD44, which is required for signaling responses through CD74 [42,43]. Accordingly, chronically elevated levels of MIF might lead to an altered or injurious response to an acute, perioperative MIF increase, and potentially explain why MIF may be renoprotective in healthy mice but deleterious in multimorbid patients with chronic, underlying inflammation. The results of the present study nevertheless remain observational and cannot explain causative pathophysiology. Further studies investigating the mechanisms by which high expression of the *MIF* genotype may mediate the observed deleterious effects may help in the development of protective strategies for high risk cardiac surgery patients.

We acknowledge several limitations of our study, including the observational design. The event rate for death was very low, and therefore the analysis addressing the association of *MIF* genotypes with mortality should be interpreted cautiously and requires validation in larger cohorts. Although we measured serum MIF in a subcohort of patients and observed a relationship with increased CATT repeat length, this observation has not been consistently observed in prior studies, in part due to limitations of the serum compartment in reflecting systemic or regional tissue *MIF* expression levels [44,45]. Moreover, the study focused on Caucasian subjects and population stratification at the *MIF* locus exists [46]. While we did not study different geographic cohorts, our homogenous study population allows generalisability across predominantly European populations. Finally, the genotyping technique employed does not allow a concise phase analysis, and single haplotypes, e.g., the co-localization of a specific CATT allele (rs3063368) with the G or C allele (rs755622), cannot be explored.

In the same study cohort, one genome-wide association study (GWAS) has been undertaken and did not identify an association of the *MIF* gene polymorphisms with postoperative outcome [47]. Therefore, our findings underscore the necessity of candidate gene studies, including of common structural variants such as microsatellite repeats that are not detectable by SNP-based GWAS platforms [47–49]. As technological advances and declining costs in next-generation sequencing technologies pave the way for the broader availability of genomic testing, the implementation of genetic susceptibility data will help to improve risk stratification and to reduce the incidence and sequelae of cardiac surgery [50].

5. Conclusions

In the setting of cardiac surgery, we identified the *MIF* promotor polymorphisms $CATT_7$ (rs3063368) and -270 (formerly -173) G>C (rs755622), to be predictive of development of postoperative AKI and death. These *MIF* promoter alleles could improve current clinical risk prediction models and thus serve as a helpful decision-making tool for clinicians and patients in the near future.

Author Contributions: Conceptualization, L.A., C.S. and K.Z.; Methodology, L.A., C.S., K.F.; Software, K.F., C.S.; Validation, K.F., L.A., C.S., Formal Analysis, K.F., L.A., C.S., J.B.; Investigation, L.A., K.F., S.M., C.S.; Resources, C.S., K.Z., R.B., J.B., G.M.; Data Curation, K.F., L.A.; Writing—Original Draft Preparation, L.A., C.S.; Writing—Review and Editing, J.B., R.B., H.S., H.-J.L., S.M., P.M., D.W., L.L., G.M., D.E.L., A.Z.; Project Administration, C.S.; Funding Acquisition, C.S., K.Z., J.B. All authors have read and agreed to the published version of the manuscript.

Acknowledgments: We are thankful for the technical support received from Christian Beckers. RIPHeart Study Collaborators: Ana Stevanovic, Rolf Rossaint, Marc Felzen, Andreas Goetzenich, Tobias Moormann, Katharina Chalk, Pascal Knuefermann, Thomas Recht, Andreas Hoeft, Michael Winterhalter, Sonja Iken, Carolin Wiedenbeck, Gerhard Schwarzmann, Simone Lindau, Andreas Zierer, Stephan Fichtlscherer, Gerold Goerlach, Matthias Wollbrueck, Ursula Boening, Markus Weigand, Julia Strauchmann, Kai U. Morsbach, Markus Paxian, Konrad Reinhard, Jens Scholz, Jochen Renner, Ole Broch, Helga Francksen, Bernd Kuhr, Hermann Heinze, Hauke Paarmann, Hans-Hinrich Sievers, Stefan Klotz, Thomas Hachenberg, Christian Werner, Susanne Mauff, Angela Alms, Stefan Bergt, and Norbert Roewer. Aachen (Department of Anesthesiology, Medical Faculty RWTH Aachen University, Aachen, Germany): Ana Stevanovic, Rolf Rossaint, Marc Felzen, (Department of Thoracic and Cardiovascular Surgery): Andreas Goetzenich; 195 patients; Berlin (Department of Anesthesiology and Intensive Care Medicine, Charité-Universitätsmedizin Berlin, Campus Charité Mitte, Berlin, Germany): Tobias Moormann, Katharina Chalk; 37 patients; Bonn (Department of Anesthesiology and Intensive Care Medicine, University Hospital Bonn, Bonn, Germany): Pascal Knuefermann, Thomas Recht, Andreas Hoeft; 73 patients; Duesseldorf (Department of Anesthesiology and Intensive Care Medicine, University Hospital Duesseldorf, Germany): Michael Winterhalter; 65 patients; Frankfurt am Main (Department of Anesthesiology, Intensive Care Medicine and Pain Therapy, University Hospital Frankfurt, Frankfurt am Main, Germany): Sonja Iken, Carolin Wiedenbeck, Gerhard Schwarzmann, Simone Lindau, (Department of Thoracic and Cardiovascular Surgery): Andreas Zierer, (Internal Medicine III: Cardiology, Angiology, Nephrology): Stephan Fichtlscherer; 117 patients; Giessen (Department of Cardiovascular Surgery, University of Giessen, Germany): Gerold Goerlach,

Matthias Wollbrueck, Ursula Boening; (Department of Anesthesiology): Markus Weigand; 148 patients; Goettingen (Department of Anesthesiology and Intensive Care Medicine, University Hospital Goettingen, Germany): Julia Strauchmann, Konrad August; 91 patients; Jena (Department of Anesthesiology and Intensive Care Medicine, Jena University Hospital, Jena, Germany): Kai U. Morsbach, Markus Paxian, Konrad Reinhard; 76 patients; Kiel (Department of Anesthesiology and Intensive Care Medicine, University Hospital Schleswig-Holstein, Campus Kiel, Germany): Jens Scholz, Jochen Renner, Ole Broch, Helga Francksen, Bernd Kuhr; 237 patients; Luebeck (Department of Anesthesiology, University Hospital Luebeck, Luebeck, Germany): Hermann Heinze, Hauke Paarmann; (Department of Cardiac and Thoracic Vascular Surgery): Hans-Hinrich Sievers, Stefan Klotz; 56 patients; Magdeburg (Department of Anesthesiology, University Hospital Magdeburg, Germany); Thomas Hachenberg; 14 patients; Mainz (Department of Anesthesiology, Medical Center of Johannes Gutenberg-University, Mainz, Germany): Christian Werner, Susanne Mauff; 116 patients; Rostock (Clinic of Anesthesiology and Intensive Care Medicine, University Hospital Rostock, Rostock, Germany): Angela Alms, Stefan Bergt; 146 patients; Wuerzburg (Department of Anesthesiology, University Hospital Wuerzburg, Wuerzburg, Germany): Norbert Roewer; 32 patients.

References

1. Brown, P.P.; Kugelmass, A.D.; Cohen, D.J.; Reynolds, M.R.; Culler, S.D.; Dee, A.D.; Simon, A.W. The Frequency and Cost of Complications Associated with Coronary Artery Bypass Grafting Surgery: Results from the United States Medicare Program. *Ann. Thorac. Surg.* **2008**, *85*, 1980–1986. [CrossRef]
2. Grover, A.; Gorman, K.; Dall, T.M.; Jonas, R.; Lytle, B.; Shemin, R.; Wood, D.; Kron, I. Shortage of Cardiothoracic Surgeons Is Likely by 2020. *Circulation* **2009**, *120*, 488–494. [CrossRef] [PubMed]
3. Roques, F.; Nashef, S.A.; Michel, P.; Gauducheau, E.; De Vincentiis, C.; Baudet, E.; Cortina, J.; David, M.; Faichney, A.; Gavrielle, F.; et al. Risk factors and outcome in European cardiac surgery: Analysis of the EuroSCORE multinational database of 19030 patients. *Eur. J. Cardio-Thorac. Surg.* **1999**, *15*, 816–823. [CrossRef]
4. Sureshbabu, A.; Ryter, S.W.; Choi, M.E. Oxidative stress and autophagy: Crucial modulators of kidney injury. *Redox Biol.* **2015**, *4*, 208–214. [CrossRef] [PubMed]
5. Stoppe, C.; Rex, S.; Goetzenich, A.; Kraemer, S.; Emontzpohl, C.; Soppert, J.; Averdunk, L.; Sun, Y.; Rossaint, R.; Lue, H.; et al. Interaction of MIF Family Proteins in Myocardial Ischemia/Reperfusion Damage and Their Influence on Clinical Outcome of Cardiac Surgery Patients. *Antioxid. Redox Signal.* **2015**, *23*, 865–879. [CrossRef] [PubMed]
6. Ozsoy, A.Z.; Karakus, N.; Tural, S.; Yigit, S.; Kara, N.; Alaylı, G.; Tumer, M.K.; Kuru, O. Influence of the MIF polymorphism −173G > C on Turkish postmenopausal women with osteoporosis. *Z. Rheumatol.* **2017**, *77*, 629–632. [CrossRef] [PubMed]
7. Vishwakarma, S.K.; Lakkireddy, C.; Sravani, G.; Sastry, B.V.S.; Raju, N.; Ahmed, S.I.; Owaisi, N.; Jaisawal, A.; Khan, M.A.; Khan, A.A. Association of CD14 and macrophage migration inhibitory factor gene polymorphisms with inflammatory microRNAs expression levels in ankylosing spondylitis and polyarthralgia. *Int. J. Immunogenet.* **2018**, *45*, 190–200. [CrossRef]
8. Benedek, G.; Meza-Romero, R.; Jordan, K.; Zhang, Y.; Nguyen, H.; Kent, G.; Li, J.; Siu, E.; Frazer, J.; Piecychna, M.; et al. MIF and D-DT are potential disease severity modifiers in male MS subjects. *Proc. Natl. Acad. Sci. USA* **2017**, *114*, E8421–E8429. [CrossRef]
9. Bae, S.-C.; Lee, Y.H. Circulating macrophage migration inhibitory factor levels and its polymorphisms in systemic lupus erythematosus: A meta-analysis. *Cell. Mol. Biol.* **2017**, *63*, 74–79. [CrossRef]
10. Baugh, J.A.; Chitnis, S.; Donnelly, S.C.; Monteiro, J.; Lin, X.; Plant, B.J.; Wolfe, F.; Gregersen, P.K.; Bucala, R. A functional promoter polymorphism in the macrophage migration inhibitory factor (MIF) gene associated with disease severity in rheumatoid arthritis. *Genes Immun.* **2002**, *3*, 170–176. [CrossRef]
11. Yao, J.; Leng, L.; Sauler, M.; Fu, W.-L.; Zheng, J.; Zhang, Y.; Du, X.; Yu, X.; Lee, P.; Bucala, R. Transcription factor ICBP90 regulates the MIF promoter and immune susceptibility locus. *J. Clin. Investig.* **2016**, *126*, 732–744. [CrossRef] [PubMed]

12. Guo, P.; Wang, J.; Liu, J.; Xia, M.; Li, W.; He, M. Macrophage immigration inhibitory factor promotes cell proliferation and inhibits apoptosis of cervical adenocarcinoma. *Tumor Biol.* **2015**, *36*, 5095–5102. [CrossRef] [PubMed]
13. Meybohm, P.; Bein, B.; Brosteanu, O.; Cremer, J.T.; Gruenewald, M.; Stoppe, C.; Coburn, M.; Schaelte, G.; Böning, A.; Niemann, B.; et al. A Multicenter Trial of Remote Ischemic Preconditioning for Heart Surgery. *N. Engl. J. Med.* **2015**, *373*, 1397–1407. [CrossRef] [PubMed]
14. Sreih, A.; Ezzeddine, R.; Leng, L.; Lachance, A.; Yu, G.; Mizuec, Y.; Subrahmanyan, L.; Pons-Estel, B.A.; Abelson, A.-K.; Gunnarsson, I.; et al. Dual effect of the macrophage migration inhibitory factor gene on the development and severity of human systemic lupus erythematosus. *Arthritis Rheum.* **2011**, *63*, 3942–3951. [CrossRef]
15. Palevsky, P.M.; Liu, K.D.; Brophy, P.D.; Chawla, L.S.; Parikh, C.R.; Thakar, C.V.; Tolwani, A.J.; Waikar, S.S.; Weisbord, S.D. KDOQI US Commentary on the 2012 KDIGO Clinical Practice Guideline for Acute Kidney Injury. *Am. J. Kidney Dis.* **2013**, *61*, 649–672. [CrossRef]
16. Thygesen, K.; Alpert, J.S.; White, H.D.; Jaffe, A.S.; Apple, F.S.; Galvani, M.; Katus, H.A.; Newby, L.K.; Jan, R.; Chaitman, B.; et al. Universal Definition of Myocardial Infarction. *Circulation* **2007**, *116*, 2634–2653. [CrossRef]
17. Ely, E.W.; Inouye, S.K.; Bernard, G.R.; Gordon, S.; Francis, J.; May, L.; Truman, B.; Speroff, T.; Gautam, S.; Margolin, R.; et al. Delirium in mechanically ventilated patients: Validity and reliability of the confusion assessment method for the intensive care unit (CAM-ICU). *JAMA* **2001**, *286*, 2703–2710. [CrossRef] [PubMed]
18. Wityk, R.J.; Pessin, M.S.; Kaplan, R.F.; Caplan, L.R. Serial assessment of acute stroke using the NIH Stroke Scale. *Stroke* **1994**, *25*, 362–365. [CrossRef]
19. Harris, J.; Morand, E.F. *Macrophage Migration Inhibitory Factor Methods and Protocols*; Methods in Molecular Biology; Springer: Berlin, Germany, 2020; Volume 2080.
20. Karczewski, K.J.; Francioli, L.C.; Tiao, G.; Cummings, B.B.; Alfoldi, J.; Wang, Q.; Collins, R.L.; Laricchia, K.M.; Ganna, A.; Birnbaum, D.P.; et al. The mutational constraint spectrum quantified from variation in 141,456 humans. *Nature* **2020**, *581*, 434–443. [CrossRef]
21. Bacher, M.; Meinhardt, A.; Lan, H.Y.; Mu, W.; Metz, C.N.; Chesney, J.A.; Calandra, T.; Gemsa, D.; Donnelly, T.; Atkins, R.C.; et al. Migration inhibitory factor expression in experimentally induced endotoxemia. *Am. J. Pathol.* **1997**, *150*, 235–246.
22. Gando, S.; Nishihira, J.; Kemmotsu, O.; Kobayashi, S.; Morimoto, Y.; Matsui, Y.; Yasuda, K. An increase in macrophage migration inhibitory factor release in patients with cardiopulmonary bypass surgery. *Surg. Today* **2000**, *30*, 689–694. [CrossRef] [PubMed]
23. Stoppe, C.; Averdunk, L.; Goetzenich, A.; Soppert, J.; Marlier, A.; Kraemer, S.; Vieten, J.; Coburn, M.; Kowark, A.; Kim, B.-S.; et al. The protective role of macrophage migration inhibitory factor in acute kidney injury after cardiac surgery. *Sci. Transl. Med.* **2018**, *10*, aan4886. [CrossRef]
24. Stoppe, C.; Grieb, G.; Rossaint, R.; Simons, D.; Coburn, M.; Götzenich, A.; Strüssmann, T.; Pallua, N.; Bernhagen, J.; Rex, S. High Postoperative Blood Levels of Macrophage Migration Inhibitory Factor Are Associated with Less Organ Dysfunction in Patients after Cardiac Surgery. *Mol. Med.* **2012**, *18*, 843–850. [CrossRef] [PubMed]
25. Liu, A.; Bao, F.; Voravuthikunchai, S.P. CATT polymorphism in MIF gene promoter is closely related to human pulmonary tuberculosis in a southwestern China population. *Int. J. Immunopathol. Pharmacol.* **2018**, *32*. [CrossRef] [PubMed]
26. Valdes-Alvarado, E.; Muñoz-Valle, J.F.; Valle, Y.; Sandoval-Pinto, E.; García-González, I.J.; Valdez-Haro, A.; De La Cruz-Mosso, U.; Flores-Salinas, H.E.; Padilla-Gutierrez, J.R. Association between the −794 (CATT)5–8 MIF Gene Polymorphism and Susceptibility to Acute Coronary Syndrome in a Western Mexican Population. *J. Immunol. Res.* **2014**, *2014*, 704854. [CrossRef] [PubMed]
27. Lan, M.-Y.; Chang, Y.-Y.; Chen, W.-H.; Tseng, Y.-L.; Lin, H.-S.; Lai, S.-L.; Liu, J.-S. Association between MIF gene polymorphisms and carotid artery atherosclerosis. *Biochem. Biophys. Res. Commun.* **2013**, *435*, 319–322. [CrossRef] [PubMed]
28. Sanchez, E.; Gómez, L.M.; Lopez-Nevot, M.A.; González-Gay, M.A.; Sabio, J.M.; Ortego-Centeno, N.; De Ramón, E.; Anaya, J.; González-Escribano, M.F.; Koeleman, B.P.; et al. Evidence of association of macrophage migration inhibitory factor gene polymorphisms with systemic lupus erythematosus. *Genes Immun.* **2006**, *7*, 433–436. [CrossRef]

29. Mitchell, R.A.; Liao, H.; Chesney, J.; Fingerle-Rowson, G.; Baugh, J.; David, J.; Bucala, R. Macrophage migration inhibitory factor (MIF) sustains macrophage proinflammatory function by inhibiting p53: Regulatory role in the innate immune response. *Proc. Natl. Acad. Sci. USA* **2001**, *99*, 345–350. [CrossRef]
30. Qian, L.; Wang, X.-Y.; Thapa, S.; Tao, L.-Y.; Wu, S.-Z.; Luo, G.-J.; Wang, L.-P.; Wang, J.-N.; Wang, J.; Li, J.; et al. Macrophage migration inhibitory factor promoter polymorphisms (-794 CATT5-8): Relationship with soluble MIF levels in coronary atherosclerotic disease subjects. *BMC Cardiovasc. Disord.* **2017**, *17*, 144. [CrossRef]
31. Payen, D.; Lukaszewicz, A.-C.; Legrand, M.; Gayat, E.; Faivre, V.; Mégarbane, B.; Azoulay, E.; Fieux, F.; Charron, D.; Loiseau, P.; et al. A Multicentre Study of Acute Kidney Injury in Severe Sepsis and Septic Shock: Association with Inflammatory Phenotype and HLA Genotype. *PLoS ONE* **2012**, *7*, e35838. [CrossRef]
32. Baron-Stefaniak, J.; Schiefer, J.; Miller, E.J.; Berlakovich, G.A.; Baron, D.M.; Faybik, P. Comparison of macrophage migration inhibitory factor and neutrophil gelatinase-associated lipocalin-2 to predict acute kidney injury after liver transplantation: An observational pilot study. *PLoS ONE* **2017**, *12*, e0183162. [CrossRef] [PubMed]
33. Brown, F.G.; Nikolic-Paterson, D.J.; Hill, P.A.; Isbel, N.M.; Dowling, J.; Metz, C.M.; Atkins, R.C. Urine macrophage migration inhibitory factor reflects the severity of renal injury in human glomerulonephritis. *J. Am. Soc. Nephrol.* **2002**, *13*, S7–S13. [PubMed]
34. Brown, F.G.; Nikolic-Paterson, D.J.; Chadban, S.J.; Dowling, J.; Jose, M.D.; Metz, C.N.; Bucala, R.; Atkins, R.C. Urine Macrophage Migration Inhibitory Factor Concentrations as a Diagnostic Tool in Human Renal Allograft Rejection. *Transplantion* **2001**, *71*, 1777–1783. [CrossRef] [PubMed]
35. Djudjaj, S.; Martin, I.V.; Buhl, E.M.; Nothofer, N.J.; Leng, L.; Piecychna, M.; Floege, J.; Bernhagen, J.; Bucala, R.; Boor, P. Macrophage Migration Inhibitory Factor Limits Renal Inflammation and Fibrosis by Counteracting Tubular Cell Cycle Arrest. *J. Am. Soc. Nephrol.* **2017**, *28*, 3590–3604. [CrossRef]
36. Herder, C.; Illig, T.; Baumert, J.; Müller-Nurasyid, M.; Klopp, N.; Khuseyinova, N.; Meisinger, C.; Martin, S.; Thorand, B.; Koenig, W. Macrophage migration inhibitory factor (MIF) and risk for coronary heart disease: Results from the MONICA/KORA Augsburg case-cohort study, 1984–2002. *Atherosclerosis* **2008**, *200*, 380–388. [CrossRef]
37. Tong, X.; He, J.; Liu, S.; Peng, S.; Yan, Z.; Zhang, Y.; Fan, H. Macrophage migration inhibitory factor -173G/C gene polymorphism increases the risk of renal disease: A meta-analysis. *Nephrology* **2015**, *20*, 68–76. [CrossRef]
38. Bruchfeld, A.; Carrero, J.J.; Qureshi, A.R.; Lindholm, B.; Bárány, P.; Heimburger, O.; Hu, M.; Lin, X.; Stenvinkel, P.; Miller, E.J. Elevated Serum Macrophage Migration Inhibitory Factor (MIF) Concentrations in Chronic Kidney Disease (CKD) Are Associated with Markers of Oxidative Stress and Endothelial Activation. *Mol. Med.* **2009**, *15*, 70–75. [CrossRef]
39. Chawla, L.S.; Kimmel, P.L. Acute kidney injury and chronic kidney disease: An integrated clinical syndrome. *Kidney Int.* **2012**, *82*, 516–524. [CrossRef]
40. Rassaf, T.; Weber, C.; Bernhagen, J. Macrophage migration inhibitory factor in myocardial ischaemia/reperfusion injury. *Cardiovasc. Res.* **2014**, *102*, 321–328. [CrossRef]
41. Tilstam, P.V.; Qi, D.; Leng, L.; Young, L.; Bucala, R. MIF family cytokines in cardiovascular diseases and prospects for precision-based therapeutics. *Expert Opin. Ther. Targets* **2017**, *21*, 671–683. [CrossRef]
42. Yoo, S.-A.; Leng, L.; Kim, B.-J.; Du, X.; Tilstam, P.V.; Kim, K.H.; Kong, J.-S.; Yoon, H.-J.; Liu, A.; Wang, T.; et al. MIF allele-dependent regulation of the MIF coreceptor CD44 and role in rheumatoid arthritis. *Proc. Natl. Acad. Sci. USA* **2016**, *113*, E7917–E7926. [CrossRef] [PubMed]
43. Ochi, A.; Chen, N.; Schulte, W.; Leng, L.; Moeckel, N.G.; Piecychna, M.; Averdunk, L.; Stoppe, C.; Bucala, R.; Moeckel, G.W. MIF-2/D-DT enhances proximal tubular cell regeneration through SLPI- and ATF4-dependent mechanisms. *Am. J. Physiol. Physiol.* **2017**, *313*, F767–F780. [CrossRef] [PubMed]
44. Herder, C.; Klopp, N.; Baumert, J.; Müller-Nurasyid, M.; Khuseyinova, N.; Meisinger, C.; Martin, S.; Illig, T.; Koenig, W.; Thorand, B. Effect of macrophage migration inhibitory factor (MIF) gene variants and MIF serum concentrations on the risk of type 2 diabetes: Results from the MONICA/KORA Augsburg Case–Cohort Study, 1984–2002. *Diabetologia* **2007**, *51*, 276–284. [CrossRef] [PubMed]
45. Matia-García, I.; Salgado-Goytia, L.; Muñoz-Valle, J.F.; García-Arellano, S.; Hernández-Bello, J.; Salgado-Bernabé, A.B.; Parra-Rojas, I. Macrophage Migration Inhibitory Factor Promoter Polymorphisms (−794 CATT5–8and −173 G > C): Relationship with mRNA Expression and Soluble MIF Levels in Young Obese Subjects. *Dis. Markers* **2015**, *2015*, 461208. [CrossRef] [PubMed]

46. Zhong, X.-B.; Leng, L.; Beitin, A.; Chen, R.; McDonald, C.; Hsiao, B.; Jenison, R.D.; Kang, I.; Park, S.-H.; Lee, A.; et al. Simultaneous detection of microsatellite repeats and SNPs in the macrophage migration inhibitory factor (MIF) gene by thin-film biosensor chips and application to rural field studies. *Nucleic Acids Res.* **2005**, *33*, e121. [CrossRef]
47. Westphal, S.; Stoppe, C.; Gruenewald, M.; Bein, B.; Renner, J.; Cremer, J.; Coburn, M.; Schälte, G.; Boening, A.; Niemann, B.; et al. Genome-wide association study of myocardial infarction, atrial fibrillation, acute stroke, acute kidney injury and delirium after cardiac surgery—A sub-analysis of the RIPHeart-Study. *BMC Cardiovasc. Disord.* **2019**, *19*, 26. [CrossRef]
48. Saw, K.M.E.; Ng, R.G.R.; Chan, S.P.; Ang, Y.H.; Ti, L.K.; Chew, T.H.S. Association of genetic polymorphisms with acute kidney injury after cardiac surgery in a Southeast Asian population. *PLoS ONE* **2019**, *14*, e0213997. [CrossRef]
49. Leaf, D.E.; Body, S.C.; Muehlschlegel, J.D.; McMahon, G.M.; Lichtner, P.; Collard, C.D.; Shernan, S.K.; Fox, A.A.; Waikar, S.S. Length Polymorphisms in Heme Oxygenase-1 and AKI after Cardiac Surgery. *J. Am. Soc. Nephrol.* **2016**, *27*, 3291–3297. [CrossRef]
50. Suwinski, P.; Ong, C.; Ling, M.H.T.; Poh, Y.M.; Khan, A.M.; Ong, H.S. Advancing Personalized Medicine Through the Application of Whole Exome Sequencing and Big Data Analytics. *Front. Genet.* **2019**, *10*, 49. [CrossRef]

15

The Preliminary Results of Bortezomib Used as a Primary Treatment for an Early Acute Antibody-Mediated Rejection after Kidney Transplantation

Aureliusz Kolonko *, Natalia Słabiak-Błaż, Henryk Karkoszka, Andrzej Więcek and Grzegorz Piecha

Department of Nephrology, Transplantation and Internal Medicine, Medical University of Silesia, 40-027 Katowice, Poland; nataliablaz@gazeta.pl (N.S.-B.); hkarkoszka@poczta.fm (H.K.); awiecek@sum.edu.pl (A.W.); g.piecha@outlook.com (G.P.)

* Correspondence: uryniusz@wp.p

Abstract: Proteasome inhibitor bortezomib has been used in the treatment of refractory cases of acute and chronic antibody-mediated rejection (AMR) in kidney transplant recipients. However, its efficacy and safety as a primary treatment for early AMR has been scarcely investigated. We herein present our preliminary experience with bortezomib- and plasmapheresis-based primary treatment for early AMR. Thirteen patients transplanted between October 2015 and September 2019 were treated (starting at median 19th post-transplant day) with bortezomib/plasmapheresis protocol for early biopsy-proven AMR. Twelve out of thirteen patients received 4 doses and one patient recieved 3 doses of bortezomib (1.3 mg/m^2 per dose). In 11/13 patients, 4–7 concomitant plasmapheresis sessions were performed, with or without intravenous immunoglobulin (IVIG). Of note, rituximab was not used in all study patients. The kidney graft and patient survival were 100%. The mean 3-month estimated glomerular filtration rate (eGFR) was 55.3 (95%CI: 44.9–65.8) mL/min/1.73m^2, 8/13 patients completed 12-month follow-up with mean eGFR 60.4 (45.4–75.4) mL/min/1.73m^2, and 6/13 patients completed a 24-month follow-up period with mean eGFR 73.9 (56.7–91.1) mL/min/1.73m^2. Neutropenia < 1 G/L was observed in one patient, third or fourth grade thrombocytopenia in two patients, and eleven patients needed a blood transfusion (median: 2 units/patient). The mid-term results of a primary bortezomib-based treatment for kidney AMR showed its non-inferiority as compared to preceding regimens and acceptable safety. However, our data should be validated in a multicenter randomized trial.

Keywords: acute humoral rejection; first-line therapy; outcomes; proteasome inhibitor

---

1. Introduction

Acute antibody-mediated rejection (AMR) accounts for 20–30% of all acute rejection episodes after kidney transplantation and is often associated with poor allograft survival [1]. It rarely occurs in unsensitized patients, but may occur in up to 50% of highly sensitized recipients [2,3]. Diagnosis of AMR is based on the histopathologic features of the graft biopsy (glomerulitis, arterial-transmural lesions, thrombotic microangiopathy, etc.) and the presence of donor-specific antibodies (DSAs), with or without positive C4d staining [4]. Nowadays, most frequently used treatment modalities for AMR include plasmaphereses (PF) or immunoadsorption (IA), intravenous immunoglobulin (IVIG), anti-T-cell therapy (antithymocyte globulin, ATG), and anti-B-cell therapy (rituximab). Unfortunately, long-term results of such therapy remain suboptimal [5,6]. The rationale for PF or IA is the removal of readily available antibodies and, therefore, limiting the acute tissue damage. Currently, PF is the standard-of-care for the treatment of AMR despite the evidence uncertainty [6].

As the plasma cells are the main source of antibody production, the proteasome inhibitor, bortezomib (Velcade®, Milennium Pharmaceuticals, Cambridge, MA, USA), had been introduced into the AMR treatment, mostly as a rescue therapy in refractory cases [7–10]. In general, kidney graft outcomes were significantly better in acute than chronic AMR [8,10–12]. In some reports, such an adjuvant therapy was effective in decreasing DSAs and stabilizing kidney graft function in mid-term observation [7,9]. Nonetheless, the rate of graft loss during longer follow-up periods was high and the excretory function of still-functioning transplanted organs was markedly decreased [7,9,13,14]. As early as 2010, Walsh et al. reported the first use of bortezomib along with a single dose of rituximab in two patients as a primary therapy in early post-transplant AMR, with a rapid DSAs elimination and excellent renal function at five and six months of observation [15]. Later on, Waiser et al. compared the effect of bortezomib- versus rituximab-based AMR therapies, but both study subgroups contained acute and chronic AMR cases with a substantial age difference between groups [16]. Since then, only a few case reports have been published [17,18]. The existing patophysiologic evidence of the potential mechanisms leading to the therapeutic effect of bortezomib indicates its ability for causing apoptosis of antibody-producing plasma cells, blocking the secretion of class IgG antibodies against human leukocyte antigens (anti-HLA) [19], and decreasing the number of plasma cells within the graft [20]. In order to maximize the bortezomib efficacy in AMR treatment, in all previously reported protocols, each dose was administered after plasmapheresis session, which aimed to decrease the amount of circulating antibodies. Therefore, we herein present the largest-to-date cohort of kidney transplant recipients with early AMR diagnosed in graft biopsy and primarily treated with bortezomib-based therapy without concomitant rituximab administration.

2. Methods

2.1. Study Group

We present a retrospective observational study, including all consecutive kidney graft recipients (KTRs) from our center, transplanted between October 2015 and September 2019 and diagnosed with early biopsy-proven AMR. All patients received their organs from deceased donors and all had negative complement-dependent cytotoxicity (CDC) crossmatch performed immediately prior to transplantation. Flow cytometric crossmatches were not performed. In our country, only patients with negative CDC crossmatch are listed for the transplant centre in order to choose the recipients of organs procured from the donor. Based on the routine pre-transplant screening and the last Luminex results, the presence of DSA with mean fluorescence intensity (MFI) $\geq$ 5000 eliminates the potential kidney transplant candidate from the ongoing procedure. A routine kidney graft early protocol biopsy was introduced at our center in the second half of 2015. Since than, all patients who were diagnosed with AMR were then assigned to primary therapy, which included bortezomib. The study was conducted in accordance with the Declaration of Helsinki. As this drug is not registered for the AMR therapy, the Bioethic Committee of the Medical University of Silesia was consulted and all patients gave their informed consent for the off-label use of bortezomib in their therapy. Notably, the guidelines for immunosuppressive therapy after kidney transplantation, issued by the Polish Transplant Society, have allowed the use of bortezomib in KTRs with AMR since 2012 [21].

2.2. Immunosuppressive Protocol

The standard immunosuppressive protocol included tacrolimus 2 $\times$ 0.1 mg/kg twice daily (with target through level 7–12 ng/mL) and mycophenolate mofetil 750 mg twice daily, both started immediately prior to operating procedure, and steroids, starting with the dose of 500 mg of methylprednisolone intravenously (i.v.) during the operation. Induction therapy was based on the rabbit antithymocyte globulin (rATG) (Thymoglobuline®, Genzyme Europe B.V., Amsterdam, Holland) in immunologically high-risk recipients (maximum panel reactive antibodies (PRA) titer > 25% and/or the presence of pre-transplant DSAs) or the anti-interleukin 2 receptor blocker basiliximab (Simulect®,

Novartis Europharm Europe, Dublin, Ireland). Pre-transplant anti-HLA antibodies were evaluated by solid-phase assays using bead arrays and a Luminex platform. Pre- and post-transplant DSAs were determined using a single-antigen bead assay and results were expressed as mean fluorescence intensity (MFI). Among 4 patients who did not receive rATG induction, in one of those patients, the pre-transplant DSA were undetermined and IL-2RB was given, one patient did not received rATG or IL-2RB induction due to the lack of information concerning the presence of DSA at the time of transplantation, and 2 others had their DSA only in HLA class I and in a relatively low titers (i.e., 1992 and 541), so IL-2RB was used. Each administration of rATG was preceded by metyloprednisolone 125 mg i.v., paracetamol 1.0 g i.v., and an antihistaminic drug, and the first dose was started preoperatively and then continued with intermittent dosing based on lymphocyte count. Additionally, routine fluconazole (100 mg), valgancyclovir (labeled dose adjusted to the kidney graft function), and sulfamethoxazole-trimethoprim (2 × 480 mg) prophylaxis was given in rATG-treated patients.

2.3. *Primary Treatment Protocol of AMR*

After diagnosis, bortezomib (four doses, each 1.3 mg/m^2) was administered subcutaneously the day after the PF session. Concomitantly, 4–8 PF sessions were performed every second/third day, with a plasma exchange rate of 2.0–2.5× patient's plasma volume. In patients who did not receive rATG induction, the routine valgancyclovir and sulfamethoxazole-trimethoprim prophylaxis was started prior to bortezomib therapy. Additionally, antibiotic prophylaxis with piperacillin/tazobactam was started and continued during the bortezomib/plasmapheresis therapy. Immediately before every subcutaneous administration of bortezomib, above i.v. metyloprednisolone, paracetamol, and an antihistaminic drug were given as a premedication.

2.4. *Kidney Graft Function and Protocol Biopsies*

Kidney graft estimated glomerular filtration rate (eGFR) was calculated based on MDRD (Modification of Diet in Renal Disease) formulation at the 3rd, 12th, and 24th post-transplant month.

Kidney graft protocol biopsies were performed usually at the 8th–11th post-transplant day. All biopsies were evaluated by one experienced pathologist according to the revised Banff classification [4,22–24]. Each kidney biopsy specimen was routinely stained for hematoxyllin and eosin, PAS, Masson trichrome, and silver methenamine. Additionally, SV40 antigen staining specific for polyoma BK virus infection and von Kossa staining for the presence of calcium-phosphate deposits within the tubular lumen or interstitium were performed. We also analyzed histologic signs of potential calcineurin inhibitor nephrotoxicity. Immunohistochemistry was routinely performed (CD4, CD8, CD20, CD68, and C4d) and described semi-quantitatively based on the grade of infiltration (as scattered cells, foci, clusters, groups, or diffused infiltration). AMR was diagnosed based on the following criteria: (1) the presence of histologic signs of microvascular injury (glomerulitis, peritubular capillaritis (PTC-itis), arteriitis, acute tubular injury/necrosis, (2) positive C4d staining, and (3) presence of DSAs. During the follow-up period, control protocol biopsies were performed and analyzed in 9 patients.

2.5. *Statistics*

Statistical analysis was performed using the Statistica software (StatSoft Polska, Cracow, Poland). Values were presented as means with 95% confidence interval (CI) or medians with Q25–Q75 quartile values. The comparison of kidney graft function before and after bortezomib treatment was performed using the Student's *t*-test. *p*-values below 0.05 were considered as statistically significant.

3. Results

3.1. *Baseline Characteristics*

Thirteen KTRs (7 males and 6 females) with early acute AMR treated with bortezomib-based primary therapy were analyzed. Their demographic and clinical characteristics are presented in

Table 1. The mean recipient age was 53 years (minimum 30, maximum 68), mean body mass index (BMI) was 26.4 (95%CI: 24.0–28.7), and the median dialysis vintage before transplantation was 43 (IQR: 27–64) months. The history of previous blood transfusions was positive in nine, negative in one, and unknown in two patients. Out of six females, four reported past pregnancies. Only three patients had historical and two patients had the last pre-transplant panel-reactive antibodies (PRA) ≥ 25%, whereas nine patients presented positive results of virtual PRA, calculated based on the Eurotransplant Reference Laboratory HLA database version 2.0. Pre-transplant DSAs were present in twelve patients, with median MFI 10,706 (IQR: 2741–11,415) (Table 2). Induction therapy was used in twelve patients, including rATG in nine and basiliximab in three patients, respectively.

3.2. AMR Diagnosis and Treatment

AMR was diagnosed based on the first protocol biopsy, performed at a median 10 (IQR: 9–10) post-transplant day (Table 2). Due to technical constraints, the histopatologic biopsy results were available after 2–5 working days. In the majority of patients, the CD4, CD8, and CD68 infiltration was predominantly seen, whereas CD20 staining revealed only single cells or scattered foci, except in three patients, in whom, CD20 clusters and/or groups were described (Figure 1). Hence, a primary AMR treatment started at median 19th post-transplant day. In eight patients, all three Banff criteria of AMR were fulfilled. In the next four patients, the suspected diagnosis was C4d-negative AMR. In one patient, results of pre-transplant single-antigen bead assay were not available, but the screening test for class II anti-HLA antibodies was positive (Table 2). Immediately after AMR diagnosis, the primary treatment was started as described above. One patient received only 3 out of 4 planned doses of bortezomib due to the observed gastrointestinal side effects. In the first three patients, PF treatment with fresh frozen plasma (FFP) was completed. In the next eight patients, FFP together with 5% human albumin was used, in the 1:1 volume proportion. The last two patients were treated with a modified protocol (bortezomib, ATG with total dose 5 mg/kg and IVIG single dose 1g/kg) as they initially received basiliximab induction, whereas we were not able to plan and perform PF sessions at that time. Besides, dialysis therapy was required in five patients before and partially also during the AMR treatment.

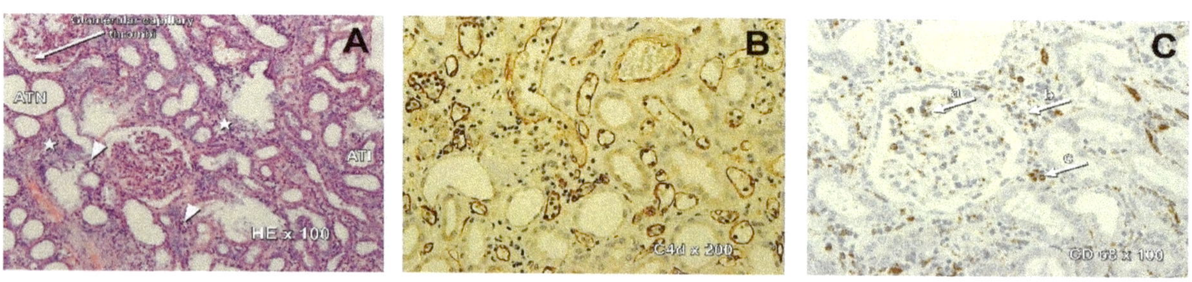

Figure 1. Microphotograph presenting typical histologic findings in kidney transplant recipients with early antibody-mediated rejection. (**A**) Hematoxylin and eosin, magnification 100×. Interstitial edema (tubules are not back to back) with inflammatory infiltrates—asterisks, acute tubular injury (ATI) with the flattening of epithelium cells with the absence of brush border, acute tubular necrosis (ATN) with the tubular basement membranes denuded of epithelial cells, peritubular capillaritis (PTC-itis)—arrowheads, and hypoperfused glomeruli with microthrombi—arrow. (**B**) A diffused C4d staining pattern around peritubular capillaries. Magnification 200×. (**C**) Immunostaining demonstrating CD68-positive macrophages within glomeruli (a), interstitial space (b), and peritubular capillaries (c). Magnification 100×.

Table 1. Baseline demographic and clinical characteristics of kidney transplant recipients with bortezomib-treated antibody-mediated rejection (AMR).

Patient	Gender	Age (years)	Cause of ESRD	KTx No	PRA (%)	PRA max (%)	vPRA Class I	vPRA Class II	vPRA Class I+II	Pre-Treatment DSA (MFI)	Induction	Early Graft Function
1	M	30	GNC	2	50	87	98.108	0	98.108	A2 (3489)	rATG	SGF
2	M	41	Unknown	1	0	15	0	0	0	A2 (15,101)	rATG	SGF
3	M	61	ADPKD	2	0	0	31.732	0	31.732	A1 (1968)	rATG	SGF
4	F	61	PNC	1	0	15	46.798	99.476	99.607	DR 4 (10,284)	rATG	IGF
5	M	68	PNC	1	0	0	n/a	n/a	n/a	n/a	IL-2RB	SGF
6	F	52	GNC	1	0	0	30.335 *	80.568	85.604	DR 13 (1500)	rATG	SGF
7	M	61	GNC	2	0	0	0	41.179	41.179	DR10 (11,509)	None	DGF
8	F	63	GNC	1	25	40	68.006	0	68.006	B18 (11,321)	rATG	SGF
9	F	56	Unknown	1	0	0	12.620	93.770	94.541	A11 (1798)	rATG	DGF
10	M	47	GNC	3	5	70	96.361	42.897	97.977	A68 (13,936)	rATG	DGF
11	F	51	ADPKD	1	0	0	75.197	48.049	86.827	B35 (4899)	rATG	DGF
12	M	47	ADPKD	1	0	0	0	0	0	A2 (1992)	IL-2RB	DGF
13	F	60	DM	1	0	0	0	0	0	A3 (541)	IL-2RB	DGF

* Only Cw antigens. AMR, acute antibody-mediated rejection; ESRD, end-stage renal disease; KTx, kidney transplantation; PRA, panel-reactive antibodies; vPRA, virtual PRA; DSA, donor-specific antibodies; MFI, mean fluorescence intensity; GNC, glomerulonephritis; PNC, pyelonephritis; ADPKD, autosomal dominant polycystic kidney disease; DM, diabetes mellitus; rATG, rabbit antithymocyte globulin; IL-2RB, interleukin-2 receptor blocker; SGF, slow graft function; IGF, immediate graft function; DGF, delayed graft function; n/a, non available.

Table 2. Protocol biopsy findings and serum creatinine concentration before primary AMR treatment and during the follow-up period.

Patient	Bx POD	Banff Biopsy Scoring										C4d	Other Diagnosis	DSA	Diagnosis	Serum Creatinine Concentration (mg/dL)				
		(g)	(t)	(i)	(v)	(ah)	(ptc)	(cg)	(ct)	(ci)	(cv)					Pre-Treatment	Post-Treatment	3 Month	12 Month	24 Month
1	10	2	0	0	0	0	2	0	0	0	0	1		1	AMR	5.7	2.2	1.1	1.1	1.1
2	8	2	0	0	0	1	2	0	0	0	0	1		1	AMR	2.5	1.8	1.2	1.3	1.3
3	9	2	0	1	1	0	1	0	1	0	0	1		1	AMR	1.8	0.8	1.1	0.9	0.8
4	10	1	0	0	0	0	1	0	0	0	0	1		1	AMR	0.9	0.7	0.8	1.1	0.8
5	9	2	0	0	0	0	1	0	0	0	0	1		0	AMR susp	1.6	1.3	1.2	1.4	1.3
6	18	0	0	2	0	0	2	0	0	0	0	1		1	AMR	6.2	1.5	0.9	0.9	0.9
7	9	3	0	3	1	0	2	0	0	0	0	0	TCMR	1	AMR susp	12.7	1.5	1.3	1.5	
8	10	0	0	0	1	1	0	0	1	0	0	0	TCMR IIA	1	AMR susp	2.7	1.7	1.5	1.6	
9	10	0	0	0	0	2	0	0	0	1	0	1		1	AMR	5.9	1.7	1.7		
10	10	2	0	0	1	0	2	2	0	0	0	1		1	AMR	8.5	3.0	1.4		
11	8	0	0	0	3	0	2	0	0	0	2	1		1	AMR	3.9	1.9	1.7		
12	11	1	1	2	0	2	2	0	0	0	1	0		1	AMR susp	4.0	1.2	1.9		
13	9	2	0	1	1	0	2	0	1	1	1	0	CNI	1	AMR susp	3.1	1.4	1.4		

AMR, acute antibody-mediated rejection; AMR susp, the suspected AMR; Bx, protocol biopsy; POD, post-operative day; DSA, donor-specific antibodies; TCMR, T-cell mediated rejection; CNI, calcineurin inhibitor toxicity.

3.3. Kidney Graft Function and Survival

After bortezomib-based primary AMR therapy, kidney graft function improved in all patients (serum creatinine concentration decreased from mean 4.6 (2.6–6.6) mg/dL before to 1.6 (1.3–1.9) mg/dL after treatment; $p < 0.001$). Mean 3-month serum creatinine concentration (S_{Cr}) was 1.35 ± 0.3 mg/dL (eGFR 55.3, 95%CI: 44.9–65.8 mL/min/1.73m^2), 8/13 patients completed 12-month follow-up with mean S_{Cr} 1.2±0.3 mg/dL (eGFR 60.4, 95%CI: 45.4–75.4 mL/min/1.73m^2), and 6/13 patients completed a 24-month follow-up period with mean S_{Cr} 1.0 ± 0.2 mg/dL (eGFR 73.9, 95%CI: 56.7–91.1 mL/min/1.73m^2) (Table 2). In post-treatment control protocol biopsies (Figure 2), four patients presented normal histology, one patient showed the partial resolution of microvascular inflammation, one patient presented mild signs of acute tubular necrosis, and one specimen was inadequate for histopatologic diagnosis. The signs of acute humoral rejection (C4d-) were still present in one patient. One patient was transferred to other transplant center and the results of her control biopsy are unknown.

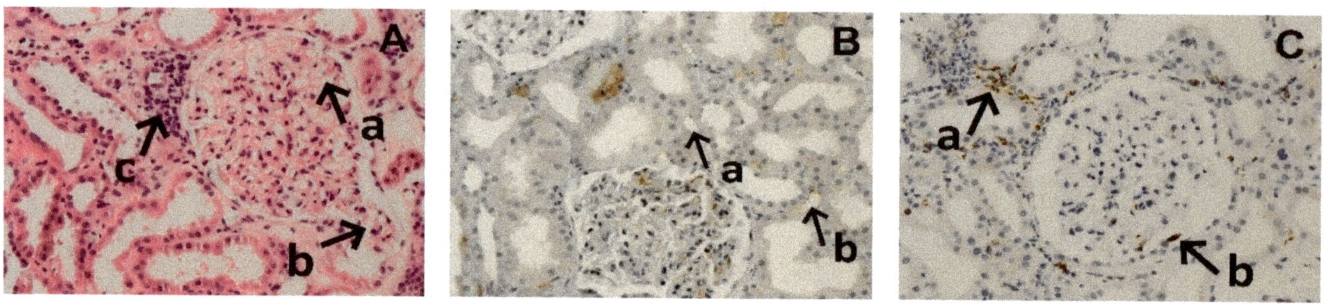

Figure 2. Microphotograph presenting histological findings after bortezomib-based therapy of acute antibody-mediated rejection. (**A**) Hematoxylin and eosin, magnification 200×. Patent capillary lamina without signs of microangiopathy or glomerulitis (a). Prolapse of capillary tuft into the lumen of proximal tubule (b). Small foci of interstitial inflammatory infiltrates (c). (**B**) Negative (a) and nonspecific (b) peritubular capillary C4d staining. Magnification 200×. (**C**) Small interstitial foci of CD68+ cells (a). Single CD68+ cells within glomeruli (b). Magnification 100×.

In the follow-up period of median 21 (IQR: 6–30) months, both patient and kidney graft survival was 100%. Post treatment DSAs were determined in nine patients and were absent in three of them. Median MFI was significantly lower (1373 (IQR: 0–3046)) than prior to treatment.

3.4. Treatment Safety

Despite the preceded induction therapy with rATG in nine patients treated with bortezomib/plasmapheresis AMR protocol approximately 2–3 weeks later, the treatment was generally well tolerated. In one patient, the last dose of bortezomib was cancelled due to gastrointestinal toxicity. Additionally, in one patient, due to the serious hemorrhage after each of the first two PF sessions and the need of reoperation due to large hematoma, the next six PF had to be performed using citrate to avoid heparin administration. In one patient, we observed ascites of unkonwn reason, which resolved thereafter, and in another, the nasal ulceration was noticed. One patient developed a urinary tract infection during AMR treatment, and another patient presented a reccurrent upper respiratory tract infection within a few post-transplant months, which finally resolved thereafter. Based on the laboratory parameters, neutropenia < 1000 cells/μL was observed in one patient, third or fourth grade thrombocytopenia (<50,000 cells/μL) was observed in two patients, and ten patients needed a blood transfusion (median: 2 units/patient). Finally, in seven patients, the transient mild elevation of liver function tests was noted. No other serious adverse events, including neurotoxicity, opportunistic infections, or malignancy, were observed during the follow-up period.

4. Discussion

In this study, we presented our results of the first-line treatment of early post-kidney transplantation AMR based on the administration of bortezomib accompanied by plasma exchange and/or rATG and IVIG. Those early and mid-term outcomes, quantified by kidney graft function, seem to be adequate, being significantly better than previously reported outcomes in KTRs with the diagnosis of early AMR, in whom the first-line treatment was based on ATG, plasmaphereses, IVIG, and/or rituximab, and then the rescue treatment with bortezomib was applied. Additionally, the overall safety profile during and after the AMR treatment was acceptable.

The use of proteasome inhibitor in the treatment of early or late AMR was postulated because it targets antibody-producing plasma cells [25]. Notably, the vast majority of AMR episodes are diagnosed during the later post-transplant period, as pre-transplant DSA titers are increasing or de novo DSAs are produced as a consequence of substantial HLA mismatch, immunosuppressive regimen minimization, non-adherence which is increasing over time, and other relevant factors [26,27]. Hence, until now, the main evidence regarding the effectiveness of multimodal AMR treatment in KTRs is based on late AMR episodes, where its success rate is only moderate. Moreover, bortezomib was usually used as a second-line therapy, after the failure of the initial treatment. Regarding its potential utility as a first-line medication, the literature evidence is scarce. To date, after the first report of two cases [15], the same group published the more comprehensive study, including ten patients who received bortezomib-based primary AMR treatment [11]. However, in all these patients, this primary treatment consisted of bortezomib, plasmapheresis, and a single dose of rituximab. The only previous evidence of the sole effect of bortezomib/plasmapheresis as a primary AMR treatment is the comparison of ten patients treated with bortezomib-based regimen with the historic control group of nine patients who received the rituximab-based AMR regimen [16]. The 18-month graft survival was 6/10 in the bortezomib group, much worse than in our present report. However, they diagnosed AMR episodes based on the indication, not protocol biopsies, which may suggest later diagnosis and treatment as compared to our study. Secondly, there were acute and chronic AMR cases mixed together in both groups and the exact post-transplant timing of AMR therapy diagnosis and treatment initiation was not given. Additionally, all PF sessions were performed using only 4% albumin, whereas in our cohort, a fresh frozen plasma constituted approximately 50% of total PF exchange volume. These particular differences, especially those involving the timing of bortezomib therapy initiation, may partly explain the considerable difference in outcomes of kidney grafts after an AMR episode.

We decided to introduce the protocol based on the four labeled doses of bortezomib associated with the concomitant plasmapheresis sessions. In two patients without plasmaphereses, rATG and IVIG were administered instead. Of note, rixutimab was not used in study patients. At the time, as well as the negative literature concerning the efficacy of rituximab in AMR treatment, we also kept in mind the relatively high cost of our previously used rituximab protocol (approximately $1352 USD/dose in patients with 1.8 m^2 of body surface). Instead, the cost of bortezomib is negligible (~$44 USD/dose in a given patient). Our present case series results suggest an adequate effectiveness of such protocol. In fact, the mean serum creatinine concentration after 12 and 24 months was just about optimal. Of note, the previously reported kidney graft outcomes after the refractory AMR treatment were noticeably worse [7,9,13,14], with several graft losses and suboptimal kidney graft excretory function. We can only hypothesize that some specific properties of bortezomib may condition its effect in the early AMR. As was shown by Perry et al. [19], bortezomib, but not rATG or rituximab, completely abolished anti-HLA antibody production against all HLA specifities. Besides, it also induced the significant increase of apoptotic plasma cells' percentage in vitro [19]. It is possible that the removal of circulating antibodies by PF results in a rebound of their production, thereby enhancing the sensitivity to proteasome [28]. It could partly explain the efficacy of our primary approach to early post-transplant AMR, with bortezomib, but not rituximab, given immediately as a first-line agent accompanied by PF. As the 12-month serum creatinine concentration was shown to be a good predictor of the long-term kidney graft survival [29], we may expect that the routine primary AMR therapy including bortezomib could also optimize the long-term results of kidney transplantations in this group of patients.

When analyzing the safety features, it is worth to notice that the spectrum of potentially bortezomib-related hematologic and gastrointestinal disturbances is generally similar to those observed after rATG induction, which was received by the majority of patients presented in this study. Thus, we may assume that the use of bortezomib did not increase the risk of adverse events in subjects who received both medications. Only one patient with leukopenia after initial rATG induction later presented aggravated leukopenia and neutropenia during the bortezomib/plasmapheresis treatment. Besides, in four patients who were not treated with rATG, but received bortezomib, we observed only mild leukopenia in two, thrombocytopenia in two, and slight elevation of liver enzymes activities in seven. Overall, the observed adverse events spectrum in our cohort was similar to the previously reported abnormalities obtained during the treatment of refractory AMR [7,9]. In patients with multiple myeloma, neurotoxicity often limits the use of bortezomib [30]. In this case series, however, we did not observe neuropathy associated with bortezomib use.

We are aware about the study limitations, namely its retrospective character and the low number of patients. However, we present the largest case series of KTRs with early diagnosed AMR, primarily treated with bortezomib. Heterogeneity of AMR treatment regimen is the another limitation, with 2/13 patients treated without plasmaphereses (but with rATG and IVIG instead), and with plasmaphereses performed in the first three patients only with sole albumin supplementation. Nevertheless, rituximab was not used in these patients, whereas the labeled dose of bortezomib was the core of the primary AMR therapy. Also, the last few patients had a shorter follow-up period and a lack of post-treatment biopsies and assessment of DSAs. Nevertheless, 6/13 patients completed the 24-month and 8/13 completed the 12-month observation period. Finally, the authors considered the lack of control group as a serious limitation.

In conclusion, the mid-term observation of primary bortezomib-based treatment of early post-kidney transplant AMR showed its non-inferiority as compared to previously proposed regimens and acceptable safety profile. It could encourage clinicians to perform early protocol biopsies, especially in patients with high immunological risk, and initiate such a therapeutic protocol as a first-line treatment. However, our data should be confirmed in a larger, multicenter randomized trial.

Author Contributions: Conceptualization, A.K. and G.P.; Methodology, G.P.; Formal analysis, A.K.; Investigation, A.K., H.K., and G.P.; Data curation, A.K. and N.S.-B.; Writing—original draft preparation, A.K. and H.K.; Writing—review and editing, G.P. and A.W. All authors have read and agreed to the published version of the manuscript.

References

1. Lefaucheur, C.; Nochy, D.; Hill, G.S.; Suberbielle-Boissel, C.; Antoine, C.; Charron, D.; Glotz, D. Determinants of poor graft outcome in patients with antibody-mediated acute rejection. *Am. J. Transplant.* **2007**, *7*, 832–841. [CrossRef] [PubMed]
2. Amico, P.; Honger, G.; Mayr, M.; Steiger, J.; Hopfer, H.; Schaub, S. Clinical relevance of pretransplant donor-specific HLA antibodies detected by single-antigen flow-beads. *Transplantation* **2009**, *87*, 1681–1688. [CrossRef] [PubMed]
3. Gloor, J.M.; Winters, J.L.; Cornell, L.D.; Fix, L.A.; DeGoey, S.R.; Knauer, R.M.; Cosio, F.G.; Gandhi, M.J.; Kremers, W.; Stegall, M.D. Baseline donor-specific antibody levels and outcomes in positive crossmatch kidney transplantation. *Am. J. Transplant.* **2010**, *10*, 582–589. [CrossRef] [PubMed]
4. Haas, M.; Sis, B.; Racusen, L.C.; Solez, K.; Glotz, D.; Colvin, R.B.; Castro, M.C.; David, D.S.; David-Neto, E.; Bagnasco, S.M.; et al. Banff 2013 meeting report: Inclusion of C4d-negative antibody-mediated rejection and antibody-associated arterial lesions. *Am. J. Transplant.* **2014**, *14*, 272–283. [CrossRef] [PubMed]

5. Budde, K.; Durr, M. Any progress in the tratment of antibody-mediated rejection? *J. Am. Soc. Nephrol.* **2018**, *29*, 350–352. [CrossRef] [PubMed]
6. Wan, S.S.; Ying, T.D.; Wyburn, K.; Roberts, D.M.; Wyld, M.; Chadban, S.J. The treatment of antibody-mediated rejection in kidney transplantation: As updated systematic review and meta-analysis. *Transplantation* **2018**, *102*, 557–568. [CrossRef]
7. Slatinska, J.; Slavcev, A.; Honsova, E.; Hruba, P.; Kratochvilova, I.; Rohal, T.; Viklicky, O. Efficacy and safety of bortezomib treatment for refractory acute antibody-mediated rejection—A pilot study. *HLA* **2018**, *92*, 47–50.
8. Oblak, T.; Lindic, J.; Gubensek, J.; Kveder, R.; Rigler, A.A.; Skoberne, A.; Veceric Haler, Z.; Bosrtnar, S.; Avgustin, N.; Ponikvar, R.; et al. Treatment of antibody-mediated rejection of kidney grafts with bortezomib and/or rituximab compared to standard regimen: Experience of Slovene Natinal Center. *Clin. Nephrol.* **2017**, *88*, S91–S96. [CrossRef]
9. De Sousa-Amorim, E.; Revuelta, I.; Diekmann, F.; Cofan, F.; Lozano, M.; Cid, J.; Palou, E.; Sole, M.; Campistol, J.M.; Oppenheimer, F. Bortezomib for refractory acute antibody-mediated rejection in kidney transplant recipients: A single-center case series. *Nephrology* **2016**, *21*, 700–704. [CrossRef]
10. Everly, M.J.; Everly, J.J.; Susskind, B.; Brailey, P.; Arend, L.J.; Alloway, R.R.; Roy-Chaudhury, P.; Govil, A.; Moquilishetty, G.; Rike, A.H.; et al. Bortezomib provides effective therapy for antibody- and cell-mediated acute rejection. *Transplantation* **2008**, *86*, 1754–1761. [CrossRef]
11. Walsh, R.C.; Brailey, P.; Girnita, A.; Alloway, R.R.; Shields, A.R.; Wall, G.E.; Sadaka, B.H.; Cardi, M.; Tevar, A.; Govil, A.; et al. Early and late acute antibody-mediated rejection differ immunologically and in response to proteasome inhibitor. *Transplantation* **2011**, *91*, 1218–1226. [CrossRef]
12. Sadaka, B.; Ejaz, N.S.; Shields, A.R.; Cardi, M.; Wadih, G.; Witte, D.; Abu Jawdeh, B.G.; Alloway, R.R.; Woodle, E.S. A Banff component scoring-based histologic assessment of bortezomib-based antibody-mediated rejection therapy. *Transplantation* **2015**, *99*, 1691–1699. [CrossRef] [PubMed]
13. Abbas, K.; Mubarak, M.; Zafar, M.N.; Musharraf, W.; Imam, M.; Aziz, T.; Rizvi, A.H. Management of plasma cell-rich acute rejection in living-related kidney transplant: Role of proteasome inhibitor. *Exp. Clin. Transplant.* **2019**, *1*, 42–46. [CrossRef] [PubMed]
14. Gubensek, J.; Buturovic-Ponikvar, J.; Kandus, A.; Arnol, M.; Lindic, J.; Kovac, D.; Rigler, A.A.; Romozi, K.; Ponikvar, R. Treatment of antibody-mediated rejection after kidney transplantation—10 years' experience with apheresis at a single center. *Ther. Apher. Dial.* **2016**, *20*, 240–245. [CrossRef] [PubMed]
15. Walsh, R.C.; Everly, J.J.; Brailey, P.; Rike, A.H.; Arend, L.J.; Mogilishetty, G.; Govil, A.; Roy-Chaudhury, P.; Alloway, R.R.; Woodle, E.S. Proteasome inhibitor-based primary therapy for antibory-mediated renal allograft rejection. *Transplantation* **2010**, *89*, 277–284. [CrossRef]
16. Waiser, J.; Budde, K.; Schutz, M.; Liefeldt, L.; Rudolph, B.; Schonemann, C.; Neumayer, H.-H.; Lachmann, N. Comparison between brtezomib and rituximab in the treatment of antibody-mediated renal allograft survival. *Nephrol. Dial. Transplant.* **2012**, *27*, 1246–1251. [CrossRef]
17. Wang, Q.; Li, X.L.; Xu, X.G.; Shi, B.Y.; Zhang, Z.M.; Li, Z.L.; Han, Y.; Zhou, W.Q.; Chen, C.Q.; Cai, M.; et al. Bortezomib-based treatment of acute antibody-mediated rejection: A case report. *Gen. Mol. Res.* **2015**, *14*, 17951–17958. [CrossRef]
18. Sureshkumar, K.K.; Hussain, S.M.; Marcus, R.J.; Ko, T.Y.; Khan, A.S.; Tom, K.; Vivas, C.A.; Parris, G.; Jasnosz, K.M.; Thai, N.L. Proteasome inhibition with bortezomib: An effective therapy for severe antibody mediated rejection after renal transplantation. *Clin. Nephrol.* **2012**, *77*, 246–253. [CrossRef]
19. Perry, D.K.; Burns, J.M.; Pollinger, H.S.; Amiot, B.P.; Gloor, J.M.; Gores, G.J.; Stegall, M.D. Proteasome inhibitor causes apoptosis of normal human plasma cells preventing alloantibody production. *Am. J. Transplant.* **2009**, *9*, 201–209. [CrossRef]
20. Tasaki, M.; Saito, K.; Nakagawa, Y.; Ikeda, M.; Imai, N.; Ito, Y.; Sudo, M.; Ikezumi, Y.; Yamada, T.; Hasegawa, H.; et al. Bortezomib eliminates plasma cells from a renal graft in plasma cell-rich acute rejection. *Transplant. Proc.* **2019**, *51*, 1732–1738. [CrossRef]
21. Durlik, M.; Klinger, M.; Lao, M.; Rutkowski, B.; Więcek, A. The treatment of antibody-mediated rejection in kidney transplantation. In *The Guidelines for Immunosuppressive Treatment in Solid Organ Transplantation*; Durlik, M., Rowiński, W., Eds.; Fundacja Zjednoczeni dla Transplantacji: Warszawa, Poland, 2012; pp. 39–40.
22. Mengel, M.; Sis, B.; Haas, M.; Colvin, R.B.; Halloran, P.F.; Racusen, L.C.; Solez, K.; Cendales, L.; Demetris, A.J.; Drachenberg, C.B.; et al. Banff 2011 meeting report: New concepts in antibody-mediated rejection. *Am. J. Transplant.* **2012**, *12*, 563–570. [CrossRef] [PubMed]

23. Loupy, A.; Haas, M.; Solez, K.; Racusen, L.; Glotz, D.; Seron, D.; Nankivell, B.J.; Colvin, R.B.; Afrouzian, M.; Akalin, E.; et al. The Banff 2015 kidney meeting report: Current challenges in rejection classification and prospects for adopting molecular pathology. *Am. J. Transplant.* **2017**, *17*, 28–41. [CrossRef] [PubMed]
24. Haas, M.; Loupy, A.; Lefaucheur, C.; Roufosse, C.; Glotz, D.; Seron, D.; Nankivell, B.J.; Halloran, P.F.; Colvin, R.B.; Akalin, E.; et al. The Banff 2017 Kidney Meeting Report: Revised diagnostic criteria for chronic active T cell-mediated rejection, antibody-mediated rejection, ad prospects for integrative endpoints for next-generation clinical trials. *Am. J. Transplant.* **2018**, *18*, 293–307. [CrossRef] [PubMed]
25. Requiao-Moura, L.R.; de Sandes-Freitas, T.V.; Marcelo-Gomes, G.; Rangel, E.B. Bortezomib in kidney transplant: Current use and perspectives. *Curr. Drug Metabol.* **2017**, *18*, 1136–1146. [CrossRef]
26. Everly, M.J.; Rebellato, L.M.; Haisch, C.E.; Ozawa, M.; Parker, K.; Briley, K.P.; Catrou, P.G.; Bolin, P.; Kendrick, W.T.; Kendrick, S.A.; et al. Incidence and impact of de novo donor-specific alloantibody in primary renal allografts. *Transplantation* **2013**, *95*, 410–417. [CrossRef]
27. Morozumi, K.; Takeda, A.; Otsuka, Y.; Horike, K.; Gotoh, N.; Narumi, S.; Watarai, Y.; Kobayashi, T. Reviewing the pathogenesis of antibody-mediated rejection and renal graft pathology after kidney transplantation. *Nephrology* **2016**, *21*, 4–8. [CrossRef]
28. Lemy, A.; Toungouz, M.; Abramowicz, D. Bortezomib: A new player in pre- and post-transplant desensitization? *Nephrol. Dial. Transplant.* **2010**, *25*, 3480–3489. [CrossRef]
29. Hariharan, S.; McBride, M.A.; Cherikh, W.S.; Tolleris, C.B.; Bresnahan, B.A.; Johnson, C.P. Post-transplant renal function in the first year predicts long-term kidney transplant survival. *Kidney Int.* **2002**, *62*, 311–318. [CrossRef]
30. Meregalli, C. An overview of bortezomib-induced neurotoxicity. *Toxics* **2015**, *3*, 294–303. [CrossRef]

Circulating Arsenic is Associated with Long-Term Risk of Graft Failure in Kidney Transplant Recipients: A Prospective Cohort Study

Camilo G. Sotomayor [1,*,†], Dion Groothof [1,†], Joppe J. Vodegel [1], Tomás A. Gacitúa [1], António W. Gomes-Neto [1], Maryse C. J. Osté [1], Robert A. Pol [2], Catterina Ferreccio [3], Stefan P. Berger [1], Guillermo Chong [4], Riemer H. J. A. Slart [5], Ramón Rodrigo [6], Gerjan J. Navis [1], Daan J. Touw [7] and Stephan J. L. Bakker [1]

1 Department of Internal Medicine, University Medical Center Groningen, University of Groningen, 9700 RB Groningen, The Netherlands; d.groothof@umcg.nl (D.G.); j.j.vodegel@umcg.nl (J.J.V.); t.a.gacitua.guzman@umcg.nl (T.A.G.); a.w.gomes.neto@umcg.nl (A.W.G.-N.); m.c.j.oste@umcg.nl (M.C.J.O.); s.p.berger@umcg.nl (S.P.B.); g.j.navis@umcg.nl (G.J.N.); s.j.l.bakker@umcg.nl (S.J.L.B.)
2 Division of Transplantation Surgery, University Medical Center Groningen, University of Groningen, 9700 RB Groningen, The Netherlands; r.pol@umcg.nl
3 Advanced Center for Chronic Diseases, Pontificia Universidad Católica de Chile, 8330033 Santiago, Chile; catferre@gmail.com
4 Department of Radiology, Clínica Alemana de Santiago, Universidad del Desarrollo, 7610658 Santiago, Chile; gchongm@yahoo.com
5 Department of Nuclear and Molecular Imaging, University Medical Center Groningen, University of Groningen, 9700 RB Groningen, The Netherlands; r.h.j.a.slart@umcg.nl
6 Institute of Biomedical Sciences, Faculty of Medicine, University of Chile, CP 8380453 Santiago, Chile; rrodrigo@med.uchile.cl
7 Department of Pharmacy and Clinical Pharmacology, University Medical Center Groningen, University of Groningen, 9700 RB Groningen, The Netherlands; d.j.touw@umcg.nl
* Correspondence: c.g.sotomayor.campos@umcg.nl
† These authors contributed equally to this work.

Abstract: Arsenic is toxic to many organ systems, the kidney being the most sensitive target organ. We aimed to investigate whether, in kidney transplant recipients (KTRs), the nephrotoxic exposure to arsenic could represent an overlooked hazard for graft survival. We performed a prospective cohort study of 665 KTRs with a functional graft ≥1 year, recruited in a university setting (2008-2011), in The Netherlands. Plasma arsenic was measured by ICP-MS, and dietary intake was comprehensively assessed using a validated 177-item food-frequency questionnaire. The endpoint graft failure was defined as restart of dialysis or re-transplantation. Median arsenic concentration was 1.26 (IQR, 1.04-2.04) μg/L. In backwards linear regression analyses we found that fish consumption (std $\beta = 0.26$; $p < 0.001$) was the major independent determinant of plasma arsenic. During 5 years of follow-up, 72 KTRs developed graft failure. In Cox proportional-hazards regression analyses, we found that arsenic was associated with increased risk of graft failure (HR 1.80; 95% CI 1.28–2.53; $p = 0.001$). This association remained materially unaltered after adjustment for donor and recipient characteristics, immunosuppressive therapy, eGFR, primary renal disease, and proteinuria. In conclusion, in KTRs, plasma arsenic is independently associated with increased risk of late graft failure.

Keywords: arsenic; diet; fish consumption; oxidative stress; kidney transplantation; graft failure

1. Introduction

Arsenic is toxic to many organ systems, the kidney being the most sensitive target organ [1,2]. Free radical mediated-oxidative damage is the cornerstone of arsenic-induced pathology [3]. Arsenic induces morphological alterations of mitochondria that lead to uncontrolled formation of free radicals [4], whilst it inhibits the production of glutathione that protects cells from oxidative damage, ultimately yielding irreversible cell damage [5,6]. The kidney being a major player in removal of arsenic from the system, it is also very much exposed to arsenic and therefore susceptible to arsenic-induced toxicity [7–10].

A large variety of arsenic compounds are known, divided into the elemental metal, inorganic, and organic compounds with a large variety of toxicity [1,2,11,12]. While an extraordinary cause for arsenic intake has been described as hydroarsenicism—contamination of drinking water with arsenic in the US, Chile, and Taiwan—arsenic in food is an increasingly recognized pathway of environmental exposure. Thus, upon background regional differences, arsenic exposure substantially derives from rice consumption, as well as vegetables, fruits, and herbal tea [13–19]. Of note, however, seafood is thought to be a major route for arsenic intake, followed by alcohol consumption, with the latter mainly due to contaminated wine, therewith representing an evident public health threat [20,21].

Basic and clinical evidence has linked arsenic exposure to nephrotoxicity, tubular necrosis, diffuse interstitial fibrosis, decline of kidney function, incident chronic kidney disease, and progress of native chronic kidney disease, among several other conditions such as hypercalciuria, albuminuria, and nephrocalcinosis [22–29]. Kidney transplant recipients (KTRs) are particularly vulnerability to the harmful effects of nephrotoxic agents. However, no study has been devoted to evaluating whether arsenic may be an otherwise overlooked modifiable risk factor in the post-kidney transplantation setting. The current study, therefore, aimed to identify independent environmental and system determinants of plasma arsenic levels and to evaluate the potential association of plasma arsenic levels with long-term risk of graft failure in a large cohort of well-characterized KTRs.

2. Methods

2.1. Design and Study Population

In this prospective cohort study, outpatient adult KTRs with a functioning graft ≥1 year, no alcohol or drug addiction, and without known systemic illnesses (i.e., malignancies, opportunistic infections) were invited to participate. The recruitment of patients took place at the University Medical Center Groningen between November 2008 and March 2011. In total, 817 KTRs were invited for the study, of whom 707 (87%) provided written informed consent to participate. All patients with missing plasma arsenic levels were excluded, resulting in 665 KTRs eligible for statistical analyses. Multiple imputations ($n = 5$) were used to account for missingness of data among variables other than data on circulating arsenic. The present study was approved by the Institutional Review Board (METc 2008/186) and was conducted in accordance with the Declaration of Helsinki.

The primary outcome of this study was death-censored graft failure, defined as end-stage kidney disease requiring dialysis or re-transplantation. The continuous surveillance system of the outpatient clinic of our university hospital, in which patients visit the outpatient clinic with declining frequency in accordance with the American Transplantation Society Guidelines, ensured updated information on patient status [30]. General practitioners or referring nephrologists were contacted in case the status of a patient was unknown. Endpoints were recorded until September 2015. No patients were lost to follow-up.

All KTRs were transplanted at the University Medical Center Groningen following the establishment of standard antihypertensive and immunosuppressive therapies. Relevant characteristics including recipient age, gender, cardiovascular history, and transplant-related information were extracted from patient records. Dietary intake, clinical parameters, and laboratory measurements were extensively assessed at baseline.

2.2. Assessment of Dietary Intake

Dietary intake was assessed using a validated semi-quantitative food frequency questionnaire (FFQ) developed and updated at Wageningen University [31]. The questionnaire consisted of 177 food items to record intake during the last month, taking seasonal variations into account. For each item, the frequency was expressed in times per day, week, or month. The number of servings was recorded in natural units (e.g., slice of bread or apple) or household measures (e.g., cup or spoon). The FFQ was self-administered and then checked by a trained researcher on the day of visit to the outpatient clinic. Inconsistent answers were verified with the patients. The results of the FFQ were converted into total energy and nutrient intake per day by using the Dutch Food Composition Table of 2006 [32].

2.3. Clinical Parameters and Definitions

All measurements were performed during a morning visit to the outpatient clinic. Blood pressure was determined with a semi-automatic device (Dinamap 1846, Critikon, Tampa, FL, USA), measuring every minute for 15 min. The last three measurements were averaged, following a strict protocol as described previously [33]. Body mass index (BMI) was calculated as weight in kilograms divided by height in meters squared (kg/m^2), and body surface area (BSA) was estimated in meters squared (m^2) by using the universally adopted formula of DuBois and DuBois [34]. Diabetes was defined as use of antidiabetic medication, fasting plasma glucose ≥ 7.0 mmol/L, and/or HbA_{1C} higher than 6.5% [35]. Kidney function was assessed by means of estimated glomerular filtration rate (eGFR) according to the Chronic Kidney Disease Epidemiology Collaboration equation [36].

2.4. Laboratory Methods and Arsenic Measurement

Blood was drawn after a fasting period of 8–12 h, which included no medication intake. Serum high-sensitivity C-reactive protein (hs-CRP), HbA_{1C}, triglycerides, low-density lipoprotein (LDL) cholesterol, high-density lipoprotein (HDL) cholesterol, and total cholesterol were measured using routine laboratory methods. Serum creatinine was determined using a modified version of the Jaffé method (MEGA AU 510, Merck Diagnostica, Darmstadt, Germany). Serum cystatin C was determined using Gentian Cystatin C Immunoassay (Gentian AS, Moss, Norway) on a modular analyzer (Roche Diagnostics, Mannheim, Germany). Class I and class II human leukocyte antigens (HLA) antibodies were assessed by ELISA (LATM20×5, One Lambda, Canoga Park, CA, USA) as described elsewhere [37]. According to a strict protocol, all participants were instructed to collect a 24 h urine sample the day before to their visit to the outpatient clinic. Total urinary protein concentration was determined using the Biuret reaction (MEGA AU 150, Merck Diagnostica, Darmstadt, Germany).

Arsenic plasma concentrations were assessed from EDTA plasma samples that were stored frozen at −80 °C. Arsenic plasma concentrations were determined using inductively coupled plasma mass spectrometry (ICP-MS, Varian 820-MS; Varian, Palo Alto, CA, USA) with a modified method for the measurement of low concentrations of heavy metals in plasma using a standard addition method. Standards were made by addition to blanc plasma known amounts of arsenic to obtain added concentrations of 0.500, 1.00, 2.00, 3.00, 4.00, and 5.00 μg/L. Control samples were made by spiking blanc plasma with known amounts of arsenic to obtain added concentrations of, respectively, 0.75 (low), 2.5 (medium), and 4.5 μg/L (high). Sample preparation consisted of diluting 100 μL sample with 1.0 mL dilution reagent. The dilution reagent contained 0.005% Triton X100, 0.005% EDTA, and 0.1 mg/L Yttrium as internal standard. Characteristics of this method are summarized in Table 1.

Table 1. Bias and precision of arsenic measurements.

Cadmium Concentration	n	µg/L	Bias (%)	Inter-Assay Coefficient	
				SD (µg/L)	CV (%)
Low	36	0.75	−13	0.26	40
Medium	36	2.5	−9.2	0.38	17
High	37	4.5	−6	0.48	11

n, number of control samples; SD, standard differentiation; CV, coefficient of variation.

2.5. *Follow-Up of Plasma Arsenic Levels in a Sample Population of the TransplantLines Cohort and Biobank Study*

Additionally, to investigate plasma arsenic levels over time, we requested follow-up plasma samples (3 months, 6 months, 1 year, and 2 years post-kidney transplantation) from 46 consecutive KTRs enrolled between February 2016 and May 2017 in the ongoing TransplantLines Prospective Cohort and Biobank Study [38]. Arsenic plasma concentrations were determined using inductively coupled plasma mass spectrometry (ICP-MS, Varian 820-MS; Varian, Palo Alto, CA, USA) with a modified method for the measurement of low concentrations of heavy metals in plasma using a standard addition method, as described hereby in the preceding section.

2.6. *Statistical Analyses*

Data analyses were performed using SPSS version 23.0 software (SPSS, Inc., Chicago, IL, USA) and R version 3.2.3 (R Foundation for Statistical Computing, Vienna, Austria). Continuous variables were summarized using mean (SD) for normally distributed data, whereas skewed distributed variables are given as median (IQR). Categorical variables were summarized as numbers (percentage). In all analyses, a two-sided $p < 0.05$ was considered significant. Linear regression analyses were performed to evaluate the association of baseline characteristics with arsenic concentrations, adjusted for (i) age and sex, and additionally (ii) eGFR. The assumption of homoscedasticity and normality of residual variance were verified, and a natural log-transformation was applied when appropriate. Std. β coefficients represent the difference (in SD) in arsenic per 1-SD increment in continuous characteristics or for categorical characteristics the difference (in SD) in arsenic compared to the implied reference group. In order to study, in an integrated manner, which baseline characteristics were independently associated with and were determinants of plasma arsenic, we performed forward selection of baseline characteristics according to preceding multivariable linear regression analyses (p for inclusion < 0.2), followed by stepwise backwards multivariable linear regression analyses (p for exclusion 0.05). Finally, we also performed a stepwise backwards multivariable linear regression with exclusion of eGFR in the initial model in order to isolate environmental determinants of plasma arsenic levels.

The prospective association of plasma arsenic with risk of graft failure during follow-up was examined incorporating time to event and accounting for death-censoring, by means of univariable and multivariable Cox proportional-hazards regression analyses with time-dependent covariates to calculate hazard ratios (HR) and 95% confidence intervals (CI). Schoenfeld residuals were calculated to assess whether proportionality assumptions were satisfied. Associations are shown with plasma arsenic as a continuous variable and according to tertiles of the plasma arsenic distribution. Following univariable analyses (model 1), we first performed multivariable adjustment for the most important environmental determinants of arsenic levels according to the results of our backwards linear regression analyses (model 2). To avoid overfitting, further models were performed with additive adjustments to model 2, defined as the primary multivariable model [39]. Thus, we performed additional adjustments for intake of fruits, vegetables, potato, rice, bread, and total energy intake (model 3); transplant characteristics (donor and recipient age, donor type, HLA mismatches, circulating anti-HLA class I antibodies, circulating anti-HLA class II antibodies, transplant vintage, and immunosuppressive therapy; model 4); risk factors of graft failure (eGFR, hs-CRP, systolic blood pressure, total cholesterol, and triglycerides concentration; model 5); and primary renal disease and proteinuria in model 6.

The intra-individual coefficient of variation (CV) for plasma arsenic levels in KTRs of the TransplantLines Cohort and Biobank Study was calculated using the formula CV = (SD/mean) × 100, in which SD is the standard deviation and mean is the mean value for plasma arsenic concentrations as measured in follow-up samples taken at 3 months, 6 months, 1 year, and 2 years post transplantation. Next, box plots were used to illustrate medians (interquartile range) of plasma arsenic levels during follow-up visits. Finally, significance of potential change during follow-up visits was tested using the Kruskal Wallis test.

3. Results

3.1. *Baseline Characteristics and Cross-Sectional Analyses*

Mean (SD) age of the 665 KTRs was 53 (13) years, of whom 383 (58%) were male. Median (IQR) plasma arsenic concentration was 1.26 (1.04––2.04) μg/L. The baseline characteristics of the study participants along with the results of age- and sex- as well as eGFR-adjusted linear regression analyses are shown in Table 2. In stepwise backward multivariable linear regression analysis, fish consumption ($\beta = 0.26$; $p < 0.001$), eGFR ($\beta = -0.11$; $p = 0.02$), and proteinuria (std $\beta = 0.18$; $p < 0.001$) were identified as independent determinants of plasma arsenic concentrations (Table 2). If analyses were performed with eGFR excluded from the initial model, fish consumption ($\beta = 0.27$; $p < 0.001$) was identified as the only independent determinant of arsenic (Table 2).

3.2. *Prospective Analyses*

During a follow-up of 5 years, 72 (11%) patients developed graft failure. Chronic allograft dysfunction was the major cause of graft failure accountable for 50 (69%) of all graft failures. Other causes for graft failure included return of primary kidney disease (11%), infection (4%), acute rejection (4%), BK nephropathy (4%), vascular complications (3%), and others (4%). From low to high tertiles of the plasma arsenic distribution, 18, 25, and 29 patients developed graft failure, respectively. Prospective analyses of the association of plasma arsenic with death-censored graft failure are shown in Table 3. Multivariable-adjusted Cox proportional hazards models showed that plasma arsenic was directly associated with graft failure (HR 1.80; 95% CI 1.28–2.53, $p = 0.001$), independent of major environmental determinants of arsenic concentration, i.e., alcohol and fish consumption. In analyses with further adjustment for potential confounders, the association remained materially unchanged (Table 3). We did not find signs of a non-linear association between plasma arsenic levels and risk of death-censored graft failure (Supplementary Materials Table S1). Figure 1 illustrates the association between plasma arsenic concentration and risk of death-censored graft failure using Cox regression analyses with mean concentration of plasma arsenic as reference, adjusted for age, sex, fish intake and alcohol consumption, and in relation to the histogram of plasma arsenic distribution.

Table 2. Baseline characteristics of 665 kidney transplant recipients (KTRs) and their association with plasma arsenic.

Baseline Characteristics	Overall KTRs $n = 665$	† Plasma Arsenic (ln), μg/L Std. β	‡ Plasma Arsenic (ln), μg/L Std. β	Backwards Linear Regression Std. β	§ Backwards Linear Regression Std. β
Plasma arsenic, μg/L, median (IQR)	1.26 (1.04–2.04)	–	–	–	–
Demographics and body composition					
Age, years, mean (SD)	53 (13)	–	–		
Sex (male), *n* (%)	383 (58)	–	–		
Diabetes mellitus, *n* (%)	160 (24)	−0.07 *	−0.07 *	~	~
Body surface area, m^2, mean (SD)	1.94 (0.22)	−0.02	−0.05		
Body mass index, kg/m^2, median (IQR)	26.0 (23.3–29.4)	−0.003	−0.02		
Waist circumference, cm, mean (SD)	99 (14)	0.003	−0.02		
Cardiovascular history and lifestyle					
History of cardiovascular disease, *n* (%)	325 (49)	−0.01	−0.01		
Heart rate, beats per minute, mean (SD)	69 (12)	0.01	0.02		
Systolic blood pressure, mmHg, mean (SD)	136 (17)	−0.04	−0.06 *	~	~
Use of antihypertensives, *n* (%)	586 (88)	0.001	−0.04		
Current or former smoker, *n* (%)	382 (57)	0.04	0.03		
Alcohol consumption > 10 g/d, *n* (%)	169 (25)	0.14 ***	0.14 ***	~	
Dietary intake					
Bread, g/day, mean (SD)	133 (59)	−0.09 **	−0.08 *	~	~
Vegetables, g/day, median (IQR)	90 (50–118)	−0.03	−0.03		
Fruit, g/day, median (IQR)	123 (61–232)	−0.04	−0.04	~	~
Potato, g/day, median (IQR)	119 (72–161)	−0.11 ***	−0.11 **	~	~
Rice, g/day, median (IQR)	15 (4–32)	0.07 *	0.06 *	~	~
Fish, g/day, median (IQR)	11 (4–21)	0.32 ***	0.31 ***	0.26 ***	0.27 ***
Coffee, mg/day, median (IQR)	500 (250–625)	−0.001	0.01		
Tea, mg/day, median (IQR)	250 (54–375)	0.03	0.01 *	~	~
Laboratory measurements					
Albumin, g/L, mean (SD)	43 (3)	−0.05	−0.03		
Calcium, mmol/L, mean (SD)	2.40 (0.15)	−0.06 *	−0.04		
Phosphate, mmol/L, mean (SD)	0.97 (0.21)	0.09 **	0.03		
eGFR, mL/min/1.73 m^2, mean (SD)	53 (20)	−0.18 ***	–	−0.11 **	–
Proteinuria, *n* (%)	150 (23)	0.12 ***	0.09 **	0.18 ***	
Alkaline phosphatase, U/L, median (IQR)	67 (54–84)	0.02	0.02		
ASAT, U/L, median (IQR)	22 (18–27)	0.06 *	0.07 *	~	~

Table 2. *Cont.*

Baseline Characteristics	Overall KTRs $n = 665$	† Plasma Arsenic (ln), µg/L Std. β	‡ Plasma Arsenic (ln), µg/L Std. β	Backwards Linear Regression Std. β	§ Backwards Linear Regression Std. β
ALAT, U/L, median (IQR)	19 (14–25)	0.01	0.04		
Gamma-GT, U/L, median (IQR)	26 (18–41)	0.05 *	0.05		
Lipids					
Total cholesterol, mmol/L, mean (SD)	5.1 (1.1)	0.03	0.02		
HDL cholesterol, mmol/L, median (IQR)	1.3 (1.1–1.6)	0.04	0.08 *	~	~
LDL cholesterol, mmol/L, mean (SD)	3.0 (0.9)	0.02	0.01		
Triglycerides, mmol/L, median (IQR)	1.7 (1.2–2.3)	−0.01	−0.04		
Inflammation and oxidative stress					
Leukocyte count, per 10^9/L, mean (SD)	8.1 (2.6)	0.01	0.01		
hs-CRP, mg/L, median (IQR)	1.6 (0.7–4.5)	−0.01	−0.02		
Malondialdehyde, µmol/L, median (IQR)	2.5 (1.9–3.7)	−0.02	−0.01		
Primary kidney disease and kidney transplantation					
Primary kidney disease					
Glomerulosclerosis, *n* (%)	190 (29)	0.02	0.01		
Glomerulonephritis, *n* (%)	51 (8)	0.01	−0.01		
Tubulointerstitial nephritis, *n* (%)	76 (11)	0.05	0.06		
Polycystic kidney disease, *n* (%)	136 (21)	−0.09	−0.07		
Kidney hypo/dysplasia, *n* (%)	29 (4)	0.02	0.02		
Renovascular disease, *n* (%)	38 (6)	−0.05	−0.04		
Diabetes, *n* (%)	32 (5)	0.04	0.04		
Other/miscellaneous, *n* (%)	113 (17)	0.02	0.02		
Donor type, living *n* (%)	229 (34)	−0.05	−0.04		
Donor age, years, median (IQR)	46 (31–54)	−0.01	−0.06 *	~	~
Transplant vintage, years, median (IQR)	5.5 (2.0–11.9)	−0.03	−0.01		
Immunosuppressive therapy					
Prednisolone dose, grams, median (IQR)	10.0 (7.5–10.0)	0.01	0.02		
Use of calcineurin inhibitor, *n* (%)	381 (57)	0.05	0.003		
Use of proliferation inhibitor, *n* (%)	553 (83)	−0.001	0.02		
Acute rejection treatment, *n* (%)	176 (26)	0.04	0.03		

* $p < 0.2$; ** $p < 0.05$; *** $p < 0.01$. † Linear regression analysis; adjusted for age, sex, ‡ and eGFR. Std β coefficients represent the difference (in SD) in arsenic per SD increment in continuous characteristics or for categorical characteristics the difference (in SD) in arsenic compared to the implied reference group. For inclusion and exclusion in stepwise backwards linear regression analyses *p* values were set at 0.2 and 0.05, respectively. § eGFR was removed from the initial model. ~ Excluded from the final models. ALAT, alanine aminotransferase; ASAT, aspartate aminotransferase; eGFR, estimated glomerular filtration rate; HDL, high-density lipoprotein; HLA, human leukocyte antigens; hs-CRP, high-sensitivity C-reactive protein; LDL, low-density lipoprotein.

Table 3. Prospective analyses of the association of plasma arsenic with death-censored graft failure in 665 kidney transplant recipients.

	Plasma Arsenic				
	Tertile 1	Tertile 2	Tertile 3	Continuous (ln)	
	Ref.	HR (95% CI)	HR (95% CI)	HR (95% CI)	p
n_{events}	18	25	29	72	
Model 1	1.00	1.41 (0.77–2.59)	1.69 (0.94–3.04)	1.47 (1.08–2.01)	0.02
Model 2	1.00	1.58 (0.86–2.92)	2.12 (1.14–3.95)	1.80 (1.28–2.53)	0.001
Model 3	1.00	1.55 (0.84–2.87)	2.05 (1.10–3.82)	1.74 (1.24–2.45)	0.001
Model 4	1.00	1.40 (0.75–2.61)	2.00 (1.06–3.77)	1.90 (1.32–2.73)	0.001
Model 5	1.00	1.32 (0.71–2.45)	1.76 (0.93–3.32)	1.56 (1.10–2.23)	0.01
Model 6	1.00	1.29 (0.70–2.40)	1.84 (0.99–3.42)	1.53 (1.09–2.14)	0.01

Cox proportional-hazards regression analyses were performed to assess the association of plasma arsenic with risk of death-censored graft failure (number of events = 72). Associations are shown with plasma arsenic concentration as a continuous variable and according to tertiles of the plasma arsenic distribution (tertile 1: ≤1.1 μg/L; tertile 2: 1.1-1.67 μg/L; tertile 3: ≥1.67 μg/L). Model 1 is univariable. Multivariable model 2 was adjusted for fish intake and alcohol consumption. Subsequently, additive adjustment was performed for intake of fruits, vegetables, potato, rice, bread, and total energy intake (model 3); donor and recipient age, donor type, human leukocyte antigen mismatches (HLA), circulating anti-HLA class I antibodies, circulating anti-HLA class II antibodies, transplant vintage, and immunosuppressive therapy (model 4); eGFR, high-sensitivity C-reactive protein, systolic blood pressure, total cholesterol, and triglyceride concentration (model 5); primary kidney disease and proteinuria (model 6).

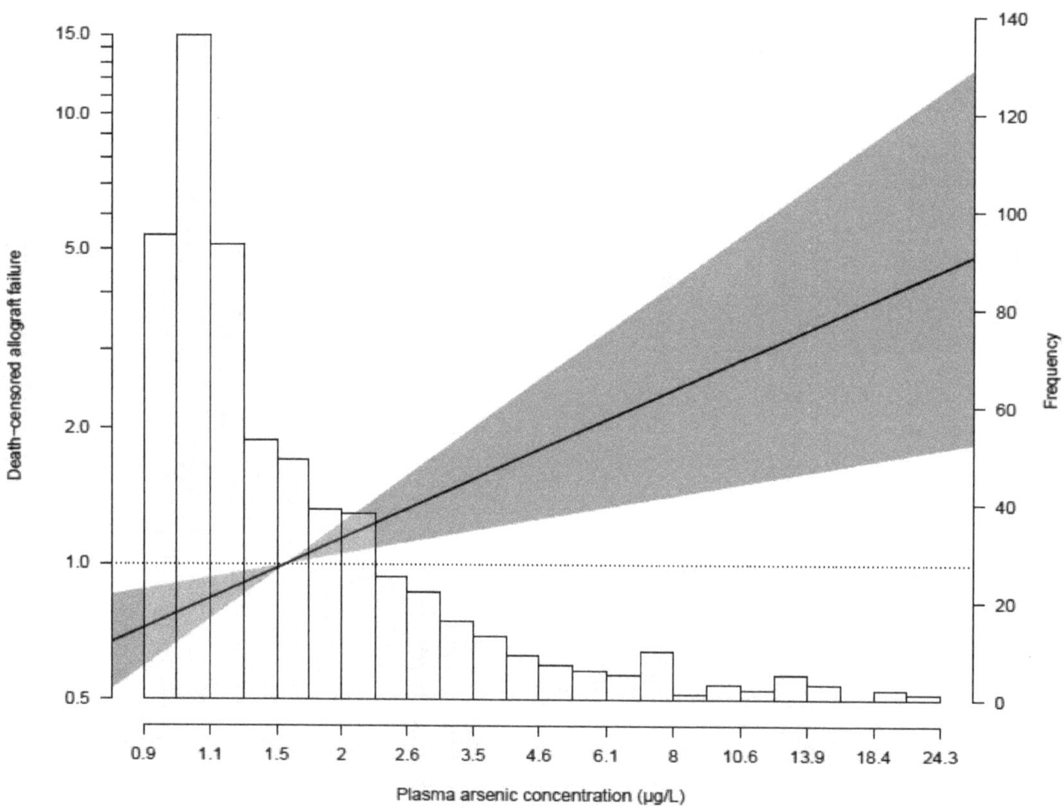

Figure 1. Association between plasma arsenic concentration and risk of death-censored graft failure using Cox regression analyses with mean concentration of plasma arsenic as reference, adjusted for age, sex, fish intake, and alcohol consumption, and in relation to the histogram of plasma arsenic distribution.

3.3. *Follow-up of Plasma Arsenic Levels in a Sample Population of the TransplantLines Cohort and Biobank Study*

In Supplementary Materials Figure S1 we show box plots with medians (IQR) of plasma arsenic concentration of 46 KTRs (mean age 52 ± 14 years-old, eGFR 43 ± 28 mL/min/1.72 m^2) from the

TransplantLines Prospective Cohort and Biobank Study, at different follow-up visits post-kidney transplantation. Median (interquartile range) plasma arsenic concentrations were 1.61 (1.51–1.99), 1.64 (1.52–2.05), 1.64 (1.43–1.94), and 1.59 (1.46–2.26) μg/L at 3 months, 6 months, 1 year, and 2 years post-kidney transplantation, respectively. Median (interquartile range) intra-individual coefficient of variation was 12.2% (6.7–28.7%), and we did not find signs of a significant change in plasma arsenic levels over time ($p = 0.64$).

4. Discussion

In these analyses of 665 well-characterized individuals from a Dutch cohort of KTRs, we identified fish consumption as the major environmental determinant of plasma arsenic levels. Prospective analyses showed that higher plasma arsenic levels are associated with increased long-term risk of graft failure, independent of donor and recipient characteristics, immunosuppressive therapy, eGFR, and proteinuria. These data pose arsenic as a potentially modifiable risk factor for late graft failure in KTRs, emphasizing the need for specific recommendations regarding arsenic exposure, as well as patient monitoring and management of arsenic-induced kidney injury, particularly in populations highly susceptible to nephrotoxic agents such as KTRs.

Being the major organ involved in arsenic clearance, the kidney is highly susceptible and the most sensitive target organ to arsenic exposure [1,2,9,10]. Arsenic-induced oxidative stress has been suggested to be the cornerstone of pathological mechanisms leading to kidney injury and development of chronic kidney disease [3,40]. On the one hand, decreased antioxidant capacity has been shown in individuals exposed to arsenic [41], wherein depletion of glutathione has been consistently described [5,42,43]. Of note, by protecting cells from oxidative damage, inhibition of glutathione production and subsequent glutathione depletion ultimately reverberates into increased vulnerability of cells to arsenic damage. On the other hand, it has been shown that arsenic induces morphological alterations of mitochondrial integrity that lead to uncontrolled free radical formation [4], which further feeds the circle of oxidative challenge and tissue injury. Indeed, basic and clinical evidence has linked arsenic exposure to nephrotoxicity, tubular necrosis, diffuse interstitial fibrosis, decline of kidney function, incident chronic kidney disease, and progress of native chronic kidney disease, amongst other conditions such as hypercalciuria, albuminuria, and nephrocalcinosis [22–29]. Subsequently, diminished kidney clearance of arsenic and enhanced production of reactive oxygen species longitudinally contribute to perpetuate tissue insult and progression of chronic kidney disease [22,23]. Previous studies have also shown an association between arsenic and hypertension and type 2 diabetes mellitus, both suggesting additional mechanisms for secondary kidney damage [44,45]. Ecological studies from the United States, Chile, and Taiwan have shown that arsenic exposure is associated with increased mortality from kidney disease [13–15,22,26,28,46–49]. KTRs are particularly vulnerable to harmful effects of nephrotoxic agents. End-stage kidney disease and maintenance immunosuppressive therapy are constant sources of oxidative challenge for the graft tissue, which shortens the capacity of oxidative stress defenses against additional environmental hazards. To our knowledge, the current study is the first to provide evidence of an independent prospective association between circulating arsenic levels and risk of late kidney graft failure.

Further supportive evidence for the key role of oxidative stress in arsenic-induced pathogenic mechanisms—and suggestive of potential management alternatives—was provided by the observation that co-administration of ascorbic acid and α-tocopherol to arsenic-exposed rats led to a reduction in the levels of lipid peroxidation, protein carbonyls, and hydrogen peroxide along with increased levels of reduced glutathione, ascorbic acid, and α-tocopherol. Investigation aimed to evaluating whether ascorbic acid and α-tocopherol supplementation may improve arsenic-induced altered microsomal functions in the kidney is warranted [50].

An increasing body of evidence supports that the kidney is a primary site of arsenic uptake and accumulation. Recently, X-ray fluorescence spectrometry allowed detection of arsenic accumulation, specifically at level of the kidney cortex [51]. X-ray fluorescence spectrometry may provide comprehensive information of bioaccumulation for biomedical and toxicological research by allowing direct measurement of the distribution of arsenic at tissue, cellular, and subcellular level. Next, X-ray absorption spectroscopy has been shown to allow in vivo assessment of whole-body distribution, which is key information for the development of chelation therapies [52]. Future studies using these analytical methods may provide essential research data to understand the sequence of specific mechanisms of nephrotoxicity and deepen the understanding of the association between long-term arsenic exposure and kidney damage [51].

The current study is etiological in nature, which needs to be separated from prediction research [53]. Whereas the latter is a distinct field of epidemiologic research aimed at predicting the risk of an outcome according to a model of statistically significant predictors, which not necessarily represents causal associations, etiological studies aim to understand a certain pathway of a disease in an attempt to prevent its onset or progression [53]. Taken together, our findings and the aforementioned studies may support an etiological role of arsenic in pathways of disease that contribute to increased risk of death-censored graft failure.

Data on the average diet-derived arsenic exposure in The Netherlands are scarce. One study reported an estimated median (range) exposure of 37.8 (20.6–70.1) μg/day [54]. This was corroborated by a more recent study of Hoogenboom et al. stating that the average diet-derived arsenic exposure is <50 μg/day. In agreement with our findings, higher intake of arsenic most frequently originates from higher fish consumption [55]. A monitoring program from the Dutch Agriculture Advisory Committee (LAC), conducted in the 1980s, demonstrated that levels of arsenic in fish landed in The Netherlands varied between 0.8 and 6.8 mg/kg wet weight, showing a slight decreasing trend over time. Likewise, the arsenic levels in shrimps decreased from 4.3 to 1.3 mg/kg wet weight during that period (LAC program, 1991, in reference [41]). However, more recent data regarding arsenic-contaminated fish landed in The Netherlands are lacking and needed to evaluate strategies aiming to reduce the dietary consumption of arsenic by the population. Next, although in The Netherlands, naturally occurring arsenic concentrations in drinking water are usually below the concentrations required by the European drinking water standard (<10 μg/L in all countries, except Denmark, where it is <5 μg/L), health risks cannot be excluded at this level, and it has been recommended to optimize water supply to arsenic levels <1 μg/L [56,57].

The current study was performed in a large cohort of extensively phenotyped KTRs, allowing us to control our main findings for several potential confounders, including donor and recipient characteristics, immunosuppressive therapy, proteinuria, and eGFR. Moreover, patients were monitored for an extensive period and patient status was updated without losses to follow-up, allowing the study of the long-term association of arsenic with graft failure. Despite considerable improvement of short-term graft survival during last decades, improvement of long-term outcomes continues to lag behind, emphasizing that future advances in the field of kidney transplantation are expected from the amelioration of long-term graft attrition [58]. Systematic description of modifiable risk factors is key to promote preventive strategies particularly addressed for this population of solid organ patients.

Our study derived from a single university center from the northern part of The Netherlands, which calls for prudence to extrapolate our results to different populations regarding potential environmental arsenic contamination and exposure. Additionally, the observational design of the current study does not allow hard conclusions on causality, nor could the potentiality of reversed causation or residual confounding be eliminated, despite the substantial number of potential confounders for which we adjusted. Furthermore, the technique used in the current study does not allow different species of arsenic to be distinguished, while arsenic species have major varieties in toxicity [1–4,11,12]. Elemental arsenic is nontoxic as the metal is insoluble in bodily fluids, and inorganic species of arsenic, e.g., arsenite and arsenate, are especially toxic to humans. Organic species vary in toxicity; the most common species, monomethylarsonic acid and dimethylarsinic acid, are less toxic compared to inorganic species, and arsenobetaine and arsenosugars have a very low toxicity [1,5,9,11,59–61]. Further studies utilizing techniques with the ability to distinguish between the different species of arsenic, e.g., high-performance liquid chromatography–inductively coupled plasma-mass spectrometry, could provide more information on the impact of the different species on graft failure in KTRs. A further limitation is that adjustment for immunological factors as potential confounders of the association was limited to adjustment for HLA matching, circulating anti-HLA class I antibodies, and circulating anti-HLA class II antibodies, since we had no data on donor-specific anti-HLA antibodies and biopsy findings. Finally, it should be acknowledged that graft failure can be the consequence of multiple, heterogenous causes. Unfortunately, in our study the numbers of cause-specific cases of death-censored graft failure was too small to allow for meaningful separate analyses [62]. Larger studies are warranted to comprehensively evaluate the association of plasma arsenic with different causes of death-censored graft failure. It should be noticed, however, that this study is the first to indicate a prospective association of arsenic with the hard endpoint graft failure, thus holding a plea for future studies which to only investigate arsenic plasma concentrations, but also take into account concentrations of arsenic in drinking water, and not only in KTRs to investigate associations with death-censored graft failure, but also in other populations, such as patients with diabetes and the general population.

5. Conclusions

In conclusion, the current study shows for the first time that circulating arsenic levels are independently associated with higher risk of late kidney graft failure, emphasizing the need for specific recommendations regarding arsenic exposure, as well as patient monitoring and management of chronic arsenic-induced kidney damage. Our findings point towards arsenic as an otherwise overlooked modifiable risk factor for adverse long-term kidney outcomes, especially in populations of vulnerability to oxidative stress challenge, *e.g.*, KTRs. Further studies are warranted to confirm our results and investigate the longitudinal association between arsenic exposure and graft failure in KTRs from populations with different dietary and environmental exposure.

Author Contributions: Conceptualization, C.G.S. and S.J.L.B.; Data curation, D.J.T.; A.W.G.-N.; Formal analysis, C.G.S., D.G., J.J.V., T.A.G., and M.C.J.O.; Funding acquisition, C.G.S. and S.J.L.B.; Investigation, C.G.S. and S.J.L.B.; Methodology, C.G.S., D.G., J.J.V., R.A.P., D.J.T., and S.J.L.B.; Project administration, S.J.L.B., A.W.G.-N.; Software, S.J.L.B.; Supervision, R.A.P., C.F., S.P.B., G.C., R.H.J.A.S., R.R., G.J.N., and D.J.T.; Writing—original draft, C.G.S., D.G., and T.A.G.; Writing—review and editing, C.G.S., D.G., J.J.V., R.A.P., C.F., S.P.B., G.C., R.H.J.A.S., R.R., G.J.N., D.J.T., and S.J.L.B. All authors have read and agreed to the published version of the manuscript.

References

1. Cohen, S.M.; Arnold, L.L.; Eldan, M.; Lewis, A.S.; Beck, B.D. Methylated arsenicals: The implications of metabolism and carcinogenicity studies in rodents to human risk assessment. *Crit. Rev. Toxicol.* **2006**, *36*, 99–133. [CrossRef] [PubMed]
2. Hughes, M.F.; Beck, B.D.; Chen, Y.; Lewis, A.S.; Thomas, D.J. Arsenic exposure and toxicology: A historical perspective. *Toxicol. Sci.* **2011**, *123*, 305–332. [CrossRef] [PubMed]
3. Jomova, K.; Jenisova, Z.; Feszterova, M.; Baros, S.; Liska, J.; Hudecova, D.; Rhodes, C.J.; Valko, M. Arsenic: Toxicity, oxidative stress and human disease. *J. Appl. Toxicol.* **2011**, *31*, 95–107. [CrossRef]
4. Valko, M.; Morris, H.; Cronin, M.T. Metals, toxicity and oxidative stress. *Curr. Med. Chem.* **2005**, *12*, 1161–1208. [CrossRef] [PubMed]
5. Miller, W.H.; Schipper, H.M.; Lee, J.S.; Singer, J.; Waxman, S. Mechanisms of action of arsenic trioxide. *Cancer Res.* **2002**, *62*, 3893–3903.

6. Aposhian, H.V.; Aposhian, M.M. Newer developments in arsenic toxicity. *J. Am. Coll. Toxicol.* **1989**, *8*, 1297–1305. [CrossRef]
7. Muehrcke, R.C.; Pirani, C.L. Arsine-Induced anuria. A correlative clinicopathological study with electron microscopic observations. *Ann. Intern. Med.* **1968**, *68*, 853–866. [CrossRef]
8. Uldall, P.R.; Khan, H.A.; Ennis, J.E.; McCallum, R.I.; Grimson, T.A. Renal damage from industrial arisine poisoning. *Br. J. Ind. Med.* **1970**, *27*, 372–377.
9. Peraza, M.A.; Carter, D.E.; Gandolfi, A.J. Toxicity and metabolism of subcytotoxic inorganic arsenic in human renal proximal tubule epithelial cells (HK-2). *Cell Biol. Toxicol.* **2003**, *19*, 253–264. [CrossRef]
10. Chang, Y.W.; Singh, K.P. Arsenic induces fibrogenic changes in human kidney epithelial cells potentially through epigenetic alterations in DNA methylation. *J. Cell. Physiol.* **2019**, *234*, 4713–4725. [CrossRef]
11. Duker, A.A.; Carranza, E.J.M.; Hale, M. Arsenic geochemistry and health. *Environ. Int.* **2005**, *31*, 631–641. [CrossRef] [PubMed]
12. Abernathy, C.O.; Ohanian, E.V. Non-Carcinogenic effects of inorganic arsenic. *Environ. Geochem. Health* **1992**, *14*, 35–41. [CrossRef] [PubMed]
13. Ferreccio, C.; Smith, A.H.; Durán, V.; Barlaro, T.; Benítez, H.; Valdés, R.; Aguirre, J.J.; Moore, L.E.; Acevedo, J.; Vásquez, M.I.; et al. Case-Control study of arsenic in drinking water and kidney cancer in uniquely exposed northern Chile. *Am. J. Epidemiol.* **2013**, *178*, 813–818. [CrossRef] [PubMed]
14. Ferreccio, C.; Sancha, A.M. Arsenic exposure and its impact on health in Chile. *J. Health Popul. Nutr.* **2006**, *24*, 164–175.
15. Ferreccio, C.; González, C.; Milosavjlevic, V.; Marshall, G.; Sancha, A.M.; Smith, A.H. Lung cancer and arsenic concentrations in drinking water in Chile. *Epidemiology* **2000**, *11*, 673–679. [CrossRef]
16. Gilbert-Diamond, D.; Cottingham, K.L.; Gruber, J.F.; Punshon, T.; Sayarath, V.; Gandolfi, A.J.; Baker, E.R.; Jackson, B.P.; Folt, C.L.; Karagas, M.R. Rice consumption contributes to arsenic exposure in US women. *Proc. Natl. Acad. Sci. USA* **2011**, *108*, 20656–20660. [CrossRef]
17. Baig, J.A.; Kazi, T.G. Translocation of arsenic contents in vegetables from growing media of contaminated areas. *Ecotoxicol. Environ. Saf.* **2012**, *75*, 27–32. [CrossRef]
18. Martena, M.J.; Van Der Wielen, J.C.A.; Rietjens, I.M.C.M.; Klerx, W.N.M.; De Groot, H.N.; Konings, E.J.M. Monitoring of mercury, arsenic, and lead in traditional Asian herbal preparations on the Dutch market and estimation of associated risks. *Food Addit. Contam. Part A Chem. Anal. Control. Expo. Risk Assess.* **2010**, *27*, 190–205. [CrossRef]
19. Zavala, Y.J.; Gerads, R.; Gorleyok, H.; Duxbury, J.M. Arsenic in rice: II Arsenic speciation in USA grain and implications for human health. *Environ. Sci. Technol.* **2008**, *42*, 3861–3866. [CrossRef]
20. Park, S.; Lee, B.K. Strong positive associations between seafood, vegetables, and alcohol with blood mercury and urinary arsenic levels in the Korean adult population. *Arch. Environ. Contam. Toxicol.* **2013**, *64*, 160–170. [CrossRef]
21. Choi, B.S.; Choi, S.J.; Kim, D.W.; Huang, M.; Kim, N.Y.; Park, K.S.; Kim, C.Y.; Lee, H.M.; Yum, Y.N.; Han, E.S.; et al. Effects of repeated seafood consumption on urinary excretion of arsenic species by volunteers. *Arch. Environ. Contam. Toxicol.* **2010**, *58*, 222–229. [CrossRef] [PubMed]
22. Meliker, J.R.; Wahl, R.L.; Cameron, L.L.; Nriagu, J.O. Arsenic in drinking water and cerebrovascular disease, diabetes mellitus, and kidney disease in Michigan: A standardized mortality ratio analysis. *Environ. Health* **2007**, *6*, 4. [CrossRef] [PubMed]
23. Zhang, X.; Cornelis, R.; De Kimpe, J.; Mees, L.; Vanderbiesen, V.; Vanholder, R. Determination of total arsenic in serum and packed cellsof patients with renal insufficiency. *Anal. Bioanal. Chem.* **1995**, *353*, 143–147. [CrossRef]
24. Hsueh, Y.M.; Chung, C.J.; Shiue, H.S.; Chen, J.B.; Chiang, S.S.; Yang, M.H.; Tai, C.W.; Su, C.T. Urinary arsenic species and CKD in a Taiwanese population: A case-control study. *Am. J. Kidney Dis.* **2009**, *54*, 859–870. [CrossRef] [PubMed]
25. Soderland, P.; Lovekar, S.; Weiner, D.E.; Brooks, D.R.; Kaufman, J.S. Chronic kidney disease associated with environmental toxins and exposures. *Adv. Chronic Kidney Dis.* **2010**, *17*, 254–264. [CrossRef]
26. Zheng, L.; Kuo, C.C.; Fadrowski, J.; Agnew, J.; Weaver, V.M.; Navas-Acien, A. Arsenic and chronic kidney disease: A systematic review. *Curr. Environ. Health Rep.* **2014**, *1*, 192–207. [CrossRef]

27. Kotsanis, N.; Iliopoulou-Georgudaki, J. Arsenic induced liver hyperplasia and kidney fibrosis in rainbow trout (*Oncorhynchus mykiss*) by microinjection technique: A sensitive animal bioassay for environmental metal-toxicity. *Bull. Environ. Contam. Toxicol.* **1999**, *62*, 169–178. [CrossRef]
28. Robles-Osorio, M.L.; Sabath-Silva, E.; Sabath, E. Arsenic-Mediated nephrotoxicity. *Ren. Fail.* **2015**, *37*, 542–547. [CrossRef]
29. Zhang, J.; Pan, X.; Li, N.; Li, X.; Wang, Y.; Liu, X.; Yin, X.; Yu, Z. Grape seed extract attenuates arsenic-induced nephrotoxicity in rats. *Exp. Ther. Med.* **2014**, *7*, 260–266. [CrossRef]
30. Kasiske, B.L.; Vazquez, M.A.; Harmon, W.E.; Brown, R.S.; Danovitch, G.M.; Gaston, R.S.; Roth, D.; Scandling, J.D.; Singer, G.G. Recommendations for the outpatient surveillance of renal transplant recipients. American Society of Transplantation. *J. Am. Soc. Nephrol.* **2000**, *11*, S1–S86.
31. Feunekes, G.I.; Van Staveren, W.A.; De Vries, J.H.; Burema, J.; Hautvast, J.G. Relative and biomarker-based validity of a food-frequency questionnaire estimating intake of fats and cholesterol. *Am. J. Clin. Nutr.* **1993**, *58*, 489–496. [CrossRef]
32. NEVO-Online Versie 2019/6.0, RIVM, Bilthoven. Available online: https://nevo-online.rivm.nl/ (accessed on 1 June 2019).
33. Van den Berg, E.; Geleijnse, J.M.; Brink, E.J.; Van Baak, M.A.; Homan van der Heide, J.J.; Gans, R.O.; Navis, G.; Bakker, S.J. Sodium intake and blood pressure in renal transplant recipients. *Nephrol. Dial. Transplant.* **2012**, *27*, 3352–3359. [CrossRef] [PubMed]
34. Du Bois, D.; Du Bois, E.F. A formula to estimate the approximate surface area if height and weight be known. 1916. *Nutrition* **1989**, *5*, 303–311. [PubMed]
35. Shabir, S.; Jham, S.; Harper, L.; Ball, S.; Borrows, R.; Sharif, A. Validity of glycated haemoglobin to diagnose new onset diabetes after transplantation. *Transplant Int.* **2013**, *26*, 315–321. [CrossRef] [PubMed]
36. Levey, A.S.; Stevens, L.A.; Schmid, C.H.; Zhang, Y.L.; Castro, A.F.; Feldman, H.I.; Kusek, J.W.; Eggers, P.; Van Lente, F.; Greene, T.; et al. A new equation to estimate glomerular filtration rate. *Ann. Intern. Med.* **2009**, *150*, 604–612. [CrossRef]
37. Van Timmeren, M.M.; Lems, S.P.M.; Hepkema, B.G.; Bakker, S.J.L. Anti-Human leukocyte antigen antibodies and development of graft failure after renal transplantation. *Transplantation* **2009**, *88*, 1399–1400. [CrossRef]
38. Eisenga, M.F.; Gomes-Neto, A.W.; van Londen, M.; Ziengs, A.L.; Douwes, R.M.; Stam, S.P.; Osté, M.C.J.; Knobbe, T.J.; Hessels, N.R.; Buunk, A.M.; et al. Rationale and design of TransplantLines: A prospective cohort study and biobank of solid organ transplant recipients. *BMJ Open* **2018**, *8*, e024502. [CrossRef]
39. Harrell, F.E.J.; Lee, K.L.; Mark, D.B. Multivariable prognostic models: Issues in developing models, evaluating assumptions and adequacy, and measuring and reducing errors. *Stat. Med.* **1996**, *15*, 361–387. [CrossRef]
40. Sasaki, A.; Oshima, Y.; Fujimura, A. An approach to elucidate potential mechanism of renal toxicity of arsenic trioxide. *Exp. Hematol.* **2007**, *35*, 252–262. [CrossRef]
41. Wu, M.M.; Chiou, H.Y.; Wang, T.W.; Hsueh, Y.M.; Wang, I.H.; Chen, C.J.; Lee, T.C. Association of blood arsenic levels with increased reactive oxidants and decreased antioxidant capacity in a human population of northeastern Taiwan. *Environ. Health Perspect.* **2001**, *109*, 1011–1017. [CrossRef]
42. Maiti, S.; Chatterjee, A. Effects on levels of glutathione and some related enzymes in tissues after an acute arsenic exposure in rats and their relationship to dietary protein deficiency. *Arch. Toxicol.* **2001**, *75*, 531–537. [CrossRef] [PubMed]
43. Wendt, T.; Bucciarelli, L.; Qu, W.; Lu, Y.; Yan, S.F.; Stern, D.M.; Schmidt, A.M. Receptor for advanced glycation endproducts (RAGE) and vascular inflammation: Insights into the pathogenesis of macrovascular complications in diabetes. *Curr. Atheroscler. Rep.* **2002**, *4*, 228–237. [CrossRef] [PubMed]
44. Hall, E.M.; Acevedo, J.; López, F.G.; Cortés, S.; Ferreccio, C.; Smith, A.H.; Steinmaus, C.G. Hypertension among adults exposed to drinking water arsenic in Northern Chile. *Environ. Res.* **2017**, *153*, 99–105. [CrossRef] [PubMed]
45. Eick, S.M.; Ferreccio, C.; Acevedo, J.; Castriota, F.; Cordero, J.F.; Roh, T.; Smith, A.H.; Smith, M.T.; Steinmaus, C.G. Socioeconomic status and the association between arsenic exposure and type 2 diabetes. *Environ. Res.* **2019**, *172*, 578–585. [CrossRef]
46. Tsai, S.M.; Wang, T.N.; Ko, Y.C. Mortality for certain diseases in areas with high levels of arsenic in drinking water. *Arch. Environ. Health* **1999**, *54*, 186–193. [CrossRef]

47. Chiu, H.F.; Yang, C.Y. Decreasing trend in renal disease mortality after cessation from arsenic exposure in a previous arseniasis-endemic area in southwestern Taiwan. *J. Toxicol. Environ. Health A* **2005**, *68*, 319–327. [CrossRef]
48. Smith, A.H.; Marshall, G.; Liaw, J.; Yuan, Y.; Ferreccio, C.; Steinmaus, C. Mortality in young adults following In Utero and childhood exposure to arsenic in drinking water. *Environ. Health Perspect.* **2012**, *120*, 1527–1531. [CrossRef]
49. Lewis, D.R.; Southwick, J.W.; Ouellet-Hellstrom, R.; Rench, J.; Calderon, R.L. Drinking water arsenic in Utah: A cohort mortality study. *Environ. Health Perspect.* **1999**, *107*, 359–365. [CrossRef]
50. Ramanathan, K.; Shila, S.; Kumaran, S.; Panneerselvam, C. Protective role of ascorbic acid and a-tocopherol on arsenic-induced microsomal dysfunctions. *Hum. Exp. Toxicol.* **2003**, *22*, 129–136. [CrossRef]
51. Bongiovanni, G.A.; Pérez, R.D.; Mardirosian, M.; Pérez, C.A.; Marguí, E.; Queralt, I. Comprehensive analysis of renal arsenic accumulation using images based on X-ray fluorescence at the tissue, cellular, and subcellular levels. *Appl. Radiat. Isot.* **2019**, *150*, 95–102. [CrossRef]
52. Ponomarenko, O.; La Porte, P.F.; Singh, S.P.; Langan, G.; Fleming, D.E.B.; Spallholz, J.E.; Alauddin, M.; Ahsan, H.; Ahmed, S.; Gailer, J.; et al. Selenium-Mediated arsenic excretion in mammals: A synchrotron-based study of whole-body distribution and tissue-specific chemistry. *Metallomics* **2017**, *9*, 1585–1595. [CrossRef]
53. Van Diepen, M.; Ramspek, C.L.; Jager, K.J.; Zoccali, C.; Dekker, F.W. Prediction versus aetiology: Common pitfalls and how to avoid them. *Nephrol. Dial. Transplant.* **2017**, *32*, ii1–ii5. [CrossRef]
54. Van Dokkum, W.; De Vos, R.H.; Muys, T.; Wesstra, J.A. Minerals and trace elements in total diets in The Netherlands. *Br. J. Nutr.* **1989**, *61*, 7–15. [CrossRef]
55. Hoogenboom, L.A.P.; Bovee, T.F.H.; Kloet, D.; De Waal, E.; Kleter, G.A.; Van Leeuwen, S.P.J.; Pieters, H.; De Boer, J. *Contaminanten in Vis-En Visproducten: Mogelijke Risico's Voor de Consumenten en Adviezen Voor Monotoring*; Wageningen Food Safety Research: Wageningen, The Netherlands, 2003.
56. Van Halem, D.; Bakker, S.A.; Amy, G.L.; Van Dijk, J.C. Drinking water engineering and science arsenic in drinking water: A worldwide water quality concern for water supply companies. *Drink. Water Eng. Sci.* **2009**, *2*, 29–34. [CrossRef]
57. Danish Ministry of the Environment. *BEK 1449 from 11, App. 1b*; Danish Ministry of the Environment: Copenhagen, Denmark, 2007.
58. Lamb, K.E.; Lodhi, S.; Meier-Kriesche, H.U. Long-Term renal allograft survival in the United States: A critical reappraisal. *Am. J. Transplant.* **2011**, *11*, 450–462. [CrossRef]
59. Yuan, T.H.; Ke, D.Y.; Wang, J.E.-H.; Chan, C.-C. Associations between renal functions and exposure of arsenic and polycyclic aromatic hydrocarbon in adults living near a petrochemical complex. *Environ. Pollut.* **2020**, *256*, 113457. [CrossRef]
60. Huang, M.; Choi, S.J.; Kim, D.W.; Kim, N.Y.; Park, C.H.; Yu, S.D.; Kim, D.S.; Park, K.S.; Song, J.S.; Kim, H.; et al. Risk assessment of low-level cadmium and arsenic on the kidney. *J. Toxicol. Environ. Health A* **2009**, *72*, 1493–1498. [CrossRef]
61. Feldmann, J.; Lai, V.W.; Cullen, W.R.; Ma, M.; Lu, X.; Le, X.C. Sample preparation and storage can change arsenic speciation in human urine. *Clin. Chem.* **1999**, *45*, 1988–1997. [CrossRef]
62. Gomes-Neto, A.W.; Osté, M.C.J.; Sotomayor, C.G.; van den Berg, E.; Geleijnse, J.M.; Berger, S.P.; Gans, R.O.B.; Bakker, S.J.L.; Navis, G.J. Mediterranean style diet and kidney function loss in kidney transplant recipients. *Clin. J. Am. Soc. Nephrol.* **2020**. [CrossRef]

17

Torquetenovirus Serum Load and Long-Term Outcomes in Renal Transplant Recipients

Edmund J. Gore [1,*], António W. Gomes-Neto [2], Lei Wang [3], Stephan J. L. Bakker [2], Hubert G. M. Niesters [1], Anoek A. E. de Joode [2], Erik A. M. Verschuuren [4], Johanna Westra [3] and Coretta Van Leer-Buter [1]

1. Department of Medical Microbiology, Rijksuniversiteit Groningen, University Medical Centre Groningen, 9713GZ Groningen, The Netherlands; h.g.m.niesters@umcg.nl (H.G.M.N.); c.van.leer@umcg.nl (C.V.L.-B.)
2. Department of Internal Medicine, Rijksuniversiteit Groningen, University Medical Centre Groningen, 9713GZ Groningen, The Netherlands; a.w.gomes.neto@umcg.nl (A.W.G.-N.); s.j.l.bakker@umcg.nl (S.J.L.B.); a.a.e.joode@umcg.nl (A.A.E.d.J.)
3. Department of Rheumatology and Clinical Immunology, Rijksuniversiteit Groningen, University Medical Centre Groningen, 9713GZ Groningen, The Netherlands; l.wang@umcg.nl (L.W.); johanna.westra@umcg.nl (J.W.)
4. Department of Pulmonology, Rijksuniversiteit Groningen, University Medical Centre Groningen, 9713GZ Groningen, The Netherlands; e.a.m.verschuuren@umcg.nl

* Correspondence: e.j.gore@umcg.nl

Abstract: Following transplantation, patients must take immunosuppressive medication for life. Torquetenovirus (TTV) is thought to be marker for immunosuppression, and TTV–DNA levels after organ transplantation have been investigated, showing high TTV levels, associated with increased risk of infections, and low TTV levels associated with increased risk of rejection. However, this has been investigated in studies with relatively short follow-up periods. We hypothesized that TTV levels can be used to assess long term outcomes after renal transplantation. Serum samples of 666 renal transplant recipients were tested for TTV DNA. Samples were taken at least one year after renal transplantation, when TTV levels are thought to be relatively stable. Patient data was reviewed for graft failure, all-cause mortality and death due to infectious causes. Our data indicates that high TTV levels, sampled more than one year post-transplantation, are associated with all-cause mortality with a hazard ratio (HR) of 1.12 (95% CI, 1.02–1.23) per $\log_{10}$ increase in TTV viral load, ($p = 0.02$). Additionally, high TTV levels were also associated with death due to infectious causes (HR 1.20 (95% CI 1.01–1.43), $p = 0.04$). TTV levels decrease in the years following renal transplantation, but remain elevated longer than previously thought. This study shows that TTV level may aid in predicting long-term outcomes, all-cause mortality and death due to an infectious cause in renal transplant patients sampled over one year post-transplantation.

Keywords: torquetenovirus; immunosuppression; transplantation; immunosuppressed host; outcome; renal transplantation

---

1. Introduction

Immunosuppressive therapy is vital for organ transplantation medicine; in the last 20 years, antirejection treatment has improved enormously thanks to the increased availability of new antirejection drugs. All these drugs, however, lead to some degree of immunosuppression, and subsequently increased infection risk. Measuring trough levels of antirejection drugs is currently standard of care in determining the optimal dosing of these drugs, but is well recognized that these trough levels do not accurately reflect the risk of under-immunosuppression, potentially resulting in rejection, or over-immunosuppression, potentially resulting in increased infections [1–3]. It is, therefore, important to identify the parameters that reflect the net immune status and have predictive capacities for long-term outcomes. Torquetenovirus (TTV) is a single stranded, negative sense, non-encapsulated DNA virus; it was first discovered in 1997 by Nishizawa et al. [4–6] and is present in 46%–100% of healthy people [7]. The international commission on taxonomy (ICTV) recognizes 29 different genotypes, but their relative circulation has not been researched sufficiently [8]. Attempts to discover viable antibody assays have been hampered by the hypervariable nature of the viral capsid protein [9]. A few assays have been described by various groups; however, these assays have not proven to be scalable for large-scale clinical use [9–11]. In recent years, TTV has been studied by various research groups as a potential marker of immunosuppression following transplantation. TTV levels have been shown to increase at the start of antirejection treatment, reaching a relative plateau phase between 3 and 6 months after transplantation [12]. It is currently thought that an ideal viral loads exists for each type of organ transplantation, signifying optimal antirejection dosing. Viral loads above this ideal level have been shown to increase the chance of infections, whereas low viral loads have been shown to be associated with increased chance of rejection [13]. No formal cut-off TTV levels for optimal immunosuppression have been established, however, since these levels show great variation between different research groups, even in seemingly similar patient populations. These variations may be due to differences in circulation of TTV genotypes or due to differences in the PCR test used in these studies.

Additionally, most studies have looked at longitudinal TTV measurements relatively shortly after transplantation. The follow-up periods have also been brief, usually up to one year after solid organ transplantation (SOT). The immunosuppressed condition of these patients and the increased risk of infection nevertheless persists for a lifetime. To date, very little is known about TTV levels past the first year after transplantation, and if these TTV levels are associated with increased risk of infection or rejection in the long term. In this study, we focused on TTV measurements after the first year following renal transplantation, and hypothesized that TTV levels are associated with outcome over several years. We studied this in a cohort of 666 renal transplant recipients.

2. Materials and Methods

2.1. Study Population

This cohort study was based on a previously described set of 706 renal transplant recipients [14,15]. Included were patients (aged $\geq$ 18 years) who visited the outpatient clinic of the University Medical Centre Groningen (UMCG), Groningen, the Netherlands, between November 2008 and June 2011, and who had a graft that had been functioning for at least one year with no history of alcohol and/or drug addiction. Of 706 renal transplant recipients that provided written informed consent, we excluded subjects with missing biomaterial (40 cases) from further analyses, which resulted in 666 cases eligible for study. The study protocol was approved by the UMCG institutional review board (METc 2008/186); clinical trials number NCT02811835 and adhered to the Declarations of Helsinki and Istanbul.

2.2. TTV Viral Load Measurements

Serum samples were stored at −80 °C, until analysis. One serum sample per patient was used; this was collected at enrollment. DNA was extracted from thawed serum samples using the eMAG Nucleic Acid Extraction System (bioMerieux, Marcy, France). The Argene R-Gene TTV quantification kit (bioMerieux, Marcy, France) was used to perform qPCR on an Applied Biosystems 7500 (Thermo fisher, Waltham, MA, USA) according to the manufacturer's instructions. Due to limited sample volumes, 100 μL, a 1 in 4 dilution using DMEM, was performed prior to sample extraction (ThermoFisher, Waltham, MA, USA). A control experiment (data not shown) showed no significant differences in the Ct values. The R gene assay is designed to detect TTV genotypes 1, 6, 7, 8, 10, 12, 15, 16, 19, 27 and 28 [16–18].

2.3. Clinical End Points

The primary endpoint of this study was all-cause mortality, death due to infectious causes and death-censored graft failure as secondary aims. Deaths due to infectious causes were defined using the previously specified list of International Classification of Diseases, Ninth Revision, codes 1–139 [19,20]. For example, a patient meeting the criteria, which is positive culture or PCR for *Pneumocystis jiroveci* infection, would be given the code 136.3 and would therefore be classified as dying due to an infection. Graft failure was defined as return to dialysis therapy or re-transplantation. The cause of graft failure was obtained from patient records and was reviewed by a blinded nephrologist. Endpoints were recorded until the end of September 2015 and there was no loss of subjects to follow-up.

2.4. Data Analysis

Data analyses were performed using SPSS 23.0 for Windows (SPSS Inc., Chicago, IL, USA) and R (R Foundation for Statistical Computing, Vienna, Austria). As no cut-off values for low, medium and high TTV load have been established, and to avoid bias, renal transplant recipients were stratified into three equally sized groups based on serum TTV. This created four groups, named undetectable-TTV, low-TTV, medium-TTV, and high-TTV, which were further analyzed. Differences in all-cause mortality, death due to infectious causes and graft failure between the four groups were compared using Kaplan–Meier plots and log rank tests. Data are presented as mean ± SD for normally distributed data, as median [interquartile range (IQR)] for non-normally distributed data, and as number (percentage) for nominal data. *t*-Tests, or one-way ANOVA tests with Tukey post-hoc tests, were performed on normally distributed data. Each group was compared with the other three groups. Kruskal–Wallis or Mann–Whitney U tests were performed on non-normally distributed data. Chi-square tests were used on categorical data. A two-sided $p < 0.05$ was considered to indicate statistical significance in all analyses.

Prospective associations of TTV on study endpoints were explored by means of Cox regression analysis. Risk of all-cause mortality, death due to infectious causes and graft failure are presented as HR [95% confidence interval]. In these analyses, associations were adjusted in a cumulative fashion for potential confounders, including age, sex, eGFR, proteinuria (model 1), time since transplantation (model 2) and the number of immunosuppressant medications taken (model 3). Cox regression models were built in a stepwise fashion to avoid over-fitting. The proportionality of hazards for covariates was investigated by inspecting the Schoenfeld residuals. eGFR and age were included as categorical variables with equal numbers of events in each group, as eGFR and age breached the proportionality of hazards assumption as continuous variables.

The optimal cutoff values for death due to infectious causes was identified by using Youden's Index [21] in the area under receiver operating characteristics (auROC) curve. This approach was not used for all-cause mortality as the threshold was biologically unrealistic, therefore a sensitivity of 75% was set and the threshold was calculated. Sampling by replacement was used to create 1000 bootstrapped samples of equal size from within the study population, this was then used within our multivariate Cox regression models to validate the association of the TTV DNA thresholds with risk.

To assess in further detail how TTV levels change over time, and to validate our TTV test in patients with older transplants, the patients were subdivided into two groups. The first group had had a transplant 12 to 24 months prior to analysis. The 2nd group had had transplants over 24 months prior to analysis. Cox regression analysis was also performed as previously described.

3. Results

3.1. Recipient Demographics

There was a median 4.9 [IQR 3.4–5.5] years of follow-up for our study population, with 117 (18%) of renal transplant recipients having undetectable TTV, 183 (27%) having low TTV, (median 1.52 (IQR 1.00–1.85) Log_{10}copies/mL), 184 (28%) medium TTV, (median 3.00 (IQR 2.61–3.40) Log_{10}copies/mL), and 182 (27%) high TTV, (median 5.52 (IQR 4.08–5.27) Log_{10}copies/mL) (Table 1). Median time from transplant to TTV sampling was different for each group; undetectable TTV 7.1 (IQR 4.0–12.4) years, low TTV 6.4 (IQR 3.1–11.0) years, medium TTV 5.3 (IQR 2.2–14.3) years and high TTV 3.2 (1.0–9.0) years ($p < 0.001$).

Table 1. Recipient demographics.

	Undetectable TTV	Low	Medium	High	*p*
Number of Patients (%)	117 (18)	183 (27)	184 (28)	182 (27)	
Age (years)	49 ± 14 *a	53 ± 16	53 ± 13	55 ± 12	0.01 *
Male (%)	57 (49)	103 (56)	106 (58)	112 (62)	0.18
Weight (Kg)	77 ± 15	81 ± 16	81 ± 16	81 ± 18	0.15
BMI (Kg/m^2)	26.0 ± 4.3	26.6 ± 4.5	27.0 ± 5.1	26.8 ± 5.0	0.33
Renal Function					
Serum creatine (umol/L)	132 ± 67	135 ± 63	138 ± 57	145 ± 54	0.23
eGFR (mL/1.73 m^2)	50 ± 20 *b	47 ± 20 *b	45 ± 18	40 ± 16 *b	<0.001 *
Urinary protein excretion (g/24 h)	0.18 (0.00–0.27)	0.20 (0.00–0.41)	0.19 (0.00–0.47)	0.19 (0.00–0.47)	0.49
Proteinuria present, n (%)	21 (18)	42 (23)	46 (25)	40 (22)	0.57
Albuminuria (mg/24 h)	41 (8–144)	43 (11–189)	42 (12–235)	36 (9–202)	0.94
Transplantation					
Living Donation, n (%)	45 (39)	62 (34)	69 (38)	56 (31)	0.45
Warm Ischemic Time (minutes)	42 ± 17	43 ± 15	43 ± 16	44 ± 13	0.53
Cold Ischaemic Time (hours)	13 ± 10	14 ± 10	14 ± 11	15 ± 10	0.56
HLA I Antibodies, n (%)	9 (8)	33 (18)	26 (14)	33 (18)	0.05
HLA II Antibodies, n (%)	20 (17)	37 (20)	33 (18)	25 (14)	0.43
Transplant vintage (years)	7.1 (4.0–12.4)	6.4 (3.1–11.0)	5.3 (2.2–14.3)	3.2 (1.0–9.0)	<0.001
Acute rejection, n (%)	24 (21)	54 (30)	58 (32)	38 (21)	0.04
Medication					
Mono-therapy, n (%)	4 (3)	11 (6)	4 (2)	4 (2)	0.15
Dual-therapy, n (%)	82 (70)	107 (59)	94 (51)	78 (43)	0.01
Triple-therapy, n (%)	31 (27)	65 (36)	86 (47)	100 (55)	<0.001
Prednisolone dose (mg/day)	7.5 (7.5–10)	10 (7.5–10)	10 (7.5–10)	10 (7.5–10)	0.02
MTOR inhibitors, n (%)	3 (3)	9 (5)	3 (2)	3 (2)	0.17
Cyclosporin, n (%)	24 (21)	62 (34)	82 (45)	91 (50)	<0.001
Tacrolimus, n (%)	18 (15)	24 (13)	30 (16)	46 (25)	0.03
Azathioprine, n (%)	25 (21)	27 (15)	38 (21)	23 (13)	0.15
Mycophenolate, n (%)	79 (68)	126 (69)	117 (64)	120 (66)	0.94
End Points					
All-cause mortality	6.3 (6.1–6.5)	6.2 (6.0–6.4)	6.0 (5.7–6.2)	5.7 (5.4–6.0)	0.001
Infectious Death	6.6 (6.5–6.8)	6.6 (6.5–6.8)	6.7 (6.5–6.8)	6.4 (6.2–6.6)	0.08
Graft Failure	6.1 (5.8–6.4)	6.5 (6.3–6.6)	6.3 (6.0–6.5)	6.3 (6.0–6.5)	0.5

* a Tukey post-hoc undetectable TTV vs. TTV low, medium, high groups $p = 0.01$. * b Tukey post-hoc undetectable TTV vs. TTV low group $p < 0.001$. BMI: body mass index, eGFR: estimated glomerular filtration rate, MTOR: mammalian target of Rapamycine.

The median prednisolone dose taken by the patients was different across the groups, 7.5 mg/day for the undetectable TTV group and 10 mg/day for low, medium, high groups ($p = 0.02$). The numbers of renal transplant recipients on calcineurin inhibitors (CNIs) were different across the groups with 36%, 47%, 61% and 75% for undetectable, low, medium and high ($p < 0.001$), respectively. There were comparable numbers of renal transplant recipients on proliferation inhibitors in each group ($p = 0.13$). Twenty-three recipients were on mono-therapy, 361 on dual-therapy and 282 were on triple-therapy post-transplant. Renal transplant recipients on mono-therapy had a lower median TTV 1.67 (IQR 0.71–2.68) Log_{10}copies/mL, than recipients on dual-therapy 2.1 (IQR 0.48–3.52) Log_{10}copies/mL, or on triple-therapy 3.06 (IQR 2.57–4.22) Log_{10}copies/mL.

There were no differences between the groups in regard to the type of donation (living vs. post mortal, $p = 0.45$), warm ischemic time ($p = 0.53$), cold ischemic time ($p = 0.55$) or proteinuria ($p = 0.57$). The patient demographics are represented in Table 1.

3.2. TTV and All-Cause Mortality

Patient mortality was attributed to a variety of causes, with a total of 141 patient deaths. Fifty-eight patients (41%) died due to a cardiovascular event and 40 (28%) died due to an infection. Most infectious deaths were caused by bacteria, with 29 events, five viral illness events, two fungal infections, and finally four patients died with multiple organisms. An additional 21 patients died due to malignancy and 22 due to miscellaneous causes.

We observed differences in all-cause mortality across the four categories of TTV status (log-rank test $p < 0.001$) (Figure 1A). Fourteen (12%), 30 (16%), 44 (24%), and 53 (29%) died in the undetectable group, the low group, the medium group and the high group, respectively. Time to death was shortest for the high TTV group with 5.7 (5.4–6.0) years. This compares to 6.0 (5.7–6.2) years, 6.2 (6.0–6.4) years and 6.3 (6.1–6.5) years for the medium, low and undetectable groups, respectively. As the time between transplantation and sampling was significantly shorter in the high-TTV group, it was possible that the differences in mortality and time to death were caused by disproportionally high mortality in the early years after transplantation, a period which was not observed for the patients in the low-TTV group, who were not included in the study until a median of 6.4 years after transplantation. We therefore determined the death rate within six years after transplantation and overall in the different TTV-level groups. This did not show a significant change in death rate during the follow-up period. The death rate in the first six years after transplantation was 16% in the low-TTV group and 18% overall in the follow-up period. In the high-TTV group, the mortality was 24% in the first six years after transplantation and 33% overall. It is therefore unlikely that the high all-cause mortality in the high-TTV group was attributable to the relatively early inclusion of these patients as compared to the low-TTV group. Log TTV is significantly associated with all-cause mortality in renal transplant recipients (HR 1.12 (95%CI 1.02–1.23), $p = 0.02$ per $\log_{10}$ increase in TTV), independent of potential confounders including age, gender, eGFR, time since transplantation and number of immunosuppressant medications taken (Figure 2A). Using Youden's index, we calculated the sensitivity and specificity of a single TTV measurement, using a cut-off TTV level of 3.65 Log_{10}copies/mL for identifying patients with increased chance of death; the specificity was 75% and sensitivity was 40%.

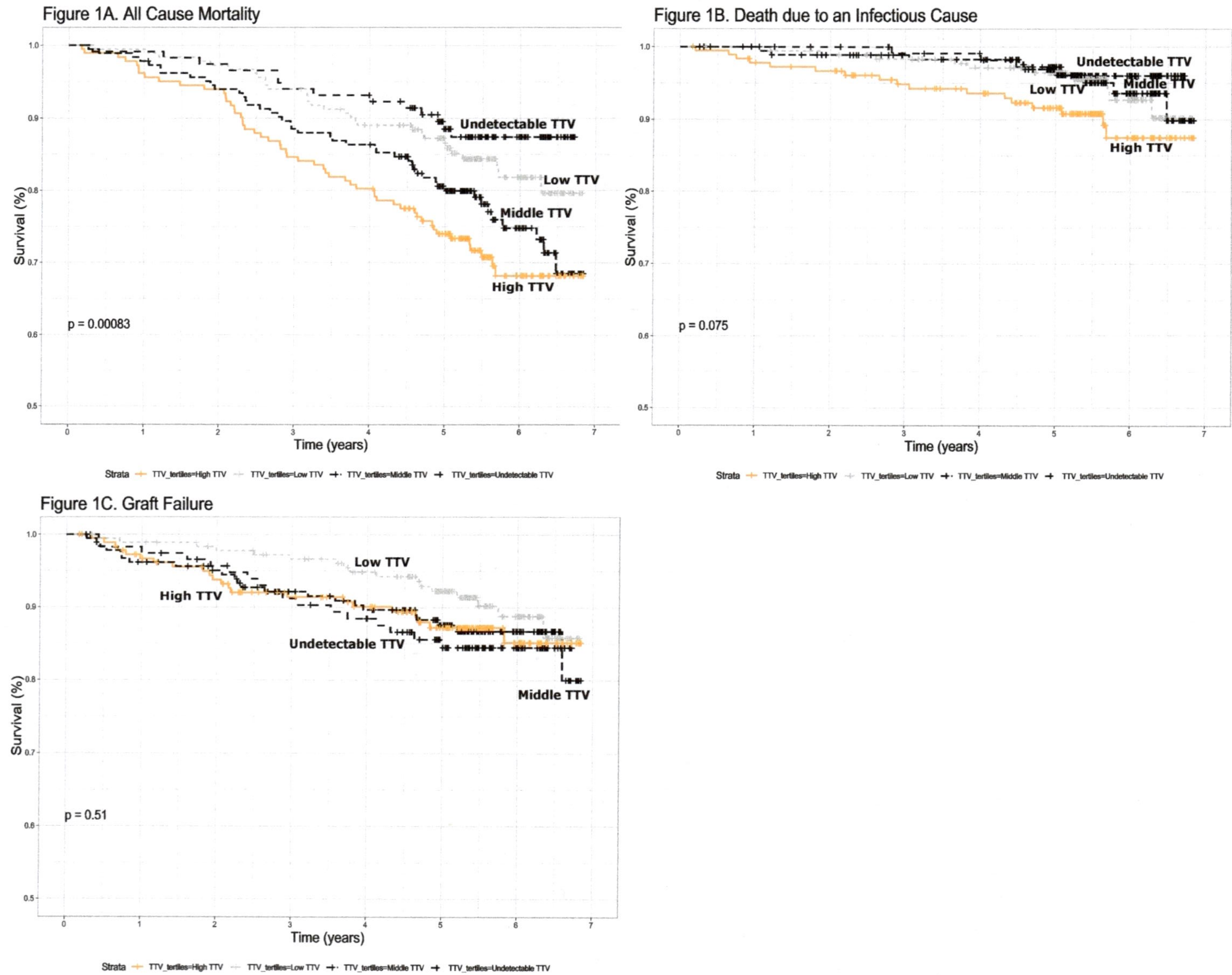

Figure 1. Kaplan–Meier plots showing differences in survival (**A**,**B**), and graft failure (**C**) over time between undetectable low torquetenovirus TTV (black), low TTV (light blue), medium TTV (red) and high TTV (orange), as measured in a serum sample tested at least 12 months after transplantation. Time from testing is displayed (**A**) All-cause mortality ($p < 0.001$, (**B**) Death due to infectious causes ($p = 0.08$), (**C**)) graft survival ($p = 0.51$).

Figure 2A.

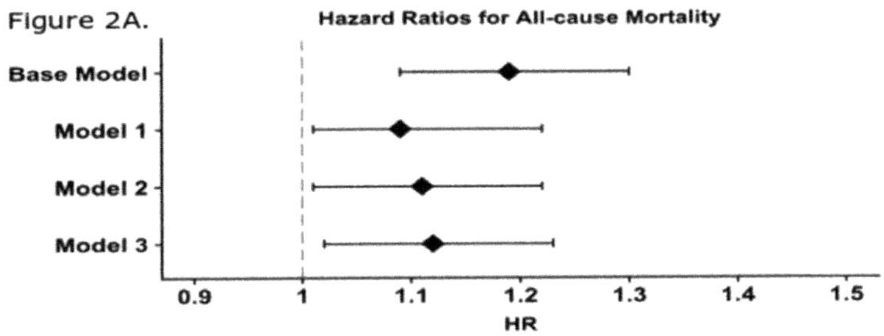

All-cause Mortality

Model Name	HR	P Value
Base Model	1.19 [1.09-1.30]	<0.001
Model 1	1.09 [1.01-1.22]	0.03
Model 2	1.11 [1.01-1.22]	0.03
Model 3	1.12 [1.02-1.23]	0.02

Figure 2B.

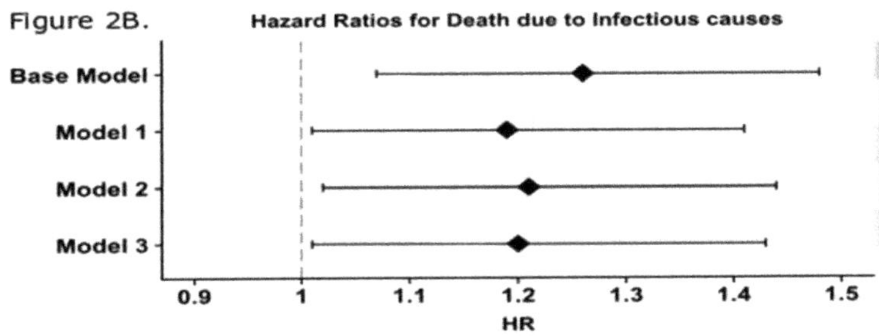

Death due to Infectious causes

Model Name	HR	P Value
Base Model	1.26 [1.07-1.48]	0.006
Model 1	1.19 [1.01-1.41]	0.07
Model 2	1.21 [1.02-1.44]	0.05
Model 3	1.20 [1.01-1.43]	0.04

Figure 2C.

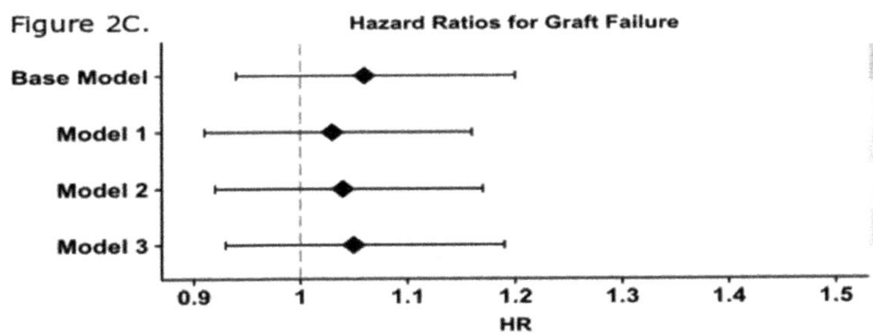

Graft Failure

Model Name	HR	P Value
Base Model	1.06 [0.94-1.20]	0.33
Model 1	1.03 [0.91-1.16]	0.68
Model 2	1.04 [0.92-1.17]	0.56
Model 3	1.05 [0.93-1.19]	0.44

Base	Log10-transformed serum TTV
Model 1	Base + Age(a), sex, eGFR(b), proteinuria
Model 2	Model 1 + time since transplantation
Model 3	Model 2 + Number of Immunosuppressants used

Figure 2. Hazard ratios calculated using Cox models and presented as a forest plot. (**A**) Log_{10} TTV is predictive of all-cause mortality after adjustment for age, gender, eGFR proteinuria, time since transplant and the number of immunosuppressant's used. This means that for each log increase in TTV, there is a 12% increase for a patient's risk of death (HR 1.12 (95% CI 1.0.2–1.23), $p = 0.02$). (**B**) Log_{10} TTV is predictive of death due to an infectious cause after adjustment for age, gender, eGFR proteinuria, time since transplant and the number of immunosuppressant's used. This means that for each log increase in TTV, there is a 20% increase for a patient's risk of death (HR 1.20 (95% CI 1.01–1.43), $p = 0.04$). (**C**) Log_{10} TTV is not predictive of graft failure after adjustment for age, gender, eGFR, proteinuria, time since transplant and the number of immunosuppressant's used. [a] Categorical variable used for death due to an infectious cause. [b] Categorical variable used for all-cause mortality and graft failure.

3.3. TTV and Death Due to a Cause

As over-immunosuppression is associated with risk of infection, we investigated the relationship between TTV levels and death due to infectious cause. In the TTV-undetectable group, four (3%) patients died from infections, whereas, 10 (6%), nine (5%) and 17 (9%) renal transplant recipients died in low group, the medium group and the high group, respectively (log-rank $p = 0.08$, Figure 1B) (Table 1). Mean time to death due to an infectious cause was not significantly different between the groups, i.e., for the undetectable group this was 6.6 (6.5–6.8) years, for the low-TTV group 6.6 (6.5–6.8) years, medium-TTV group 6.7 (6.5–6.8) years and high-TTV group 6.4 (6.2–6.6) years. Furthermore, we observed that log TTV is significantly associated with death due to infections (HR 1.20 (95% CI 1.01–1.43), $p = 0.04$), independent of potential confounders (Figure 2B). Using Youden's index, we determined that a single TTV measurement with a level over 3.38 Log_{10}copies/mL identified patients at risk of death due to infections with a sensitivity of 55%, and a specificity of 67%.

3.4. *TTV and Graft Failure*

We also observed no difference in mean graft survival across the four groups, ($p = 0.51$, Figure 1C). The numbers of patients with graft failure was not significantly different across the four groups, with 17 (15%), 17 (9%), 23 (13%) and 22 (12%) for the undetectable group, the low group, the medium group and the high group respectively ($p = 0.57$). This result is replicated when looking at the Cox model data (HR 1.01 (95% CI 0.93–1.19) $p = 0.44$, Figure 2C).

3.5. *Time since Transplantation and TTV*

Because there is limited data on TTV levels in renal transplant recipients beyond the first year after transplantation, we divided our transplant population into two groups. One group which were sampled 12–24 months post-transplant ($n = 164$ patients) and the other over 24 months since transplant ($n = 502$ patients). This showed that TTV levels up to 24 months from transplantation were significantly higher than TTV levels in patients 2–3 years, 3–4 years, 4–5 years and over five years from transplantation ($p < 0.05$) (Figure 3).

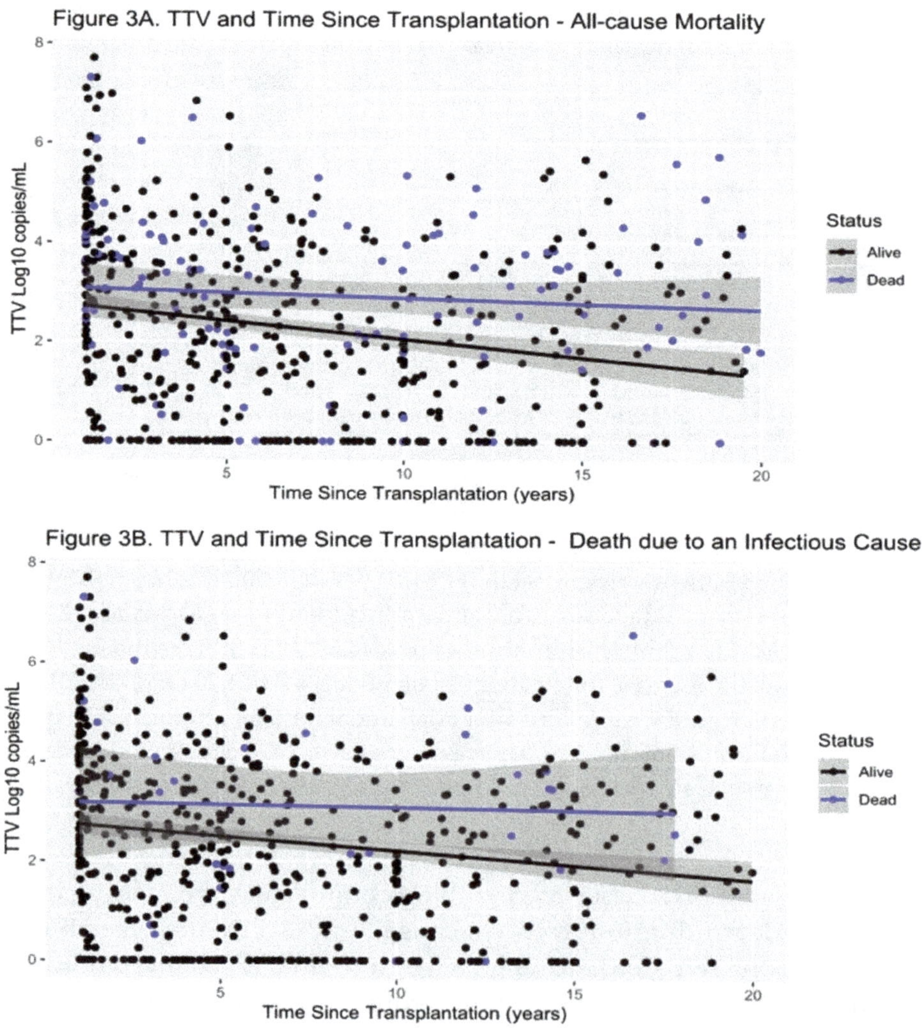

Figure 3. Scatter plot showing levels of TTV in our transplant patients and their outcomes in all-cause mortality (**A**), and death due to infectious causes (**B**). TTV levels are higher in the first years after transplantation than in later years. Patients with worse outcome show a trend of higher TTV levels over the entire follow-up period.

TTV measured within 24 months of transplantation was not associated with an increased risk of death by all causes of due to an infectious cause (Figure 4).

Figure 4A. Within 24 months of transplant
Hazard Ratios for All-cause Mortality

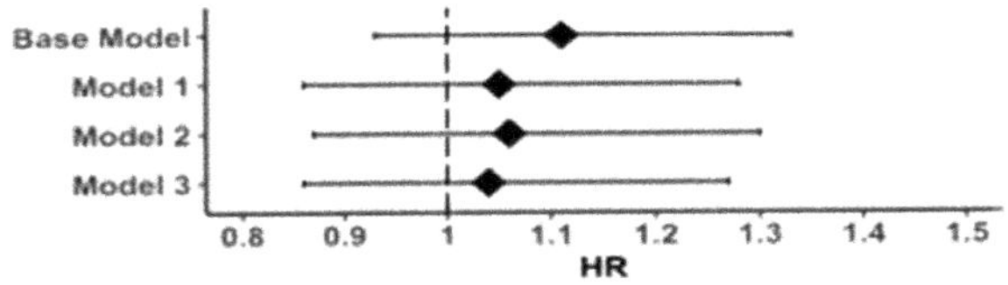

Model Name	HR	P Value
Base Model	1.11 [0.93-1.33]	0.25
Model 1	1.05 [0.86-1.28]	0.62
Model 2	1.06 [0.87-1.30]	0.35
Model 3	1.04 [0.86-1.27]	0.69

Figure 4B. Over 24 months since transplantation
Hazard Ratios for All-cause Mortality

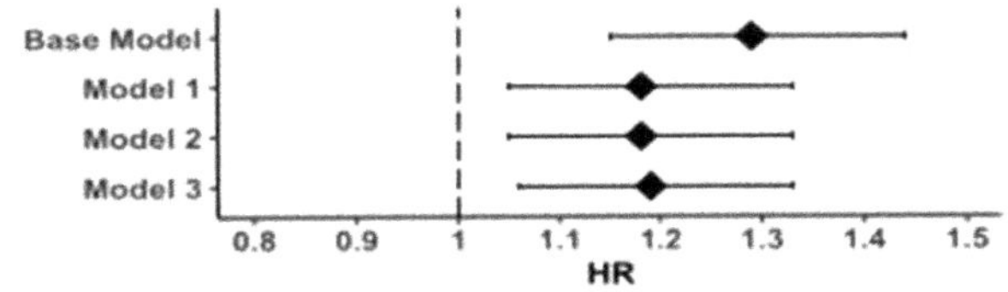

Model Name	HR	P Value
Base Model	1.29 [1.15-1.44]	<0.001
Model 1	1.18 [1.05-1.33]	<0.01
Model 2	1.18 [1.05-1.33]	<0.01
Model 3	1.19 [1.06-1.33]	<0.01

Figure 4C. Within 24 months of transplant
Hazard Ratios for Infectious Mortality

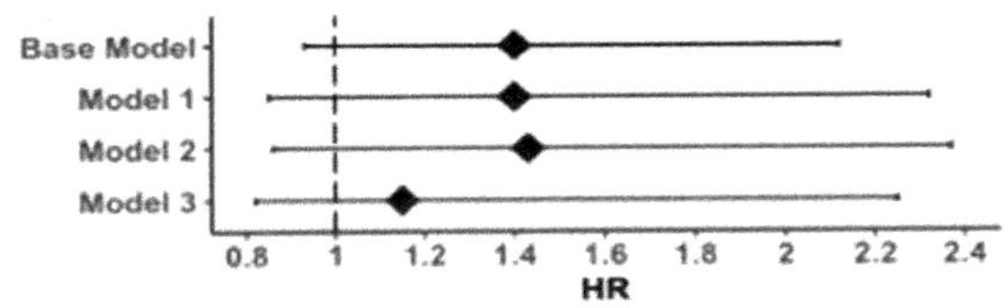

Model Name	HR	P Value
Base Model	1.40 [0.93-2.12]	0.11
Model 1	1.40 [0.85-2.32]	0.19
Model 2	1.43 [0.86-2.37]	0.16
Model 3	1.15 [0.82-2.25]	0.86

Figure 4D. Over 24 months since transplantation
Hazard Ratios for Infectious Mortality

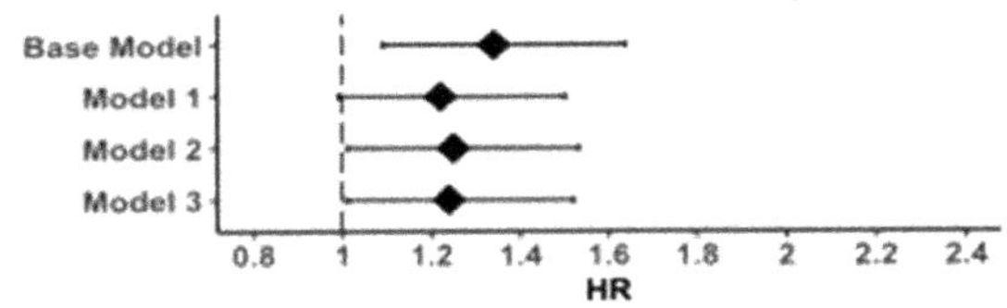

Model Name	HR	P Value
Base Model	1.34 [1.09-1.64]	0.005
Model 1	1.22 [0.99-1.50]	0.06
Model 2	1.25 [1.01-1.53]	0.04
Model 3	1.24 [1.01-1.52]	0.04

Base	Log10-transformed serum TTV
Model 1	Base + Age(a), sex, eGFR(b), proteinuria
Model 2	Model 1 + time since transplantation
Model 3	Model 2 + Number of Immunosuppressants used

Figure 4. Forest plots with hazard table of Cox models after adjustment for age, gender, eGFR proteinuria, and the number of immunosuppressant's used. (**A**) All-cause mortality in patients transplanted within 24 months of TTV analysis; this includes 31 events. Log_{10} TTV cannot be used to predict risk of death transplanted within 24 months of TTV analysis. (**B**) All-cause mortality in patients tested over 24 months after transplantation, this includes 110 events. Log_{10} TTV is highly predictive of the risk of death for patients with elevated TTV (HR 1.19 (95%CI 1.06–1.33), $p < 0.01$). (**C**) Log_{10} TTV is not predictive of death due to an infectious cause in patients tested over 24 months since transplantation (HR 1.15 (95% CI 0.82–2.25), $p = 0.86$). (**D**) Log_{10} TTV is predictive of death due to an infectious cause in patients 24 months after transplantation (HR 1.24 (95%CI 1.01–1.52), $p = 0.04$). [a] Categorical variable used for death due to an infectious cause. [b] Categorical variable used for all-cause mortality.

On the contrary, TTV measured in patients over 24 months from transplantation show that there is a significant difference in survival between patients with high, medium, low or undetectable TTV ($p < 0.001$, Figure 4). Cox modeling also shows an increased all-cause mortality when adjusting for age, gender, eGFR, and number of immunosuppressant medications taken (HR 1.18 (95% CI 0.05–1.33), $p < 0.004$). Time to death due to death due infectious causes is also shorter in the high-TTV population that are over 24 months post-transplant ($p = 0.04$, Figure 4C). This conclusion is supported by Cox analysis (HR 1.24 (1.01–1.52), $p = 0.04$). Graft failure again shows no relationship with measured TTV either within 24 months after transplantation or thereafter.

4. Discussion

In recent years, the use of TTV levels as a means to gauge immunosuppression has been investigated by several groups. Most of this research has used longitudinal samples taken relatively shortly after transplantation and has been aimed to predict either infection risk, due to over-immunosuppression, or rejection, due to under-immunosuppression, during the first post-transplant year. These studies have shown mixed results, with some reporting elevated TTV in patients who subsequently died of sepsis and a higher risk of CMV reactivation in patients with high TTV levels [22–25], while others showed no connection between TTV and the overall risk of infection [26]. A reason for this apparent discrepancy may be that non-specified "risk for infection" is difficult to assess, because infections are diverse and may not be observed by the transplantation center but by referring hospitals and general practitioners instead, but may also be because TTV levels are only related to certain types of infections. Because we were interested in the relationship between TTV levels and long-term outcome after renal transplantation, we focused on all-cause mortality and death due to infectious causes, as this information can be traced reliably. We found that high TTV levels are associated with both all-cause mortality and with death due to infections. The excess mortality in the high TTV group was not attributable to other factors such as age, gender, eGFR, number of immunosuppressive medications used, proteinuria and years after transplantation. Our findings suggest that TTV-levels may be predictive of much longer-term outcomes then have been investigated thus far. Other studies have shown that a relative plateau phase in TTV levels is reached in most patients, after a first period of increasing TTV levels caused by induction immunosuppression, and subsequent tapering to maintenance therapy [17]. Our study suggests that sampling during this relative plateau phase could be useful in identifying patients at risk of adverse outcomes. However, our study also suggests the relative plateau phase is relative indeed, as the TTV-levels show a decreasing trend after this first year which continues until a final stable phase develops after 24 months, and that high TTV levels are especially predictive of long-term adverse outcome if samples are taken after 24 months.

Several papers have been published looking at the role of TTV in graft failure in different types of organ transplantation [22,27–31]. A role for TTV measurements in predicting antibody mediated rejection in renal transplantation was suggested, with lower levels of TTV found to correlate with this type of rejection [31–33]. Likewise, TTV levels were also shown to be significantly lower before the diagnosis of chronic lung allograft dysfunction in lung transplant patients [31]. These results support the theory that lower levels of TTV are a risk factor for graft failure. In our study, we did not find an association between TTV and graft failure. The main reason for this may be that we looked at patients a minimum of 12 months after transplantation, past the period which represents the highest risk for acute rejection [2,34,35]. This means we likely removed several patients with a risk of rejection, reducing our power to detect rejection. Another reason for the lack of association between TTV levels and graft failure is may be that graft failure is also caused by non-immunogenic factors such as vascular damage, which TTV is unlikely to be associated with.

Although our study investigated the use of a single TTV measurement for predicting outcome after renal transplantation, and was able to show a relationship in a large group, we do not consider this method accurate enough for use in individual patients. The sensitivity and specificity of a single measurement in identifying patients with increased risk of death is so low that no real conclusions could be drawn. The cut-off TTV level which should alert clinicians to potential over immunosuppression has not become clear from this study. Our calculated cut-offs for mortality risk and infectious mortality risk are similar to the ones calculated by Fernandez-Ruiz. et al. for increased risk of infections (i.e., 3–4 Log copies/mL) [36] but are much lower than the values suggested by other authors by several orders of magnitude [22,37]. These differences stress the need for TTV assay standardization and make it difficult to draw a consensus opinion as to clinically relevant TTV viral load measurements, which would warrant action.

Nevertheless, our study results show that time since transplantation is a consideration when attempting to evaluate TTV levels as a marker for optimal immunosuppression. What may be eventually be considered a marker for either infectious risk or rejection risk may depend on when the patient is sampled.

The group of TTV-negative renal transplant recipients in our study and their collective favorable outcome after transplantation deserves attention in future research. In all studies investigating the use of TTV after transplantation, TTV-negative recipients are found. This group logically includes patients without TTV, as well as patients whose immune systems are able to suppress TTV effectively. The fact that this group has the lowest risk of death due to infections and the lowest all-cause mortality, is not surprising. However, in studies investigating TTV levels within the first year after transplantation, this group appeared to have a higher rejection risk and more graft failure. We were not able to show a connection between graft failure and TTV level. Although the set-up of our study, with a single sample taken at least one year after renal transplantation, was not inappropriate to assess acute rejection risk, the fact that there is no association between negative TTV and graft failure stresses that more investigation is needed to determine TTV level cut-offs for optimal immunosuppression after the first year post-transplantation.

When writing it was interesting to note that many studies on TTV in transplantation medicine, including this study, have come from Central and Western Europe, while the exact geographic variation of TTV has not been fully elucidated. These are also studies that, in general, have shown a correlation between TTV and various outcomes. With the advent of a minimum of four available PCR detection methods, including one commercial kit, capable of detecting various TTV genotypes with varying levels of efficiency, it would be interesting to know exactly which TTV genotype is being detected by each kit. Several authors have noted a correlation between genogroup 4 and specifically genotype 21, which has been associated with arthritis and acute respiratory disease in children [25,38]. It may be time rethink our detection strategies by using specific PCR reactions or by using sequencing more readily.

In conclusion, our data suggest a use for TTV viral load monitoring in renal transplant recipients for long term follow-up. While cut-off values remain to be determined, high TTV levels are associated with increased all-cause mortality and increased risk of death due to infections.

Author Contributions: Conceptualization: A.A.E.d.J., S.J.L.B., E.A.M.V., J.W., C.V.L.-B.; Methodology: S.J.L.B., H.G.M.N.; Validation: H.G.M.N., C.V.L.-B., E.J.G., L.W.; Formal analyses: E.J.G., A.W.G.-N.; Investigation: E.J.G., C.V.L.-B.; Resources: H.G.M.N., S.J.L.B., J.W., E.A.M.V.; Data validation: E.J.G., A.W.G.-N.; Writing—original draft preparation: E.J.G., C.V.L.-B.; Writing—review and editing: J.W., S.J.L.B., E.A.M.V., H.G.M.N.; Supervision: C.V.L.-B., J.W., E.A.M.V. All authors have read and agreed to the published version of the manuscript.

Acknowledgments: The cohort on which the study was based is registered at clinicaltrials.gov as "TransplantLines Food and Nutrition Biobank and Cohort Study (TxL-FN)" with number NCT02811835.

References

1. Meier-Kriesche, H.-U.; Schold, J.D.; Srinivas, T.R.; Kaplan, B. Lack of Improvement in Renal Allograft Survival Despite a Marked Decrease in Acute Rejection Rates Over the Most Recent Era. *Am. J. Transplant.* **2004**, *4*, 378–383. [CrossRef] [PubMed]
2. Chand, S.; Atkinson, D.; Collins, C.; Briggs, D.; Ball, S.; Sharif, A.; Skordilis, K.; Vydianath, B.; Neil, D.; Borrows, R. The Spectrum of Renal Allograft Failure. *PLoS ONE* **2016**, *11*, e0162278. [CrossRef] [PubMed]
3. Morrissey, P.E.; Reinert, S.; Yango, A.; Gautam, A.; Monaco, A.; Gohh, R. Factors Contributing to Acute Rejection in Renal Transplantation: The Role of Noncompliance. *Transplant. Proc.* **2005**, *37*, 2044–2047. [CrossRef] [PubMed]
4. Maggi, F.; Bendinelli, M. Human Anelloviruses and the Central Nervous System. *Rev. Med. Virol.* **2010**, *20*, 392–407. [CrossRef] [PubMed]
5. Nishizawa, T.; Okamoto, H.; Konishi, K.; Yoshizawa, H.; Miyakawa, Y.; Mayumi, M. A Novel DNA Virus (TTV) Associated with Elevated Transaminase Levels in Posttransfusion Hepatitis of Unknown Etiology. *Biochem. Biophys. Res. Commun.* **1997**, *241*, 92–97. [CrossRef] [PubMed]

6. Okamoto, H.; Nishizawa, T.; Ukita, M. A Novel Unenveloped DNA Virus (TT Virus) Associated with Acute and Chronic Non-A to G Hepatitis. *Intervirology* **1999**, *42*, 196–204. [CrossRef]
7. Spandole, S.; Cimponeriu, D.; Berca, L.M.; Mihaescu, G. Human Anelloviruses: An Update of Molecular, Epidemiological and Clinical Aspects. *Arch. Virol.* **2015**, *160*, 893–908. [CrossRef]
8. Focosi, D.; Antonelli, G.; Pistello, M.; Maggi, F. Torquetenovirus: The Human Virome from Bench to Bedside. *Clin. Microbiol. Infect.* **2016**, *22*, 589–593. [CrossRef]
9. Ott, C.; Duret, L.; Chemin, I.; Trepo, C.; Mandrand, B.; Komurian-Pradel, F. Use of a TT Virus ORF1 Recombinant Protein to Detect Anti-TT Virus Antibodies in Human Sera. *J. Gen. Virol.* **2000**, *81*, 2949–2958. [CrossRef]
10. Mankotia, D.S.; Irshad, M. Cloning and Expression of N22 Region of Torque Teno Virus (TTV) Genome and Use of Peptide in Developing Immunoassay for TTV Antibodies. *Virol. J.* **2014**, *11*, 96. [CrossRef]
11. Nishizawa, T.; Okamoto, H.; Tsuda, F.; Aikawa, T.; Sugai, Y.; Konishi, K.; Akahane, Y.; Ukita, M.; Tanaka, T.; Miyakawa, Y.; et al. Quasispecies of TT Virus (TTV) with Sequence Divergence in Hypervariable Regions of the Capsid Protein in Chronic TTV Infection. *J. Virol.* **1999**, *73*, 9604–9608. [CrossRef] [PubMed]
12. Kulifaj, D.; Essig, M.; Meynier, F.; Pichon, N.; Munteanu, E.; Moulinas, R.; Joannes, M.; Heckel, D.; Combrissson, J.; Barranger, C.; et al. Torque Teno Virus (TTV) in Immunosuppressed Host: Performances Studies of TTV R-Gene Registered Kit and Donors and Recipients Kidney Samples Genotyping: Presentation at ESCV 2016: Poster 166. *J. Clin. Virol.* **2016**, *82*, S103–S104. [CrossRef]
13. Rezahosseini, O.; Drabe, C.H.; Sørensen, S.S.; Rasmussen, A.; Perch, M.; Ostrowski, S.R.; Nielsen, S.D. Torque-Teno Virus Viral Load as a Potential Endogenous Marker of Immune Function in Solid Organ Transplantation. *Transplant. Rev.* **2019**, *33*, 137–144. [CrossRef] [PubMed]
14. Minović, I.; Eisenga, M.F.; Riphagen, I.J.; van den Berg, E.; Kootstra-Ros, J.E.; Frenay, A.-R.S.; van Goor, H.; Rimbach, G.; Esatbeyoglu, T.; Levy, A.P.; et al. Circulating Haptoglobin and Metabolic Syndrome in Renal Transplant Recipients. *Sci. Rep.* **2017**, *7*, 14264. [CrossRef]
15. Eisenga, M.F.; Kieneker, L.M.; Soedamah-Muthu, S.S.; van den Berg, E.; Deetman, P.E.; Navis, G.J.; Gans, R.O.B.; Gaillard, C.A.J.M.; Bakker, S.J.L.; Joosten, M.M. Urinary Potassium Excretion, Renal Ammoniagenesis, and Risk of Graft Failure and Mortality in Renal Transplant Recipients. *Am. J. Clin. Nutr.* **2016**, *104*, 1703–1711. [CrossRef]
16. Kulifaj, D.; Durgueil-Lariviere, B.; Meynier, F.; Munteanu, E.; Pichon, N.; Dubé, M.; Joannes, M.; Essig, M.; Hantz, S.; Barranger, C.; et al. Development of a Standardized Real Time PCR for Torque Teno Viruses (TTV) Viral Load Detection and Quantification: A New Tool for Immune Monitoring. *J. Clin. Virol.* **2018**, *105*, 118–127. [CrossRef]
17. Solis, M.; Velay, A.; Gantner, P.; Bausson, J.; Filiputti, A.; Freitag, R.; Moulin, B.; Caillard, S.; Fafi-Kremer, S. Torquetenovirus Viremia for Early Prediction of Graft Rejection after Kidney Transplantation. *J. Infect.* **2019**, *79*, 56–60. [CrossRef]
18. Macera, L.; Spezia, P.G.; Medici, C.; Rofi, E.; Re, M.D.; Focosi, D.; Mazzetti, P.; Navarro, D.; Antonelli, G.; Danesi, R.; et al. Comparative Evaluation of Molecular Methods for the Quantitative Measure of Torquetenovirus Viremia, the New Surrogate Marker of Immune Competence. *J. Med. Virol.* **2019**. [CrossRef]
19. World Health Organisation; Centre for Disease Control; Prevention. *ICD-9-CM CDC Copy*; National Center for Health Statistics: Hyattsville, MD, USA, 2015.
20. World Health Organisation. *ICD 9 001-139*; Pan American Health Organization: Washington, DC, USA, 2012; ISBN 9241540044.
21. Youden, W.J. Index for Rating Diagnostic Tests. *Cancer* **1950**, *3*, 32. [CrossRef]
22. Görzer, I.; Haloschan, M.; Jaksch, P.; Klepetko, W.; Puchhammer-Stöckl, E. Plasma DNA Levels of Torque Teno Virus and Immunosuppression after Lung Transplantation. *J. Hear. Lung Transplant.* **2014**, *33*, 320–323. [CrossRef]
23. Walton, A.H.; Muenzer, J.T.; Rasche, D.; Boomer, J.S.; Sato, B.; Brownstein, B.H.; Pachot, A.; Brooks, T.L.; Deych, E.; Shannon, W.D.; et al. Reactivation of Multiple Viruses in Patients with Sepsis. *PLoS ONE* **2014**, *9*, e98819. [CrossRef] [PubMed]
24. Maggi, F.; Focosi, D.; Statzu, M.; Bianco, G.; Costa, C.; Macera, L.; Spezia, P.G.; Medici, C.; Albert, E.; Navarro, D.; et al. Early Post-Transplant Torquetenovirus Viremia Predicts Cytomegalovirus Reactivations In Solid Organ Transplant Recipients. *Sci. Rep.* **2018**, *8*, 15490–15498. [CrossRef] [PubMed]

25. Maggi, F.; Pifferi, M.; Fornai, C.; Andreoli, E.; Tempestini, E.; Vatteroni, M.; Presciuttini, S.; Marchi, S.; Pietrobelli, A.; Boner, A.; et al. TT Virus in the Nasal Secretions of Children with Acute Respiratory Diseases: Relations to Viremia and Disease Severity. *J. Virol.* **2003**, *77*, 2418–2425. [CrossRef] [PubMed]
26. Nordén, R.; Magnusson, J.; Lundin, A.; Tang, K.-W.; Nilsson, S.; Lindh, M.; Andersson, L.-M.; Riise, G.C.; Westin, J. Quantification of Torque Teno Virus and Epstein-Barr Virus Is of Limited Value for Predicting the Net State of Immunosuppression After Lung Transplantation. *Open Forum Infect. Dis.* **2018**, *5*, ofy050. [CrossRef] [PubMed]
27. Shang, D.; Lin, Y.H.; Rigopoulou, I.; Chen, B.; Alexander, G.J.M.; Allain, J.-P. Detection of TT Virus DNA in Patients with Liver Disease and Recipients of Liver Transplant. *J. Med. Virol.* **2000**, *61*, 455–461. [CrossRef]
28. Burra, P.; Masier, A.; Boldrin, C.; Calistri, A.; Andreoli, E.; Senzolo, M.; Zorzi, M.; Sgarabotto, D.; Guido, M.; Cillo, U.; et al. Torque Teno Virus: Any Pathological Role in Liver Transplanted Patients? *Transpl. Int.* **2008**, *21*, 972–979. [CrossRef]
29. Béland, K.; Dore-Nguyen, M.; Gagné, M.-J.; Patey, N.; Brassard, J.; Alvarez, F.; Halac, U. Torque Teno Virus in Children Who Underwent Orthotopic Liver Transplantation: New Insights About a Common Pathogen. *J. Infect. Dis.* **2014**, *209*, 247–254. [CrossRef]
30. Görzer, I.; Jaksch, P.; Kundi, M.; Seitz, T.; Klepetko, W.; Puchhammer-Stöckl, E. Pre-Transplant Plasma Torque Teno Virus Load and Increase Dynamics after Lung Transplantation. *PLoS ONE* **2015**, *10*, e0122975. [CrossRef]
31. Görzer, I.; Jaksch, P.; Strassl, R.; Klepetko, W.; Puchhammer-Stöckl, E. Association between Plasma Torque Teno Virus Level and Chronic Lung Allograft Dysfunction after Lung Transplantation. *J. Hear. Lung Transplant.* **2017**, *36*, 366–368. [CrossRef]
32. Schiemann, M.; Puchhammer-Stöckl, E.; Eskandary, F.; Kohlbeck, P.; Rasoul-Rockenschaub, S.; Heilos, A.; Kozakowski, N.; Görzer, I.; Kikić, Ž.; Herkner, H.; et al. Torque Teno Virus Load-Inverse Association with Antibody-Mediated Rejection after Kidney Transplantation. *Transplantation* **2017**, *101*, 360–367. [CrossRef]
33. Strassl, R.; Doberer, K.; Rasoul-Rockenschaub, S.; Herkner, H.; Görzer, I.; Kläger, J.P.; Schmidt, R.; Haslacher, H.; Schiemann, M.; Eskandary, F.A.; et al. Torque Teno Virus for Risk Stratification of Acute Biopsyproven Alloreactivity in Kidney Transplant Recipients. *J. Infect. Dis.* **2019**, *219*, 1934–1939. [CrossRef] [PubMed]
34. El-Zoghby, Z.M.; Stegall, M.D.; Lager, D.J.; Kremers, W.K.; Amer, H.; Gloor, J.M.; Cosio, F.G. Identifying Specific Causes of Kidney Allograft Loss. *Am. J. Transplant.* **2009**, *9*, 527–535. [CrossRef] [PubMed]
35. Sellarés, J.; De Freitas, D.G.; Mengel, M.; Reeve, J.; Einecke, G.; Sis, B.; Hidalgo, L.G.; Famulski, K.; Matas, A.; Halloran, P.F. Understanding the Causes of Kidney Transplant Failure: The Dominant Role of Antibody-Mediated Rejection and Nonadherence. *Am. J. Transplant.* **2012**, *12*, 388–399. [CrossRef] [PubMed]
36. Fernández-Ruiz, M.; Albert, E.; Giménez, E.; Ruiz-Merlo, T.; Parra, P.; López-Medrano, F.; San Juan, R.; Polanco, N.; Andrés, A.; Navarro, D.; et al. Monitoring of Alphatorquevirus DNA Levels for the Prediction of Immunosuppression-Related Complications after Kidney Transplantation. *Am. J. Transplant.* **2019**, *19*, 1139–1149. [CrossRef] [PubMed]
37. Strassl, R.; Schiemann, M.; Doberer, K.; Görzer, I.; Puchhammer-Stöckl, E.; Eskandary, F.; Kikic, Ž.; Gualdoni, G.A.; Vossen, M.G.; Rasoul-Rockenschaub, S.; et al. Quantification of Torque Teno Virus Viremia as a Prospective Biomarker for Infectious Disease in Kidney Allograft Recipients. *J. Infect. Dis.* **2018**, *218*, 1191–1199. [CrossRef]
38. Rocchi, J.; Ricci, V.; Albani, M.; Lanini, L.; Andreoli, E.; Macera, L.; Pistello, M.; Ceccherini-Nelli, L.; Bendinelli, M.; Maggi, F. Torquetenovirus DNA Drives Proinflammatory Cytokines Production and Secretion by Immune Cells via Toll-like Receptor 9. *Virology* **2009**, *394*, 235–242. [CrossRef]

Permissions

All chapters in this book were first published by MDPI; hereby published with permission under the Creative Commons Attribution License or equivalent. Every chapter published in this book has been scrutinized by our experts. Their significance has been extensively debated. The topics covered herein carry significant findings which will fuel the growth of the discipline. They may even be implemented as practical applications or may be referred to as a beginning point for another development.

The contributors of this book come from diverse backgrounds, making this book a truly international effort. This book will bring forth new frontiers with its revolutionizing research information and detailed analysis of the nascent developments around the world.

We would like to thank all the contributing authors for lending their expertise to make the book truly unique. They have played a crucial role in the development of this book. Without their invaluable contributions this book wouldn't have been possible. They have made vital efforts to compile up to date information on the varied aspects of this subject to make this book a valuable addition to the collection of many professionals and students.

This book was conceptualized with the vision of imparting up-to-date information and advanced data in this field. To ensure the same, a matchless editorial board was set up. Every individual on the board went through rigorous rounds of assessment to prove their worth. After which they invested a large part of their time researching and compiling the most relevant data for our readers.

The editorial board has been involved in producing this book since its inception. They have spent rigorous hours researching and exploring the diverse topics which have resulted in the successful publishing of this book. They have passed on their knowledge of decades through this book. To expedite this challenging task, the publisher supported the team at every step. A small team of assistant editors was also appointed to further simplify the editing procedure and attain best results for the readers.

Apart from the editorial board, the designing team has also invested a significant amount of their time in understanding the subject and creating the most relevant covers. They scrutinized every image to scout for the most suitable representation of the subject and create an appropriate cover for the book.

The publishing team has been an ardent support to the editorial, designing and production team. Their endless efforts to recruit the best for this project, has resulted in the accomplishment of this book. They are a veteran in the field of academics and their pool of knowledge is as vast as their experience in printing. Their expertise and guidance has proved useful at every step. Their uncompromising quality standards have made this book an exceptional effort. Their encouragement from time to time has been an inspiration for everyone.

The publisher and the editorial board hope that this book will prove to be a valuable piece of knowledge for researchers, students, practitioners and scholars across the globe.

List of Contributors

Charat Thongprayoon and Api Chewcharat
Division of Nephrology, Department of Medicine, Mayo Clinic, Rochester, MN 55905, USA

Wisit Kaewput
Department of Military and Community Medicine, Phramongkutklao College of Medicine, Bangkok 10400, Thailand

Karthik Kovvuru, Swetha R. Kanduri, Maria L. Gonzalez-Suarez and Wisit Cheungpasitporn
Division of Nephrology, Department of Medicine, University of Mississippi Medical Center, Jackson, MS 39216, USA

Panupong Hansrivijit
Department of Internal Medicine, University of Pittsburgh Medical Center Pinnacle, Harrisburg, PA 17105, USA

Tarun Bathini
Department of Internal Medicine, University of Arizona, Tucson, AZ 85721, USA

Napat Leeaphorn
Department of Nephrology, Department of Medicine, Saint Luke's Health System, Kansas City, MO 64111, USA

Gentzon Hall, Liming Wang and Robert F. Spurney
Division of Nephrology, Department of Medicine, Duke University; Durham, NC 27710, USA

Carolien P. J. Deen
Department of Internal Medicine, University of Groningen, University Medical Center Groningen, 9713 GZ Groningen, The Netherlands
Department of Laboratory Medicine, University of Groningen, University Medical Center Groningen, 9713 GZ Groningen, The Netherlands
TiFN, 6709 PA Wageningen, The Netherlands

Anna van der Veen, M. Rebecca Heiner-Fokkema and Ido P. Kema
Department of Laboratory Medicine, University of Groningen, University Medical Center Groningen, 9713 GZ Groningen, The Netherlands

António W. Gomes-Neto
Department of Internal Medicine, University of Groningen, University Medical Center Groningen, 9713 GZ Groningen, The Netherlands
Transplant Lines Food and Nutrition Biobank and Cohort Study, University of Groningen, University Medical Center Groningen, 9713 GZ Groningen, The Netherlands

Johanna M. Geleijnse and Karin J. Borgonjen-van den Berg
Division of Human Nutrition and Health, Wageningen University, 6708 PB Wageningen, The Netherlands

Stephan J. L. Bakker
Department of Internal Medicine, University of Groningen, University Medical Center Groningen, 9713 GZ Groningen, The Netherlands
Department of Internal Medicine, Division of Nephrology, University Medical Center Groningen, University of Groningen, 9700 RB Groningen, The Netherlands
TiFN, 6709 PA Wageningen, The Netherlands
Transplant Lines Food and Nutrition Biobank and Cohort Study, University of Groningen, University Medical Center Groningen, 9713 GZ Groningen, The Netherlands

Eun Seop Seo, Se In Sung, So Yoon Ahn, Yun Sil Chang and Won Soon Park
Department of Pediatrics, Samsung Medical Center, Sungkyunkwan University School of Medicine, 06351 Seoul, Korea

Frank Klont, Péter Horvatovich and Rainer Bischoff
Department of Analytical Biochemistry, Groningen Research Institute of Pharmacy, University of Groningen, 9713 AV Groningen, The Netherlands

Lyanne M. Kieneker, Suzanne P. Stam and Else van den Berg
Department of Internal Medicine, Division of Nephrology, University Medical Center Groningen, University of Groningen, 9700 RB Groningen, The Netherlands

Nick H. T. ten Hacken
Department of Pulmonary Diseases, University Medical Center Groningen, University of Groningen, 9700 RB Groningen, The Netherlands

Ido P. Kema
Department of Laboratory Medicine, University Medical Center Groningen, University of Groningen, 9700 RB Groningen, The Netherlands

André P. van Beek
Department of Endocrinology, University Medical Center Groningen, University of Groningen, 9700 RB Groningen, The Netherlands

Yukari Mae, Tomoaki Takata, Ayami Ida, Masaya Ogawa, Sosuke Taniguchi, Marie Yamamoto, Takuji Iyama, Satoko Fukuda and Hajime Isomoto
Division of Medicine and Clinical Science, Faculty of Medicine, Tottori University, Yonago, Tottori 683-8504, Japan

Sooin Choi
Department of Laboratory Medicine, Soonchunhyang University Hospital Cheonan, Soonchunhyang University College of Medicine, Cheonan 31151, Korea

Kyo Won Lee and Jae Berm Park
Department of Surgery, Samsung Medical Center, Sungkyunkwan University School of Medicine, Seoul 06351, Korea

Kyunga Kim
Statistics and Data Center, Research Institute for Future Medicine, Samsung Medical Center, Seoul 06351, Korea

Hye-Ryeon Jang and Wooseong Huh
Division of Nephrology, Department of Medicine, Samsung Medical Center, Sungkyunkwan University School of Medicine, Seoul 06351, Korea

Eun Suk Kang
Department of Laboratory Medicine and Genetics, Samsung Medical Center, Sungkyunkwan University School of Medicine, Seoul 06351, Korea

Caroline Jadlowiec, Kunam Reddy and Adyr Moss
Division of Transplant Surgery, Mayo Clinic, Phoenix, AZ 85054, USA

Maxwell Smith
Division of Anatomic Pathology, Mayo Clinic, Phoenix, AZ 85054, USA

Matthew Neville
Instructor in Biostatistics, Mayo Clinic College of Medicine, Phoenix, AZ 85054, USA

Shennen Mao
Division of Transplant Surgery, Mayo Clinic, Jacksonville, FL 32224, USA

Dina Abdelwahab
Division of Nephrology, Mayo Clinic, Phoenix, AZ 85054, USA

Bashar Aqel
Division of Transplant Hepatology, Mayo Clinic, Phoenix, AZ 85054, USA

Timucin Taner
Division of Transplant Surgery, William J von Liebig Transplant Center, Rochester, MN 55902, USA

Michele F. Eisenga, Maarten A. De Jong and Martin H. De Borst
Division of Nephrology, Department of Internal Medicine, University of Groningen, University Medical Center Groningen, 9700 RB Groningen, The Netherlands

David E. Leaf
Division of Renal Medicine, Brigham and Women's Hospital, Harvard Medical School, Boston, MA 02215, USA

Ilja M. Nolte
Department of Epidemiology, University of Groningen, University Medical Center Groningen, 9700 RB Groningen, The Netherlands

Carlo A. J. M. Gaillard
Division of Nephrology, Department of Internal Medicine, University of Groningen, University Medical Center Groningen, 9700 RB Groningen, The Netherlands
Department of Internal Medicine and Dermatology, University of Utrecht, University Medical Center Utrecht, 3508 GA Utrecht, The Netherlands

Dominik J. G. Flothow, Barbara Suwelack, Hermann Pavenstädt, Katharina Schütte-Nütgen and Stefan Reuter
Department of Medicine D, University Hospital of Muenster, 48149 Münster, Germany

Joana Gameiro and José António Lopes
Division of Nephrology and Renal Transplantation, Department of Medicine, Centro Hospitalar Lisboa Norte, EPE, Av. Prof. Egas Moniz, 1649-035 Lisboa, Portugal

Tiago Branco
Department of Medicine, Centro Hospitalar Lisboa Norte, EPE, Av. Prof. Egas Moniz, 1649-035 Lisboa, Portugal

Oyuntugs Byambasukh
Department of Epidemiology, University Medical Center Groningen, University of Groningen, 9713 GZ Groningen, The Netherlands
Department of Internal Medicine, Mongolian National University of Medical Sciences, 976 Ulaanbaatar, Mongolia

Maryse C. J. Osté, Else van den Berg and Gerjan Navis
Department of Nephrology, University Medical Center Groningen, University of Groningen, 9700 RB Groningen, The Netherlands

Eva Corpeleijn
Department of Epidemiology, University Medical Center Groningen, University of Groningen, 9713 GZ Groningen, The Netherlands

Fabio Fabbian and Roberto Manfredini
Clinica Medica Unit, Azienda Ospedaliero-Universitaria, I-44121 Ferrara, Italy
Department of Medical Sciences, University of Ferrara, I-44121 Ferrara, Italy

Alfredo De Giorgi, Emanuele Di Simone and Benedetta Boari
Clinica Medica Unit, Azienda Ospedaliero-Universitaria, I-44121 Ferrara, Italy

Rosaria Cappadona
Department of Medical Sciences, University of Ferrara, I-44121 Ferrara, Italy

Nicola Lamberti
Department of Biomedical and Specialty Surgical Sciences, University of Ferrara, I-44121 Ferrara, Italy

Fabio Manfredini
Department of Biomedical and Specialty Surgical Sciences, University of Ferrara, I-44121 Ferrara, Italy
Neuroscience and Rehabilitation Department, Azienda Ospedaliero-Universitaria, I-44121 Ferrara, Italy

Alda Storari
Nephrology and Dialysis Unit, Azienda Ospedaliero-Universitaria, I-44121 Ferrara, Italy

Luisa Averdunk
Department of Intensive Care Medicine, University Hospital Aachen, Rheinisch Westphälische Technische Hochschule Aachen, 52074 Aachen, Germany
Institute of Human Genetics and Department of Pediatrics, Medical Faculty, Heinrich Heine University, 40225 Düsseldorf, Germany

Jürgen Bernhagen
Department of Vascular Biology, Institute for Stroke and Dementia Research, Klinikum der Universität München, Ludwig-Maximilians-University Munich, 80333 Munich, Germany
German Center for Cardiovascular Research (DZHK), Partner Site Munich Heart Alliance, 10785 Berlin, Germany
Munich Cluster for Systems Neurology (EXC 2145 SyNergy), 81377 Munich, Germany

Karl Fehnle
Algora: Statistics and Clinical Research GmbH, 85540 Haar, Germany

Harald Surowy, Hermann-Josef Lüdecke and Dagmar Wieczorek
Institute of Human Genetics and Department of Pediatrics, Medical Faculty, Heinrich Heine University, 40225 Düsseldorf, Germany

Sören Mucha
Institute of Clinical Molecular Biology, Christian Albrechts University of Kiel, 24118 Kiel, Germany
Institute for Cardiogenetics, University of Lübeck, Ratzeburger Allee 160, 23562 Lübeck, Germany

Patrick Meybohm and Kai Zacharowski
Department of Anesthesiology, Intensive Care Medicine & Pain Therapy, University Hospital Frankfurt, Goethe University, 60323 Frankfurt, Germany

Lin Leng and Richard Bucala
Department of Internal Medicine, Yale University School of Medicine, New Haven, CT 06510, USA

Gernot Marx
Department of Intensive Care Medicine, University Hospital Aachen, Rheinisch Westphälische Technische Hochschule Aachen, 52074 Aachen, Germany

David E. Leaf
Division of Renal Medicine, Brigham and Women's Hospital, Boston, MA 02115, USA
Harvard Medical School, Boston, MA 02115, USA

Alexander Zarbock
Intensive Care and Pain Medicine, Department of Anesthesiology, University of Münster, 48149 Münster, Germany

Christian Stoppe
Department of Intensive Care Medicine, University Hospital Aachen, Rheinisch Westphälische Technische Hochschule Aachen, 52074 Aachen, Germany
Department of Anesthesiology, Intensive Care Medicine and Pain Therapy, University Hospital Würzburg, 97080 Würzburg, Germany

Aureliusz Kolonko, Natalia Słabiak-Błaż, Henryk Karkoszka, Andrzej Więcek and Grzegorz Piecha
Department of Nephrology, Transplantation and Internal Medicine, Medical University of Silesia, 40-027 Katowice, Poland

Camilo G. Sotomayor, Dion Groothof, Joppe J. Vodegel, Tomás A. Gacitúa, Maryse C. J. Osté, Stefan P. Berger and Gerjan J. Navis
Department of Internal Medicine, University Medical Center Groningen, University of Groningen, 9700 RB Groningen, The Netherlands

Robert A. Pol
Division of Transplantation Surgery, University Medical Center Groningen, University of Groningen, 9700 RB Groningen, The Netherlands

Catterina Ferreccio
Advanced Center for Chronic Diseases, Pontificia Universidad Católica de Chile, 8330033 Santiago, Chile

Guillermo Chong
Department of Radiology, Clínica Alemana de Santiago, Universidad del Desarrollo, 7610658 Santiago, Chile

Riemer H. J. A. Slart
Department of Nuclear and Molecular Imaging, University Medical Center Groningen, University of Groningen, 9700 RB Groningen, The Netherlands

Ramón Rodrigo
Institute of Biomedical Sciences, Faculty of Medicine, University of Chile, CP 8380453 Santiago, Chile

Daan J. Touw
Department of Pharmacy and Clinical Pharmacology, University Medical Center Groningen, University of Groningen, 9700 RB Groningen, The Netherlands

Edmund J. Gore, Hubert G. M. Niesters and Coretta Van Leer-Buter
Department of Medical Microbiology, Rijksuniversiteit Groningen, University Medical Centre Groningen, 9713GZ Groningen, The Netherlands

Anoek A. E. de Joode
Department of Internal Medicine, Rijksuniversiteit Groningen, University Medical Centre Groningen, 9713 GZ Groningen, The Netherlands

Lei Wang and Johanna Westra
Department of Rheumatology and Clinical Immunology, Rijksuniversiteit Groningen, University Medical Centre Groningen, 9713GZ Groningen, The Netherlands

Erik A. M. Verschuuren
Department of Pulmonology, Rijksuniversiteit Groningen, University Medical Centre Groningen, 9713GZ Groningen, The Netherlands

Index

Printed in the USA
CPSIA information can be obtained
at www.ICGtesting.com
LVHW080046211023
761596LV00010BA/1932

9 781646 466092